HIV/AIDS Prevention, Management and Strategy

1st Edition

Author: Dr Prince Efere

(The author is the principal of the College of Venereal Disease Prevention, London)

Edited by: Janet Kale and Dr Prince Efere

College of Venereal Disease Prevention

Printed in Victoria, Canada

Note for Librarians: a cataloguing record for this book that includes Dewey Classification and US Library of Congress numbers is available from the National Library of Canada. The complete cataloguing record can be obtained from the National Library's online database at:
www.nlc-bnc.ca/amicus/index-e.html
ISBN 1-4120-2672-5

TRAFFORD

This book was published on-demand in cooperation with Trafford Publishing.
On-demand publishing is a unique process and service of making a book available for retail sale to the public taking advantage of on-demand manufacturing and Internet marketing. On-demand publishing includes promotions, retail sales, manufacturing, order fulfilment, accounting and collecting royalties on behalf of the author.

Suite 6E, 2333 Government St., Victoria, B.C. V8T 4P4, CANADA
Phone 250-383-6864   Toll-free 1-888-232-4444 (Canada & US)
Fax 250-383-6804   E-mail sales@trafford.com   Web site www.trafford.com
TRAFFORD PUBLISHING IS A DIVISION OF TRAFFORD HOLDINGS LTD
Trafford Catalogue #04-0500   www.trafford.com/robots/04-0500.html

13   12   11   10   9   8   7   6   5   4   3

Contents

Foreword

This book is part of the Simplified Series and readers do not have to have any background knowledge in the subject area to understand the contents of this book.

College of Venereal Disease Prevention, London UK.

Preface

This is a definitive guide to the effective prevention and management of HIV/AIDS. It is a comprehensive and excellently written book, that will be of interest to anyone who is already involved in or is interested in HIV/AIDS prevention. HIV/AIDS is playing havoc on humanity, with tens of millions already dead from AIDS and tens of millions more destined to die.

This book is suitable for health professionals, social workers, policy makers, managers, personnel officers, as well as undergraduate and post-graduate students in the following disciplines:

a) public health
b) health services management
c) social policy/sociology
d) health education and promotion
e) health sciences
f) epidemiology
g) environmental health
h) social care
i) sexual health
j) nursing
k) social work
l) midwifery
m) social sciences
n) research
o) human resource management

Although comprehensive, this book is written in a style that makes you want to continue to read without stopping. This is because it is presented in a way that simplifies this supposedly complex area of knowledge. It is a truly unique and unparalled book that deals with the most important areas of HIV/AIDS prevention, management and strategy. This book can also be used as a reference and training manual in colleges, universities, offices and other institutions.

I hope that you find the content of this book relevant, useful and practical.

Dr Prince Efere
Principal, College of Venereal Disease Prevention, London

March 2004

Chapter 1

Poverty & Healthcare

Contents of this Chapter

1. Poverty – Introduction

According to the United Nations Centre for Human Settlements (HABITAT):

> "Poverty implies deprivation or human needs that are not met. It is generally understood to arise from lack of income or assets".

2. Absolute and Relative Poverty

Using the concept of the poverty line to measure the level of poverty in society, HABITAT explains the concepts of absolute and relative poverty:-

> "The absolute poverty line remains and seeks to identify people who are destitute for instance lacking an income or asset base and the access to social services that mean that individuals or households cannot obtain sufficient food to eat, shelter and health care. In effect, their life is threatened by this level of deprivation.

The secondary poverty line, to identify those living in 'relative poverty' defines a minimum 'basket' of goods and services about which there is some agreement within a society that all citizens should have. People are relatively deprived if they cannot obtain the conditions of life, that is the diets, amenities, standards and services, which allow them to play the roles, participate in the relationships and follow the customary behaviour which is expected of them by virtue of their membership of society.

The range of goods and services within this socially determined level of need will vary greatly, not only related to the wealth and structure of a society but also to societal attitudes. There are usually minor disagreements within any society as to what constitutes need and the income and level of service provision required to meet this need.

However, there is general agreement that poverty lines or other means to identify those suffering from deprivation have to be determined within each country so that the needs defined match the real needs in that particular society and culture."

Poverty has become a familiar subject in the United Kingdom to the extent that as many as over thirteen million people can be considered as "poor" in the UK.

The report, which is the foundation stone of the present welfare state in the UK, was published by William Beveridge in 1942. It was intended to bring to an end poverty, disease, poor housing, unemployment and lack of education in society.

Despite the good intentions and provisions of the Beveridge report, poverty continues to plague not only people in the United Kingdom but the world at large, so that no nation is immune from it.

Indeed, in some cases, the level of poverty in society actually increases along with increase in societal development.

In this regard The Robert Schalkenbach Foundation (The Henry George Institute), USA comments on the work of American Economist; Henry George (1839-1897) – 'Progress and Poverty':

"George was endowed for his job. He was curious and he was alertly attentive to all that went on around him. He had that rarest of all attributes in the scholar and historian - that gift without which all education is useless.

He had mother wit. He read what he needed to read, and he understood what he read.

What is more, he saw what was before his eyes, exactly, with the clear vision of an artist and the approval of a scientist. And he was fortunate.

He lived and worked, in a rapidly developing society in which his environment changed daily.

George had the unique opportunity of studying the formation of a civilisation - the change of an encampment into a thriving metropolis. He saw a city of tents and mud change into a fine town of paved streets and decent housing, with tramways and buses.

And as he saw the beginning of wealth, he noted the first appearance of pauperism. He saw the coming of the first beggars the West had ever known in its entire history. He saw degradation forming as he saw the advent of leisure and affluence. It was his personal characteristic that he felt compelled to discover why they arose concurrently.

The result of his inquiry, PROGRESS AND POVERTY...."

Henry George was right. Today, the Los Angeles that he saw while it changed and rapidly developed, is like many other cities in the world - a city of extreme contrasts, a city where there is extreme wealth and extreme poverty.

"Probably the most famous poverty study was conducted in 1899 by Joseph Rowntree.

The research was done in York, in the United Kingdom where Rowntree's chocolate and Cocoa factory was a major employer. Rowntree established the idea of a 'poverty line'. This concept, which is still in use, sets a level of income, below which people are considered to be living in poverty.

Rowntree considered that people were poor if their income was so low that the resulting deprivation affected their health.

For example, to calculate the amount of money required for food, Rowntree worked out the number of calories necessary for physical efficiency. He then found an inexpensive diet which provided the calorie requirement and established the cost.

Rowntree admitted that the poverty line was based on as extremely austere scale and explained that he had designed it in this way to offset possible accusations of exaggeration.

For example, no allowance was made for bus or rail fares, for newspapers or stamps to write to children living away from home. The poverty line excluded money for toys or sweets, tobacco or alcohol.

In considering poverty, Rowntree distinguished between 'primary' and 'secondary' poverty. Families were in primary poverty if their income was not sufficient to maintain their physical existence. Secondary poverty meant that the income would have been sufficient, were it not that some was spent on items not in the scale, whether useful or wasteful.

Even on the basis of a far from generous definition of poverty, Rowntree found that 10 per cent of the population of York were living in primary poverty and a further 18 per cent in secondary poverty.

Rowntree conducted two later surveys, one in 1936 and one in 1950. He changed his definition of poverty to some extent, recognising that poverty could not be defined simply as the lack of necessities for physical survival.

This led to an acceptance of the social dimension of poverty, in terms of the inability to participate in the life of the community.

As a result, the 1936 study included allowance for a radio, books, newspapers, beer, tobacco, presents and a holiday.

Rowntree's work set a precedent for more recent research into poverty. It also influenced Beveridge in the design, in 1942, of the social security system. Rowntree himself was a member of a committee appointed to calculate the rates for social security benefits.

In 1983 a major survey on poverty in Britain was carried out for a London Weekend Television series called Breadline Britain. The results were written up in a book by Joanna Mack and Stewart Lansley called Poor Britain.

In 1990 the survey was repeated to update it for a new decade. The survey defines poverty as 'an enforced, lack of socially perceived necessities'.

.....There is no official poverty line in Britain, however, it is possible to use government statistics on income to create an unofficial measure of poverty. This done by calculating the average income for the country, excluding housing costs, and halving the figure.

Those people whose income falls below this point are considered to be living in poverty. Figures released by the government in 1994 showed there to be 13.9 million people living on less than half of the average income.

This is one in four of the population. Of these people 4.1 million are children, representing 31 percent of all children. The figures show a big increase in poverty over the last 10 years."
(Pat Young - Mastering Social Welfare - 1995)

Furthermore, the Lothian Anti Poverty Alliance (Dec 2000) provides the following statistics about poverty in the United Kingdom:

- *Between 1979 and 1999 the numbers living on a low income (Below Half Average Income) in the UK increased from **5 million** (9% of the population) to over **14 million** (26% of the population). The proportion of children living in poverty is even higher with 33% living in low income households*

- *More people are now living in poverty than at any other time in the past 20 years*

- *In the 1990s more than 60,000 households, equivalent to the number of homes in a city the size of Brighton or Milton Keynes – joined the poor each year*

- *Of the 56 million Britons, about 15 million or 26% of the population live without what many would regard as the basic necessities of life*

- *8 million cannot afford one or more essential household goods such as a fridge, a telephone or carpets for the living areas in their homes*

- *7.5 million people are so poor that they cannot afford social activities (such as Christmas, birthdays, visiting relatives in hospital) considered necessary by the rest of the population*

- *2 million British children go without at least two things they need (such as 3 meals a day, toys or adequate clothes)*

- *6.5 million adults go without essential clothing, such as a warm, waterproof coat, because of a lack of money*

- *Over 10.5 million suffer from financial insecurity*

- *Between 1995/6 and 1997/8 the number of people living on less than 40% of the national average income grew from 7 to 8 million*

- *The numbers of children and pensioners living in poverty in the UK increased between 1997 and 1999 (by 200,000 and 100,000 respectively) despite the primary aim of Government welfare policy being to reduce poverty amongst these two groups. However, it should be remembered that the effect of the increases in Minimum Income Guarantee and the introduction of Working Families Tax Credit had not been felt at that time*

- *A Unicef report found that in a league table of 23 industrialised nations Britain was 4th worst in terms of the proportion of children living in 'relative' poverty and 6th worst in terms of children living in 'absolute' poverty. In Britain 30% of children live in 'absolute' poverty whilst in Sweden it is less than 5%.*

- *The gap between the richest and poorest sections of society is getting wider*

- *At the start of the 1970s the incomes of the richest 10% were 3 times higher than the poorest 10%*

- *In the 1990s they were 4 times higher*

- *Real income – that is how much your money can buy – fell for the poorest tenth of the population between 1979 and 1995/96 by 9%. That meant the poorest tenth were on average £13 a week worse off. During the same period the real income of the richest tenth of the population rose by 70%.*

- *The proportion of income taken in taxes from the poorest fifth of the population rose from 27% in 1983 to 39% in 1995. meanwhile the proportion of income taken from the richest fifth of the population fell from 41% to 36%. This was largely due to the shift from direct taxation through income tax to indirect taxation of goods and services*

- *The richest 1% became £908 a week better off due to cuts in direct taxation*

- *The distribution of wealth has altered little in the past 20 years and is now even more unevenly shared*

- *In 1996 1% of the population owned 20% of the wealth – approximately £388 billion*

- *Over 50% of the total wealth was owned by 10% of the population*

- *The wealthiest 50% owned almost all the wealth, 93%*

- *In 1997 – 98 about 30% of households said that they had no savings*

- *Over 50% had savings of less than £1,500*

- *Only 14% had savings of more than £20,000*

- *80% of households in social housing had a weekly income of less than £200*

Poverty is a global problem, but particularly in Asia, Africa and South America. United Nations statistics shows that **over 1 billion** people are in absolute poverty on earth and the problem is getting worse coupled with the problems of increasing urbanisation and the increasing global population that is now 6 billion in September 1999.

Furthermore, the WORLD BANK (September 2000) states that:

a)   3 billion people live on less than $2 a day and 1.3 billion on less than $1 a day,

b)   40,000 die of preventable diseases every day

c)   130 million never have the opportunity to go to school, and

d)   1.3 billion do not have clean water to drink

According to one report, bad drinking water accounts for almost 80% of diseases in developing countries.

The diagrams below illustrate the extent of poverty in the United Kingdom and some selected countries in the world.

Proportion of the population below the poverty line in the world

Country or Region	In urban areas	In rural areas	In whole nation	Date	Separate rural/ urban poverty lines
Africa	**29.0**	**58.0**	**49.0**	**1985**	
Botswana	30.0	64.0	55.0	1985/6	
Cote d'Ivoire	30.0	26.0	28.0	1980/86	
Egypt	34.0	33.7	33.8	1984	Yes
Gambia	63.8	57.7		1989	Yes
Ghana			59.5	1985	
Morocco	28.0	32.0		1985	
Mozambique	40.0	70.0	55.0	1980/89	
Swaziland	45.0	50.0	49.0	1980	Yes
Tunisia	7.3	5.7	6.7	1990	Yes
Uganda	25.0	33.0	32.0	1989/90	
Zambia	40.0		80.0	1993	
Asia (excluding China)	**34.0**	**47.0**	**43.0**	**1985**	
Bangladesh	58.2	72.3		1985/86	Yes
China	0.4	11.5	8.6	1990	Yes
India	37.1	38.7		1988	
Indonesia	20.1	16.4	17.4	1987	Yes
Korea, Republic of	4.6	4.4	4.5	1984	
Malaysia	8.3	22.4	17.3	1987	
Nepal	19.2	43.1	42.6	1984/85	
Pakistan	25.0	31.0		1984/85	
Philippines	40.0	54.1	49.5	1988	
Sri Lanka	27.6	45.7	39.4	1985/6	Yes
Europe					
France			16.0	c.1990	
Germany			10.0	c.1990	
Hungary			15.4	1991	
Ireland			19.0	c.1990	
Italy			15.0	c.1990	
Poland			22.7	1987	
Spain			19.0	c.1990	
United Kingdom			18.0	c.1990	
Latin America	**32.0**	**45.0**		**1985**	
Argentina	14.6	19.7	15.5	1986	Yes
Brazil	37.7	65.9	45.3	1987	Yes
Columbia	40.2	44.5	41.6	1986	Yes
Costa Rica	11.6	32.7	23.4	1990	
El Salvador	61.4			1990	
Guatemala	61.4.	85.4	76.3	1989	

Haiti	65.0	80.0	76.0	1980-86	
Honduras	73.9	80.2	77.5	1990	
Mexico	30.2	50.5	29.9	1984	Yes
Panama	29.7	51.9	41.0	1986	Yes
Peru	44.5	63.8	51.8	1986	Yes
Uruguay	19.3	28.7	20.4	1986	Yes
Venezuela	24.8	42.2	26.6	1986	Yes
North America					
Canada			15.0	c.1990	
United States of America			13.0		

Source: UN Global Report on Human Settlements - 1996

3. Poverty, Hunger and Cannibalism

Hunger or starvation is one of the possible consequences of poverty. History and well-documented evidence shows that amongst other things, extreme hunger could lead to cannibalism.

While the evidence illustrated below shows no direct link between poverty and cannibalism, it shows a clear link between hunger and cannibalism – hunger, a factor of which poverty is one of the causes.

One such documented evidence is the case of **R v Dudley and Stephens (1884)** in English Criminal Law.

> *"The defendants, a third man, and cabin boy were cast adrift in a boat following a shipwreck. They were some 1,600 miles from land, and had endured over a week without food and water. Dudley and Stephens agreed that as the cabin boy was already weak, and looked likely to die soon, they would kill him and live off his flesh and blood for as long as they could, in the hope that they would be rescued before they themselves die of starvation. Dudley carried out the killing and all three surviving crew members ate the boy's flesh. A few days later they were rescued by a passing ship. On returning to England, the defendants were charged with murder, the jury returning a special verdict to the effect that if the defendants had not eaten the boy they would probably have died; that the boy would have died in any event, and that at the time of the killing the defendants had no reasonable prospect of being rescued; but that there had been no greater reason to take the life of the cabin boy than that of any other member of the crew. The special verdict was referred for consideration by the judges of the Queen's Bench Division, where it was held that the defendants were guilty of murder in killing the cabin boy.*
>
> *Lord Coleridge C.J, having referred to Hale's assertion that a man was not to be acquitted of theft of food on account of his extreme hunger, doubted that the defence of necessity could ever be extended to a defendant who killed another to save his own life. After referring to the Christian doctrine of actually giving up one's own life to save others, rather than taking another's life to save one's own, he referred to the impossibility of choosing between the value of one person's life as against another's:*
>
> > *'Who is to be the judge of this sort of necessity? By what measure is the comparative value of lives to be measured? Is it to be strength, or intellect, or what? It is plain that the principle leaves to him who is to profit by it to determine*

the necessity which will justify him in deliberately taking another's life to save his own. In [the present case] the weakest, the youngest, the most unresisting life was chosen. Was it more necessary to kill him than one of the grown men? The answer be, NO.....'

The defendants were sentenced to death, but this was commuted to six months imprisonment"
(HLT CRIMINAL LAW - 1996)

A much more recently documented case is depicted in the 1993 Hollywood movie **"ALIVE"** directed by Frank Marshall. It is a real life story of a rugby team from Uruguay whose plane crashed in the Andes Mountains in South America in October 1972. They were stranded on the mountains for over two months and some survived by resorting to cannibalism.

It is worth noting that documented evidence of the link between hunger and cannibalism goes back as far as 2,600 years ago; an account contained in the Bible in Lamentations (2:20) where Jeremiah lamented about how normally caring and loving parents were eating their own children in Jerusalem out of starvation caused by the siege and destruction of Jerusalem by the Babylonians.

4. Those worst hit by poverty

Some of those who are worst hit by poverty in society are:

a) The unemployed

b) The elderly

c) Single parent families

d) People with disabilities

e) The homeless

f) Ethnic minority groups

g) Immigrant communities

h) People on low incomes

5. The consequences of poverty

Poverty can have very adverse effects on those afflicted and also on society at large. Some of the negative consequences identified by Pat Young are:

a) Domestic violence

b) Frustration, anxiety and discrimination

c)   Mental and physical illness

d)   Humiliation and loss of confidence

e)   Shame and feelings of failure

f)   Alcoholism and drug addiction

g)   Feelings of powerlessness and inability to participate fully in society.

h)   Crime and juvenile delinquency

i)   Poor communities become run-down physically and are characterised by feelings of despair.

j)   Negative effects on children's' upbringing

k)   Poor housing conditions

l)   Poor educational upbringing

m)   Stigma and lack of status

n)   Lack of leisure

o)   Stress

p)   Hopelessness, violence, riots, community unrests and wars

q)   Premature death

Furthermore, poverty is now known to be a major cause of wars, social unrest, intolerance, communal conflicts and political unrest as people fight to get a little bit more or to protect the little they have. This, in turn, causes bloodshed, despair and even greater poverty. It is basically like an unending, dangerous revolving door, which traps its victims, taking them with it.

6. Healthcare Implications of Poverty

Poverty can have a profound negative effect on a person's state of mind, healthcare and hygiene. The poorer a person is, the less good his state of healthcare is likely to be. This is because:

a) poorer people are less likely to be well-informed about healthcare as they are likely to be less educated

b) even where they are informed, a lot of them cannot afford proper healthcare

c) Or they may be too preoccupied with the daily search for survival so much that healthcare is not considered a priority

d) This daily search for survival makes many poor people take unnecessary health risks

e) They are more likely to attract diseases that are attributable to:

- Malnutrition
- Bad housing and living conditions
- Bad drinking water
- Unhealthy food

f) This in turn may weaken their immune system

g) They are less likely to have healthcare insurance and advice

h) They have shorter life expectancy

i) Also, as poorer governments are less able to provide proper healthcare, the physical and mental health of the people declines

Poverty is indeed an evil that kills on a massive scale.

Conclusion

Although the precise definition of poverty is open to interpretation, it is clear that the numbers of poor in the UK run into millions, whereas in the rest of the world, billions of people can be categorised as in either absolute or relative poverty. The wider health implications of this are massive. Not only will people's lives be at risk through hunger and malnutrition, but there are many and varied associated health risks because of limited access to healthcare, medicine and safe housing.

Self-Assessment Questions

1. How would you define 'poverty'?

2. What is the difference between 'absolute' and 'relative' poverty?

3. What is the link between increasing urbanisation and poverty?

4. Study the list of consequences of poverty in section 5. Which of these factors do you think also lead to health problems?

5. How widespread is poverty?

6. What is the relationship between poverty and healthcare?

7. Do you think there is any relationship between poverty and cannibalism? Give reasons for your answer.

Chapter 2

The Nature of HIV/AIDS

Contents of this Chapter

1. Introduction

HIV stands for **Human Immuno-deficiency Virus.** The HIV virus belongs to a group of viruses that are known as **retroviruses** or the family named **retoviridae.**

Broadly, retroviruses are made up of the following groups:

a) **Lenti-Viruses**
The characteristics of these viruses include:
immune-deficiency, pneumonia, arthritis and anaemia.

b) **Onco-Viruses**
These are leukaemia and sarcoma (cancer or tumour) based retroviruses.

c) **Spuma-Viruses**
Also known as "foamy" retroviruses. They are not known to cause any disease.

2. The Nature of the Virus

HIV belongs to the species of **Lenti-Viruses** which means 'slow' viruses.

The human body has an in-built immune system (the body's defence mechanism) that prevents germs and viruses from taking a hold on it by attacking them. Without this defence mechanism, humans would be prone to attack from all sorts of diseases and illnesses, which may eventually lead to death.

What the HIV does is to gradually damage the body's immune system so that a point may be reached when the entire system collapses. This then attracts infections and diseases that may kill the person. The point at which the entire immune system collapses is when the virus has progressed to the stage of the disease called AIDS **(Acquired Immune-Deficiency Syndrome)**.

In a more medical terminology, a person has AIDS when his body's CD4 + T lymphocyte (also known as T-4 cells) count per micro litre of blood - which normally ranges between 500 to 1,600 - drops to below 200. T-4 cells are a type of lymphocyte (white blood cells) that is an important part of the immune system. Also known as 'Helper' Cells, T-4 cells are at the forefront in preventing germs and viruses from taking hold on the body.

The higher a person's CD4 + count, the stronger his immune system. It is believed that HIV replication in the body doubles when the CD4 + count drops below 500 microlitres of blood. The virus gradually reduces the CD4 + T-cells in the blood until a point, when the immune system collapses, leading to AIDS.

The surface of these T-cells, have receptors that are called CD4. Thus, the name CD4 + T-cells. HIV has a spiky surface. These spikes are known as **gp120**. The virus is able to enter the helper cells by using gp120 to attach to the receptors (CD4).

While the CD4 + T-cells are suppose to prevent the body from being invaded by viruses and diseases, there are other T lymphocytes known as **Cytotoxic T Lymphocytes (CTLs) or CD8 + (also called Killer T-cells)** that attack and destroy any invader. This cooperation between the T-cells is important for the body to effectively fight off viruses and diseases. However, HIV incapacitates the CD4 + T-cells leaving only CD8 + (killer cells) to do the impossible job of controlling HIV, which makes **10 billion copies** of itself in one person in a single day.

HIV enters the helper cell, by latching itself to CD4 and copying itself into the DNA of the cell. HIV propagates it offspring, by splitting the infected cell into many more HIV infected cells, which will eventually get killed by the killer cells. This replicated virus will infect another cell, and the process is repeated. As the number of T-Cells count per micro litre of blood decreases, the immune system weakens, which then attracts **opportunistic infections** that may kill the person. As HIV replicates faster than the spread or killing mechanism of the killer cells, the virus prevail over the killer cells in the end.

Thus, one way to tame the HIV might be to produce a vaccine that can slow its ability to replicate, so that that the virus can be kept under control by the killer cells. Another mean might be a vaccine that can drastically increase the number of killer cells and improve their fighting power, in order to overtake and subdue the replication of HIV. Still, another possibility might be to produce a vaccine that can block gp120 from attaching itself to CD4.

Although it replicates very quickly, HIV is not very good at copying accurately. Thus, it copies slight variances of itself, any time that it replicates, making the virus much more difficult to be identified and controlled by CD8 +. HIV is a very varied virus with many different types, subtypes and strains.

Though all viruses change over time, none is as prolific as HIV, which mutates in minutes, hours, days and weeks, rather than in years. Indeed, gp120 is the most variable part of the virus; changing itself in minutes.

A person may have the virus, but the condition may never lead to AIDS. Such persons may be referred to as **CARRIERS** - that is, they are capable of passing the virus to others (who may then develop AIDS and eventually die), but their own condition may never progress to AIDS at all. Surprisingly, some are not infected by the virus at all, even though they have been exposed to it on several occasions. This may be because of their unusually strong immune system (CD4 +) and/or the great fighting and killing power (i.e. the quantity and quality) of their CD8 + T-cells.

However, it is worth pointing out that even people with high numbers of killer cells can get AIDS. Nevertheless, there is documented evidence that some sex workers in Africa have been infected with HIV for a long time, but the infection is not progressing to AIDS. It was discovered that they have a very high number of killer cells. Similar cases have been reported in other parts of the world; prompting some scientists to believe the killer cell solution to HIV/AIDS. Others believe that the solution will be found when scientists have full understanding of the virus and its exploits. They have a limited understanding of it at the moment.

Others who are already infected, may be able to prevent the virus from progressing to full blown AIDS, by taking specialist HIV medication known as **anti-retroviral drugs** that are now readily available. These can, however, be very expensive and not everyone can afford them without government support. Costs could be in the region of £5,000 to £8,000 per year.

However, something unprecedented occurred in April 2001 that is gradually changing this situation for good. The **South African government threatened** to either manufacture by itself or import cheaper anti-retroviral drugs from sources other than the big drug companies who have the patent right to produce and distribute the drugs for 20 years, based on the World Trade Organisation's (WTO) patent rules. The drug companies sued the South African government, but as a result of global pressure and adverse publicity, they later abandoned their legal action before the case was heard. This paved the way for possible cheaper drugs to counter this appalling disease.

Concerning the possibility of cheaper drugs, the Guardian newspaper of 16th June 2001 comments:

> "...African governments began threatening to import cheap generic anti-retrovirals and the western companies which had sewn up the market started cutting their prices. By April, prices had halved. After the South Africa's court victory over the companies later that month, they were slashed by up to 85%.

> Most patented AIDS drugs now cost about the same as their generic versions: around £2 a day. But the governments are still threatening; and the prices are still falling..."

But there are already serious worries about the possible proliferation of fake HIV drugs being peddled by fraudsters in developing countries. The Guardian of that same day writes under the heading **"FAKE MEDICINES THREATEN POOR":**

> "Large amounts of fake and substandard drugs are being sold through bona fide distributors in the developing world, according to evidence published this week.

> This could have serious implications for the treatment of HIV/AIDS in poor countries, since strains of the virus could become resistant to drugs.

> There is growing pressure on the UN global health fund, established by the Secretary General, Kofi Annan, to help countries improve their hospital and clinic services as well as

to buy medicines. Some argue that the anti-retroviral drugs will quickly become useless if they are wrongly used, badly copied or faked.

In one of two studies published in the Lancet this week, researchers in South-East Asia found that 38% of the samples they bought of artesunate used to treat drug-resistant strains of malaria contained no trace of the drug.

"The recent emergence of counterfeit artesunate in this region has led to the death of many patients who would have survived if given the genuine drug." The group from Oxford University and Bangkok wrote.

They urged the authorities to test the medicines.

The second group from Robert Gordon University in Aberdeen, examined the quality of drugs on sale in pharmacies in Lagos and Abuja in Nigeria. Nearly half the 581 samples they tested were substandard, which, they point out, could lead to a greater likelihood of drug-resistant strains of the virus...."

However, the report concluded that the sub-standard drugs were largely due to lack of effective quality control during manufacture rather than deliberately faking the drugs.

There seems to be **good news** for developing countries as there are moves by some big drug companies to provide anti-retroviral drugs free of charge to patients in some poor countries where HIV/AIDS infection rates are high. According to The Independent newspaper on Sunday 5th October 2003, under the heading "Drugs Giants close to HIV Giveaway for Third World":

"Seven of the world's biggest pharmaceutical companies, including GlaxoSmithKline and Pfizer, are in talks with a leading international workers' organisation that could result in HIV drugs being given free to some of the world's poorest nations.

The talks are being held between the International Federation of Chemical, Energy, Mine and General Workers' Unions (ICEM) and the main producers of HIV drugs. Besides Pfizer, the world's largest drugs company and Glaxo, they include US firms Bristol-Myers Squibb and Abbott Laboratories; Swiss-based Merck and Roche; and the family owned German business Boehringer Inglheim.

The talks got under way six months ago after a US-based consultant, acting for many of the pharmaceutical companies, approached the ICEM about supplying HIV drugs to poor countries where the virus is rampant. The aim is to provide individual patients with a tailor-made cocktail of anti-retroviral HIV drugs, either for free or at affordable prices. The talks are focussed on Sub-Saharan Africa and on those nations on the UN's list of the world's 49 least developed countries.

The issue has been a controversial one, and many of the drug companies have been heavily criticised over their apparent refusal to provide affordable treatments. But the ICEM's general-secretary, Fred Higgs, is confident the talks will be successful.

'I'm optimistic that we will get a good result,' said Mr Higgs. 'I don't believe that, if the companies are serious, it will take us any longer than the end of the quarter of next year for something beneficial to come out of it.'

HIV and AIDS have become a devastating problem for Sub-Saharan Africa, where life expectancy has dropped to below 40 in some countries. The main problem is that the drugs are highly expensive and beyond the reach of the bulk of the population. HIV and AIDS treatments are also protected by long patents, meaning cheaper generic versions are not currently available. Some pharmaceutical companies have stopped charging poorer countries for a variety of treatments, but these are mainly for the symptoms of Aids and do not include the crucial anti-retroviral drugs used in the treatment of HIV, which can significantly delay the onset of Aids. Many of the drugs companies do sell these at cheap rates, but the ICEM is keen to bring the prices down further under a single agreement with the producers.

The ICEM has 20 million members and 400 affiliated unions. It represents chemical workers in the pharmaceutical industry and in sectors hard hit by HIV, such as energy and mining in developing regions of sub-Saharan Africa, Asia and Latin America. Said Mr Higgs: ' We feel the ICEM is strategically positioned to make a difference.'

A spokesman for Glaxo, which has already cut the price it charges developing countries for HIV drugs said: 'Our ambition is to provide our medicines on a not-for-cost basis both to countries and to employers in those countries.'"

A person who is tested and found to have the HIV virus in their blood is referred to as being **HIV Positive** and the phrase **HIV Negative** is used if the HIV virus is not present in the person.

The incubation period from initial HIV infection to when the symptoms of AIDS start to show ranges from **6 months to over 10 years**. Thus, some HIV positive persons would not be aware of their infection for a very long time, during which period they may continue to infect others.

3. Retroviruses in other Creatures

Retroviruses are not peculiar to humans. Different types of retroviruses can be found in several animals, primates and other creatures. Some of these are shown in the table below:

Types of Retrovirus	Host found
1. HIV	Humans
2. Simian Immunodeficiency Virus (SIV)	Primates (e.g. monkeys, chimpanzees)
3. Visna Maedi	Sheep and goats
4. a) Bovine Immunodeficiency Virus (BIV) b) Bovine Leukemia Virus (BLV)	Cows and sheep
5. Equine Infectious Anaemia Virus (EIAV)	Horses and donkeys
6. Feline leukaemia virus (FIV)	Cats
7. Porcine Endogenous Retroviruses (PERV)	Pigs
8. Canine Immunodeficiency Virus (CIV)	Dogs
9. Walleye Dermal Sarcoma Virus (WDSV). This is a tumour-based virus.	Walleye Fish
10. a) Avian Leukosis Sarcoma Virus (ALSV) b) Reticuloendotheliosis Viruses (REV). These are tumour-based viruses	Chickens and Turkeys

This makes cross-species organ transplantation seem a frightening prospect.

4. Picture of the HIV Virus

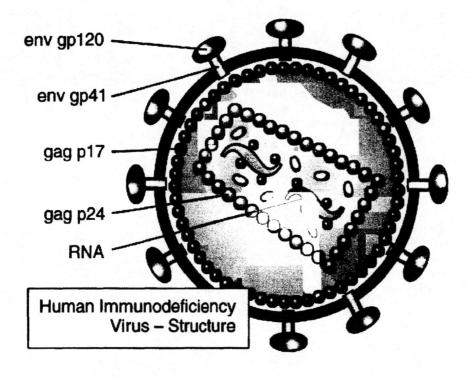

env gp120

env gp41

gag p17

gag p24

RNA

Human Immunodeficiency
Virus – Structure

Source: AVERT, UK (2002)

5. Some Symptoms of HIV/AIDS

You cannot tell merely by looking, who is infected with HIV/AIDS. However, where there are symptoms they may include some of following:

a)   Severe Weight loss

b)   Persistent Diarrhoea

c)   Chronic tiredness and loss of appetite

d)   Night sweats and fever

e)   Persistent rashes and patches on the face and body

f)   Persistent Joint and muscle pain

g)   Persistent cough

h)   Tuberculosis

i)   Swollen lymph glands and persistent sore throat

j)   Persistent vaginal yeast infection (candidiasis) in women

k)   Persistent candidiasis infection in the form of patches on the tongue and in the mouth.

l)   Several recurring viral, bacterial, parasitic and fungal infections one after the other

m)   Unpredictable mood changes

n)   Cervical cancer

o)   Anaemia

p)   Memory loss

q)   Dementia

r)   Blurred and slow speech

s)   Many other unexplained illnesses one after the other

According to the National Institute of Allergy and Infectious Diseases, USA (1992):

"Some may have flu-like symptoms within months of infection. They may have fever, headaches, malaise and enlarged lymph nodes. These symptoms usually disappear within a week to a month and are often mistaken for those of another viral infection.

More persistent or severe symptoms may not surface for a decade or more after HIV first enters the body in adults, or within two years in children born with HIV infection...

Some may begin to have symptoms in as soon as a few months, whereas others may by symptom-free for more than 10 years. However, within this period, the virus is actively infecting and killing cells of the immune system"

These HIV/AIDS related infections are generally known as **opportunistic infections** as they take advantage of the opportunities created by the weakened and compromised immune system.

It is worth pointing out, however, that not everyone who has one or more of these symptoms is suffering from HIV/AIDS. Only an HIV test can reveal whether or not a person is infected.

6. AIDS is not the Direct Killer

It is important to note that neither the HIV virus nor AIDS is the direct killer. It is the many opportunistic diseases and illnesses that the now completely deficient immune system attracts (as a result of HIV/AIDS infection) that kill.

Sadly, there is not yet any known cure for AIDS, but for people infected with HIV there are now drugs to prevent the infection from progressing into full-blown AIDS.

HIV is not an air-borne disease. To contract it, there has to be contact with infected blood, semen, vaginal secretions or other body fluids. The virus cannot survive for a long time outside the human fluid system.

A test should show HIV antibodies where there is an infection. It may, however, take several weeks or months before the results are known.

In some developing countries, HIV/AIDS is now referred to as the **Slim Disease**, because of the severe weight loss that many infected persons experience.

7. How Long does HIV survive outside the Human Body

This is a question that many people ask. The answer is that HIV is a very fragile virus and does not survive long outside body fluid. Some laboratory experiments have shown that in a dry state the virus can only survive outside body fluid for 2 to 5 seconds.

Even in a wet state outside body fluid, HIV can disintegrate very fast on exposure to:

a)   heat or high temperatures
b)   hydrogen peroxide
c)   bleach
d)   disinfectants
e)   detergents
f)   alcohol based products

The virus is very fragile when outside body fluid, because its genome (i.e. the total gene complement of a set of chromosomes) is made of an enveloped RNA which is not as tough as DNA. The shell of the envelope is made of a very thin cell membrane, thus, it is not hard and water-tight enough to withstand the conditions outside the human body fluid system.

However, HIV can survive up to 7-21 days or more outside the human body, if stored at temperatures of 4°C/39°F. It could survive up to months or years if stored frozen.

Conclusion

Because HIV and AIDS disable the body's immune system, a whole range of diseases and viruses are able to attack the body, in many cases leading to death. This is one of the reasons that AIDS is so hard to treat: a combination of many possible infections or diseases and a body that cannot fight it off. It is not surprising that so many people die in developing countries once HIV turns into **full-blown AIDS**.

There are steps underway to produce an effective vaccine for HIV prevention; but vaccine takes time to develop.

Self-Assessment Questions

1. *What does HIV stand for?*

2. *What does AIDS stand for?*

3. *What is the difference between HIV and AIDS?*

4. *How complex is HIV?*

5. *Who is a 'Carrier'?*

6. *Why can it sometimes be difficult for a person to know that they are infected with HIV?*

7. *What is the best way of confirming whether a person is HIV – Positive or negative?*

8. *Is there hope for the reduction of prices of HIV drugs? Give your reasons.*

9. *How long can HIV survive outside the human body?*

10. *Why is HIV/AIDS referred to as Slim Disease?*

Chapter 3

Different Types of HIV

Contents of this Chapter

1. Introduction

HIV is one of the most complex and varied viruses, with a ferocious ability to mutate into different subtypes and strains.

There are now known to be two main types of the Human Immuno-deficiency Virus (HIV) namely **HIV–1 and HIV-2**. However, when a person mentions the word 'HIV', without distinguishing which type, it is generally assumed that he is referring to HIV-1, as it is by far the most prevalent of the two viruses. Thus HIV–1 is referred to as the global HIV.

However, HIV-1 is far from being uniform. It is in fact a very variable virus itself with different strains that are made up of two main groups, namely **groups 'M' and 'O'**. These two groups are in turn made up of several different subtypes (see diagram below) that are unevenly distributed and found in different unconnected regions/countries of the world. All these subtypes and strains are both biologically and genetically different.

2. Types of HIV

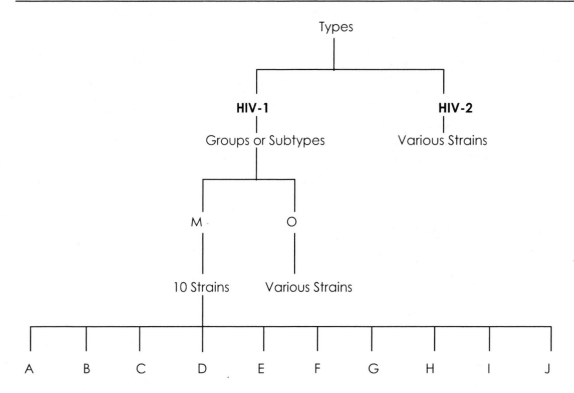

Although the modes of transmission and the effects of being infected by HIV-1 or HIV-2 are exactly the same, HIV-2 (which was first identified in May 1986) is less easily transmitted and, even where it is transmitted, the incubation period is generally longer than with HIV-1.

HIV-2 is referred to as the West African HIV as it is predominant in Western Africa and is found mostly in Gambia, Senegal, Guinea, Ivory Coast, Burkina Faso, Guinea-Bissau and Cape Verde Islands, Nigeria, Cameroon, Ghana and Ivory Coast. HIV-1 group O was first found in Cameroon and Gabon. However, some persons are infected with both HIV-1 and HIV-2 at the same time.

The diagram below shows the regional distribution of the HIV-1 group M subtypes (A-J).

HIV-1: Different Strains of Group M (ranging from A-J)

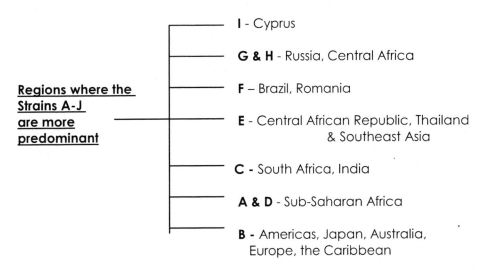

Regions where the Strains A-J are more predominant

- **I** - Cyprus
- **G & H** - Russia, Central Africa
- **F** – Brazil, Romania
- **E** - Central African Republic, Thailand & Southeast Asia
- **C** - South Africa, India
- **A & D** - Sub-Saharan Africa
- **B** - Americas, Japan, Australia, Europe, the Caribbean

Source: AVERT – 2003

These are countries and regions where different subtypes predominate. It is of course, possible for these subtypes to be found in other regions as a result of cross-infection. Besides, HIV-1 is now found in almost every part of the earth.

Furthermore, a strain of HIV-1 (apart from groups M and O) was found in three women in Cameroon in 1998 by French researchers. Some scientists now believe that even more strains and subtypes of the virus are likely to be discovered in the future.

Finally, some scientists are worried that the genetic and biological variations in different types, strains and subtypes of HIV might prevent an early development of an effective vaccine and possible cure for the disease.

HIV is a virus that is a lot more complex than many first thought.

Conclusion

From the above it can be seen that there are distinct strains of the HIV virus, which are prevalent in different regions of the world. Although the risk of cross-infection could delay the search for a cure, this knowledge seems sure to be beneficial, as it will help researchers to more clearly categorise the virus.

Self-Assessment Questions

1. What are the 2 main types of the HIV virus?

2. Which of the 2 types is the most prevalent globally?

3. Where is HIV-2 most prevalent?

4. Why do scientists believe that finding a cure for HIV might take longer than was originally thought?

Chapter 4

How HIV is Transmitted

Contents of this Chapter

1. Introduction

For effective HIV prevention to be possible, it is important that we fully understand the means by which HIV is transmitted. HIV is not the easiest virus to transmit. It is for instance, not as infectious as tuberculosis or influenza. Certain specific circumstances have to occur before HIV transmission is possible. This chapter examines the main methods of transmitting HIV.

2. Methods of Transmitting HIV

HIV is not an air or water-borne disease but a virus transmitted through contact with blood and other body fluids such as semen and vaginal fluids. HIV has also been found in saliva, tears, urine, faeces, breast milk and bone marrow.

Thus, the virus has to have contact with a person's blood or body fluid for transmission to be possible. The virus cannot survive for long outside the human body, as it is very fragile.

Certain factors facilitate the **rapid spread of HIV infection** in society. These are:

- Poverty

- Illiteracy/Ignorance

- Lack of Proper Health Care and Health Advice

- Easy Mobility/Mobile Society

- Promiscuity, Prostitution and Commercial Sex

- Political Instability

- Wars and Conflicts

Regarding the relationship between poverty and HIV infection, the Guardian Newspaper of 6th June 2001 comments in an article "AIDS Plays Havoc with Africa's Children":

"HIV/AIDS has reached a "catastrophic" proportion and is unravelling decades of gains in child survival and development, especially in sub-Saharan Africa, the UN Secretary General Kofi Annan, warns in a new report.

The social profile of the AIDS pandemic has been gradually shifting, the report warns, with the disease increasingly affecting the young, poor and illiterate. Above all, its victims are adolescent girls.

Elsewhere too, deepening poverty and "increasingly obscene disparities" shame commitments made by the world community at a summit a decade ago to improve children's lives across the world, the report says.

In a major study prepared by UNICEF for a UN special session on children in September which will bring dozens of heads of state to New York, Mr Annan challenges them to find it "unacceptable that 600 million children in developing countries have to struggle to survive on less than $1 a day.....

...10 million children still die every year from often readily preventable causes, an estimated 150 million are malnourished and more than 100 million are out of school – 60% of them girls.

Rising numbers of children are also the victims of abuse, neglect and exploitation. Sexual abuse occurs in the home, in communities and across societies. But worst of all, it is commercialised. "The worst forms of exploitation include prostitution and child slavery, often in the guise of household domestic work. The trafficking of children for sexual exploitation has reached alarming levels" the report states. As many as 30 million children are victimised by traffickers, largely with impunity.

The International Labour Organisation estimates that 250 million children work, with 50 – 60 million of them "engaged in intolerable forms of labour". These children work in plantations, factories and homes, often with no contact with their families, no shelter and no access to education....

The gulf between rich and poor countries continues to widen – between 1960 and 1995, the disparity in per capita income between industrialised and developing countries has more than tripled. Never in history have we seen such numbers. And never have we seen overall aid to the world's neediest countries fall to levels as low as they have in recent years....

The report's data on Africa over the last decade is chilling: the already minimal incomes fell further, immunisation coverage decreased, the total number of malnourished children increased and the weakness of public health systems was reflected in the resurgence of cholera. Less than half of children under one are fully immunised against diphtheria, whooping cough and tetanus. Forty per cent of the world's children out of school are Africans, and they are increasingly vulnerable to all forms of exploitation and abuse.

Some 95% of AIDS orphans live in Africa. Faced with social stigma, isolation and discrimination, and deprived of basic care and financial resources, AIDS orphans are less likely to be immunised, more likely to be malnourished, less likely to go to school and more vulnerable to abuse and exploitation".

Poverty is indeed an evil that every government should sincerely work hard to destroy.

Below is an AIDS and Child Mortality table in some African countries:

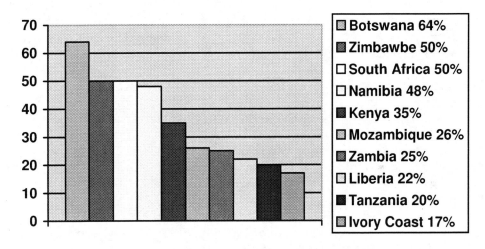

**% Under 5 Child Mortality Due to AIDS
2000 – 2005 Projection**

Source: UN population division.

The following are the best known modes of transmission of HIV:

1.   **By having sexual intercourse** with an infected person, whether:

a)   Vaginal Sex

b)   Oral Sex, or

c)   Anal Sex

HIV affects heterosexuals, bisexuals and homosexuals alike. Though it was first identified among homosexuals (as mentioned earlier), by far the most common mode of transmission of the disease now (especially in developing countries), is heterosexual intercourse.

2.   **By blood transfusion** – this may occur when HIV infected blood is transfused into a person during illness or accident.

3. **By an infected mother** – an HIV infected mother can pass the virus to her foetus during pregnancy or to her baby at birth.

4. **By sharing syringes and needles** – this is quite common amongst hard drug users, who frequently share needles which may be contaminated and infected by the virus. This mode of transmission is also of particular concern in some developing countries where sharing needles (although not for hard drugs) is practised during the giving of routine medication or vaccination. People should also be aware of body piercing or tattoo needles which may be contaminated.

5. **By Sharing razors and blades** – it is possible to transmit HIV by sharing HIV-contaminated razors and blades during circumcision and hair cutting or shaving.

6. **By body tissue or organ transplantation** – this mode of transmission may occur where body tissue or organs (such as a liver or kidney) was transplanted to a person and the organs were taken from an HIV infected person.

7. **By artificial insemination** – Artificial insemination is a process where sperm taken from a man is injected or deposited into a woman's womb (by artificial means) in order to make her pregnant. This may occur where a woman is finding it difficult to be pregnant through the conventional means.

The disease may be transmitted to the woman if the donated sperm was infected with HIV.

8. **By Occupational Exposure** – Some occupations such as those of doctors, dentists or nurses can cause exposure to the HIV infection, for example, if they prick or injure themselves with an infected needle or metal or while treating an infected person.

9. **By an infected doctor** – similar to (7) above. An infected doctor, surgeon or midwife could also transmit the virus to their patient if there was contact with infected fluids, needles or syringes.

10. **By breast-feeding** – it is possible for an infected mother to transmit the virus to a baby through breast-feeding. This mode of transmission as well as the one mentioned under (3) above, is sometimes referred to as **vertical transmission**. On the other hand, or the other mode can be referred to as **horizontal transmission**.

3. HIV is <u>not</u> transmitted in the Following ways:

Though misinformed people may think otherwise, HIV is <u>not</u> transmitted by:

a)   Sneezing, coughing, talking or laughing

b)   Shaking hands with an infected person

c)   Hugging or cuddling an infected person

d)   Swimming in the same pool or bathing in water with an infected person

e)   Sharing cups, plates or other cooking utensils with an infected person

f)   Sharing seats or sofas with an infected person

g)   Using the same toilet seat as an infected person

h)   Contact with the clothes of an infected person

i)   Being in the same room as an infected person

j)   Mosquitoes or other insects – there is no evidence that this is possible

k)   Kissing – even though the HIV virus has been found in saliva, kissing is not a conventional mode of transmission. However, it is advisable for a person who has a deep cut or sores in the mouth to abstain from mouth-to-mouth kissing since the possibility of transmission will be greater.

It is clear from the foregoing, that any means which makes it possible for the virus to have contact with a person's blood or body fluid is a potential mode of HIV transmission.

The **HIV TRANSMISSION TREE** below shows how the disease can spread to many others from just one person who is referred to as person 1:

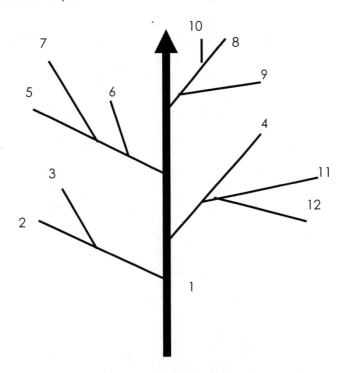

If uncontrolled, the spread of HIV could be endless. Prevention therefore, is the most effective way of controlling the disease.

4. Women and HIV/AIDS

There is growing evidence that women, especially in developing countries are increasingly becoming more vulnerable to the HIV epidemic. In this regard, the World Health Organisation provides the following information:

Facts and Figures

- 33.6 million people are living with HIV/AIDS, 14.8 million of whom are women

- 5 million adults were newly infected in 1999, 1.1 million of whom were women

- 2.1 million people died of AIDS in 1999, 1.1 million of whom were women

- 12-13 African women are currently infected for every 10 African men

- There are half a million infections in children (under 15), most of which have been transmitted from mother to child

- 55% of adult infections in sub-Saharan Africa are in women, 30% in South East Asia, 20% in Europe and the USA

Modes of Transmission

The AIDS epidemic in women is overwhelmingly heterosexual – almost entirely so in Africa and South-East Asia.

In other areas, a proportion of women are infected through:

- Sex with a bisexual or drug injecting partner

- Their own injecting drug use

- Heterosexual sex without these factors

- Blood transfusion (in developing countries where blood is not routinely screened)

Why are Women Vulnerable to HIV infection?

a) Biologically

- Larger mucosal surface; microlesions which can occur during intercourse may be entry points for the virus; very young women are even more vulnerable in this respect

- More virus are contained in sperm than in vaginal secretions

- As with Sexually Transmitted Infections (STIs), women are at least four times more vulnerable to infection; the presence of untreated STIs is a risk factor for HIV infection

- Coerced sex increases risk of microlesions

b) Economically

- Financial or material dependence on men means that women often cannot control when and in what circumstances they have sex

- Many women have to exchange sex for material favours, for daily survival. There is formal sex work but there is also this exchange which, in many poor settings, is many women's only way of providing for themselves and their children

c) Socially and Culturally

- Women are not expected to discuss or make decisions about sexual matters

- They cannot request (let alone insist) on using condoms or any other form of protection during sex

- If they require sex or request condom use, they often risk abuse, as there may then be a suspicion of infidelity

- The many forms of violence against women mean that sex is often coerced which is itself a risk factor for HIV infection

- For married and unmarried men, multiple partners (including sex workers) are culturally accepted

- Women are expected to have relations with or marry older men, who are more experienced, and more likely to be infected. Men are seeking younger and younger partners in order to avoid infection and in the false belief that sex with a virgin cures AIDS and other diseases.

5. Other Sexually Transmitted Diseases and HIV

There is clear evidence that the presence of other Sexually Transmitted Diseases (STDs) in a person increases the likelihood of HIV infection.

This is particularly the case in so many infected persons in developing countries, where the open sores caused by untreated or improperly treated STD infections become the source of entry for the HIV infection.

The fact that these people are poor means that they cannot afford antibiotics for the proper treatment of the STDs, and the open sores then becomes the route for the HIV infection to enter their bodies.

Furthermore, it is also now suspected that not only does the presence of other STDs in a person attract additional white cells and macrophages, but that they may also significantly change the protective mucosa of the vagina, urethra or the rectum, thus increasing the risk of HIV infection.

6. HIV and Alcohol

It is increasingly becoming clear that many people, especially teenagers and young persons engage in unwanted and unprotected sex because they were drunk and so risk being infected with HIV. They may never have engaged in such behaviour if not for the alcohol or other drugs which can adversely affect their judgement and their ability to refuse unwanted sexual advances.

The advice is, therefore to stay away from alcohol if you cannot drink and be sober enough to avoid being persuaded to take such risks.

7. HIV and Other Risk Factors

Apart from the ones discussed above, there are other risk factors that increase the risk of HIV infection; some of which are discussed below.

i)   Bleeding during sexual activities

Bleeding caused by open sores or lesions during sexual activities, however minor, increases the risk of HIV infection.

Sexual intercourse during menstruation also increases the risk of infection.

ii)   Circumcision

It is believed that an uncircumcised man is at greater risk of hosting viruses thus, is at greater risk of being infected and transmitting HIV.

iii)   Number of Sexual Partners

It is quite clear that the more the number of sexual partners that a person has unprotected sex with, the greater the risk of HIV infection.

iv)   Infection Stage

Some experts believe that the HIV is most infectious at certain stages of the infection. They believe that the early stages of being infected and the stage that the person becomes unwell as a result of the infection are the most infectious stages of the virus.

v)   Amount of Virus

Another risk factor is the amount of the HIV virus that a person is exposed to. The larger the amount of virus present at the time that the individual was exposed to it, not only increases the risk of HIV infection but is also more likely to hasten progression to AIDS.

vi)   Type of Virus

As discussed in the chapter on "Different Types of HIV", it is clear that HIV is a very varied virus with different types, sub-types and strains some of which are less infectious than others. Thus, the risk of being infected is to some extent dependent on the type or strain of the virus that a person was exposed to.

vii)   <u>Sex Between Men</u>

One of the most effective means of transmitting the virus is sex between two men by the way of anal sex.

Thus people engaging in such sexual activities have a very high risk of being infected with HIV.

Nevertheless, by far the most common means of HIV infection in developing countries is unprotected sexual activities between men and women, be they vaginal or anal.

Conclusion

There are several different and clearly understood ways of contracting HIV, which all involve contact with an infected person's body fluids. This means that although it is an infectious virus, it cannot be passed on by simple body contact or being in close proximity to an infected person. A clear understanding of these distinctions will certainly help prevent people catching the virus through ignorance.

Self-Assessment Questions

1.   *How is HIV transmitted?*

2.   *What are the 5 main factors which allow HIV to spread in society?*

3.   *List the 9 best known methods of transmitting the HIV virus.*

4.   *List 4 ways HIV cannot be transmitted.*

5.   *Why are women in developing countries considered more vulnerable to HIV infection that men?*

6.   *What connection do you think exists between poverty and HIV infection?*

7.   *Imagine a friend comes to you for help. He has just found out that a visitor who is staying with him has the HIV virus. The visitor has been using the same kitchen, lounge and bathroom facilities as your friend and he is now terrified that he will also catch the HIV virus. Advise the friend.*

8.   *What is the relationship between STDs and HIV infection?*

Chapter 5

Global Epidemic of HIV/AIDS

Contents of this Chapter

1. **HIV/AIDS: Global Prevalence**
2. **Next Wave of the Pandemic**
3. **Regional HIV/AIDS Statistics**
4. **Global Country Specific HIV/AIDS Statistics**
5. **Conclusion**
6. **Self-Assessment Questions**

1. HIV/AIDS: Global Prevalence

With its vicious and ferocious exploits on humanity, the disease has graduated from an epidemic to a pandemic. Always remember that HIV/AIDS statistics are so fluid and they change in days and weeks rather than in months and years.

HIV and AIDS have become pandemics of global proportions, with over **71 million** cases of infection worldwide, 29 million of whom are known to have died. There are over **42 million** people now living with HIV infection globally, with over 70% of them in Sub-Saharan Africa.

A UN report states that the fastest rate of infection is now in the Caribbean, South Africa and the former Soviet Union. However, in terms of the percentage of people infected in a particular country, Botswana is worse hit with 1 in every 3 persons (one third of the population) infected in December 2001.

In the United Kingdom, about 50,000 people are living with HIV in September 2003. According to the US Centers for Disease Control and Prevention, 282,000 people were living with HIV in the USA by 2002.

Every day as many as **17,000** people are infected by HIV in the world, amounting to over **6 million** people being infected each year.

However, the rate of new infections in the developed world is declining as education and better awareness of the disease is making more and more people take precautionary measures, especially regarding their sexual behaviour. On the other hand, there is a frightening increase in the prevalence of HIV infections in developing countries and South Africa is leading the way with 5.3 million living with HIV by the end of 2002.

During 2002, there were **15,000** HIV related deaths in the world every day, out of which over, 10,000 were from the African continent.

It is now estimated that between **7 – 10 billion US dollars** is needed to begin to have an impact on AIDS in Africa.

Furthermore, it is estimated that poorer nations would require **US$9.2 billion** a year to tackle AIDS, half of which would be needed for Sub-Saharan Africa.

As a result of the massive prevalence of HIV, life expectancy in Africa has recently been re-evaluated and is now estimated to be just 30 years in June 2000. Furthermore, by 2005, life expectancy in South Africa is expected to plummet by 17 years.

In a heart-moving article entitled "Health Warning" (March 2000), the BBC magazine 'FOCUS ON AFRICA' comments on the prevalence of AIDS in Africa:

"Funerals have become one of the most common social events in Africa in the late 1990s. Elderly parents are burying their sons and daughters, and are left to care for their grandchildren. Workers are burying their bosses or their colleagues, and are left to fill the gaps in the production process...

In the last two decades of the 20th century, AIDS rocketed from being a disease thought to be irrelevant to sub-Saharan Africa – a disease of gay white men and drug addicts – to being the number-one cause of death across the continent. The United Nations AIDS programme, UNAIDS, estimates that some 14 million people have died of AIDS in the last two decades of the century in 40 or so countries in Africa south of the Sahara. Twenty-three million more are currently infected with HIV, the virus that causes AIDS. Most of these men, women and children will die within the next decade. And they will not be the last.

Every day of 1999, another 10,000 people became infected with the fatal disease in sub-Saharan Africa. In fact, over 100 people will probably be infected in the time it takes you to read this article.

The overwhelming majority of these infections are transmitted between men and women during sex without a condom. Most of the rest are the indirect consequence of sex: infections passed on by mothers to their children in the womb, at the time of birth or during breastfeeding. In Africa, around a third of mothers infected with HIV will pass the virus on to their infants. Over three million African children have already died of HIV-related illnesses, and nearly a million more are living with the virus right now.

While heterosexual infection dominated in sub-Saharan Africa, the pattern of spread differs from region to region. At the moment, West Africa is in general least affected by HIV and AIDS. East Africa, the focal point for HIV infection in the 1980s and early 1990s, has recently been overtaken by a massive rise in HIV in southern Africa. It is estimated that close to one person in five aged between 15 and 49 is infected with HIV in Botswana, Lesotho, Namibia, South Africa, Swaziland, Zambia and Zimbabwe. In some of those countries the rate is as high as one in three. That makes these countries far and away the worst-hit in the world.

A number of new studies conducted in randomly chosen households in various countries confirmed what has long been feared – young girls are being infected by older men, and in huge numbers. By the time they were 19, a third of all girls were infected with HIV in a recent study in western Kenya. Even as young as 15, one girl in every 12 tested HIV positive. Among boys the same age, infection rates are far, far lower.

On average eight times as many teenage girls as boys are infected with HIV in studies in nine African countries. If boys their own age are not infected, girls must be getting infected during sex with older men. In one study after another, young girls say they have sex with older men because those men have money for school fees, for clothes or just for a good evening out. If current patterns of infection continue, more than half of the girls now in their teens in several African countries will die before they reach 40.

Needless to say, the massive rise in young adult death is taking its toll on society and the economy. Most visible are the orphans. Because of AIDS, close to 11 million African children had, by the end of the 20th century, been to their mother's funeral before their 15th birthday. Many of these children will have seen their father die as well.

Factories and farms in badly hit areas have recorded a halving in productivity as key staff die, take sick leave, or take time off to care for ailing family members and attend funerals. Some companies have been bankrupted by HIV-related medical expenses, leading to job losses for surviving workers. These are blows that Africa's fragile economies are ill-equipped to withstand.

Why is Africa so much worse affected by this disease than other continents? There are several reasons, all of them unpalatable. First, despite the predominantly Christian moral rhetoric preached by many African leaders, studies of sexual behaviour show that pre-marital and extra-marital sex is extremely common in many areas of the continent. Secondly (perhaps in part because of the same rhetoric), condom use is very low in most countries.

On top of that, most governments in Africa have done less to fight the spread of AIDS than governments in other parts of the world. Not one head of state turned up to a major international conference on the disease, held in Zambia in September 1999. A few countries, led by Uganda, Senegal and – belatedly – South Africa, are speaking openly about HIV, the sex that spreads it and the condoms that can prevent it. They are also trying to make condoms and HIV tests available to anyone who wants them. Uganda has been rewarded with a dramatic fall in new infections in young people, and Senegal, which started its prevention campaign early, still has one of the lowest infection rates in sub-Saharan Africa.

Why don't other governments want to follow these examples? Some leaders are elderly and conservative. Kenya's Daniel Arap Moi, for example, is just beginning to talk about the "scourge of AIDS" but is still too squeamish to talk about the sex that spreads it. Others, such as Zimbabwe's Robert Mugabe, appear to fear that an open admission of widespread sexual networking would alienate strong conservative Christian lobbies.

Their silence echoes through society. Row after row of young faces stare out of the death announcements in African newspapers, men and women who dies of "a long illness" or "a short illness". Asked if HIV is a problem in their community, the children of these dead men and woman say, yes, a big problem. Asked what their own parents died of, many will say witchcraft. Few, if any, will say AIDS.

The social stigma attached to the disease is so great that a woman in South Africa was recently beaten to death just for admitting publicly that she was HIV positive. Elders accused her of bringing shame on the community, even though statistics suggest that more than one in five adults are infected nationwide.

In a way, this silence serves those in power well. People who are not willing to recognize that AIDS exists in their own communities, their own families, their own lives are unlikely to demand that the government provide services for those affected. Even in the wealthier countries of Africa, the sophisticated combination of drugs widely available in the West is out of reach for most people. Indeed, the cheapest combination therapy costs South Africa's average per capital income and over 100 times Mozambique's.

But because most people with HIV die of diseases that feed on a weakened immune system but are relatively cheap and easy to treat – diarrhoea or tuberculosis, for example – there is a lot that could be done within current health budgets to deliver extra years of healthy life to young parents and breadwinners in the next millennium. This will not happen unless people throughout the continent make it impossible for political leaders to ignore the epidemic that is decimating their populations, their economies and their families"

In a detailed article under the heading "A Global Disaster" The Economist of 2nd January 1999 adds:

"...In rich countries, AIDS is no longer a death sentence. Expensive drugs keep HIV-positive patients alive and healthy, perhaps indefinitely. Loud public-awareness campaigns keep the number of infected Americans, Japanese and West Europeans to relatively low levels. The sense of crisis is past.

In developing countries, by contrast, the disease is spreading like nerve gas in a gentle breeze. The poor cannot afford to spend $10,000 a year on wonder-pills. Millions of Africans are dying. In the longer term, even greater numbers of Asians are at risk. For many poor countries, there is no greater or more immediate threat to public health and economic growth. Yet few political leaders treat it as a priority.

...It now claims many more lives each year than malaria, a growing menace, and is still nowhere near its peak. If India, China and other Asian countries do not take it seriously, the number of infections could reach "a new order of magnitude", says Peter Piot, head of the UN's AIDS programme.

The human immuno-deficiency virus (HIV) which causes acquired immune deficiency syndrome (AIDS), is thought to have crossed from chimpanzees to humans in the late 1940s or early 1950s in Congo. It took several years for the virus to break out of Congo's dense and sparsely populated jungles but, once it did, it marched with rebel armies through the continent's numerous war zones, rode with truckers from one rest-stop brothel to the next, and eventually flew, perhaps with an air steward, to America, where it was discovered in the early 1980s. As American homosexuals and drug injectors started to wake up to the dangers of bath-houses and needle-sharing, AIDS was already devastating Africa.

*So far, the worst-hit areas are east and **southern Africa**. In **Botswana, Namibia, Swaziland and Zimbabwe**, between a fifth and a quarter of people aged 15-49 are afflicted with HIV or AIDS. In Botswana, children born early in the next decade will have a life expectancy of 40; without AIDS, it would have been nearer 70. Of the 25 monitoring sites in Zimbabwe where pregnant women are tested for HIV, only two in 1997 showed prevalence below 10%. At the remaining 23 sites, 20-50% of women were infected. About a third of these women will pass the virus on to their babies.*

The region's giant, South Africa, was largely protected by its isolation from the rest of the world during the apartheid years. Now, it is host to one in ten of the world's new infections - more than any other country. In the country's most populous province, KwaZulu-Natal, perhaps a third of sexually active adults are HIV-positive.

Asia is the next disaster-in-waiting. Already, 7m Asians are infected. India's 930m people look increasingly vulnerable. The Indian countryside, which most people imagined relatively AIDS-free, turns out not to be. A recent study in Tamil Nadu found over 2% of rural people to be HIV-positive: 500,000 people in one of India's smallest states. Since 10% had other sexually transmitted diseases (STDs), the avenue for further infections is clearly open. A survey of female STD patients in Poona, in Maharashtra, found that over 90% had never had sex with anyone but their husband; and yet 13.6% had HIV. China is not far behind.

No one knows what AIDS will do to poor countries' economies, for nowhere has the epidemic run its course. An optimistic assessment, by Alan Whiteside of the University of Natal, suggests that the effect of AIDS on measurable GDP will be slight. Even at high prevalence, Mr Whiteside thinks it will slow growth by no more than 0.6% a year. This is because so many people in poor countries do not contribute much to the formal economy. To put it even more crudely, where there is a huge over-supply of labour, the dead can easily be replaced. Some people argue that those who survive the epidemic will benefit from a tighter job market. After the Black Death killed a third of the population of medieval Europe, labour scarcity forced landowners to pay their workers better.

Other researchers are more pessimistic. AIDS takes longer to kill them than did the plague, so the cost of caring for the sick will be more crippling. Modern governments, unlike medieval ones, tax the healthy to help look after the ailing, so the burden will fall on everyone. And AIDS, because it is sexually transmitted, tends to hit the most energetic and productive members of society. A recent study in Namibia estimated that AIDS cost the country almost 8% of GNP in 1996. Another analysis predicts that Kenya's GDP will be 14.5% smaller in 2005 than it would have been without AIDS, and that income per person will be 10% lower.

In general, the more advanced the economy, the worse it will be affected by a large number of AIDS deaths. South Africa, with its advanced industries, already suffers a shortage of skilled manpower, and cannot afford to lose more. In better-off developing countries, people have more savings to fall back on when they need to pay medical bills. Where people have health and life insurance, those industries will be hit by bigger claims. Insurers protect themselves by charging more or refusing policies to HIV-positive customers. In Zimbabwe, life-insurance premiums quadrupled in two years because of AIDS. Higher premiums force more people to seek treatment in public hospitals: in South Africa, HIV and AIDS could account for between 35% and 84% of public-health expenditure by 2005, according to one projection.

Little research has been done into the effects of AIDS on private business, but the anecdotal evidence is scary. In some countries, firms have had to limit the number of days employees may take off to attend funerals. Zambia is suffering power shortages because so many engineers have died. Farmers in Zimbabwe are finding it hard to irrigate their fields because the brass fittings on their water pipes are stolen for coffin handles. In South Africa, where employers above a certain size are obliged to offer generous benefits and paid sick leave, companies will find that many of their staff, as they sicken, becoming more expensive and less productive. Yet few firms are trying to raise awareness of AIDS among their workers, or considering how they will cope.

In the public sector, where pensions and health benefits are often more generous, AIDS could break budgets and hobble the provision of services. In South Africa, an estimated 15% of civil servants are HIV-positive, but government departments have made little effort to plan for the coming surge in sickness. Education, too, will suffer. In Botswana, 2-5% of teachers die each year from AIDS. Many more take extended sick leave.

At a macro level, the impact of AIDS is felt gradually. But at a household level, the blow is sudden and catastrophic. When a breadwinner develops AIDS, his (or her) family is impoverished twice over: his income vanishes, and his relations must devote time and money to nursing him. Daughters are often forced to drop out of school to help. Worse, HIV tends not to strike just one member of the family. Husbands give it to wives, mothers to babies. This correspondent's driver in Kampala lost his mother, his father, two brothers and their wives to AIDS. His story is not rare."

2. Next Wave of the Pandemic

Southern and eastern Africa have so far, been disproportionally affected by the HIV/AIDS pandemic. However, it is now projected by the US National Intelligence Council (which reports to the CIA) that the next wave of the pandemic will badly hit the following countries:

a)   China
b)   Ethiopia
c)   India
d)   Nigeria; and
e)   Russia

The following table shows the projected level of the problem.

Country	Projected number of people living with HIV by 2010
China	10-15 million
Ethiopia	7-10 million
India	20-25 million
Nigeria	10-15 million
Russia	5-8 million

Source: US National Intelligence Council, (2002)

These five countries, which make up 40% of the world's population, will have a total of 50 - 75 million infected persons by 2010.

It is projected that Ethiopia and Nigeria will be worse hit by all of this, as they lack infrastructure, proper healthcare and resources to combat the problem.

China is already feeling the pinch of the HIV/AIDS epidemic. The Guardian Newspaper of 11th June 2001 provides the following information concerning HIV spread in China:

Causes of HIV's Spread in China

1.   Drug abuse, mostly inland frontier provinces; Xinjiang and Unnan.

2.   Commercial sex, especially along the south-east coast.

3.   Unhygienic blood collection in rural areas where people sold their plasma.

4.   Transfusions of contaminated blood, an emerging threat in urban areas

HIV Statistics in China

1.   Official number of HIV cases is 500,000

2.   Internal estimate: up to 4 million

3.   31 provinces report HIV infections (1998)

4.   of those infected 80% are in 20-49 age group

5.   Expert warning: "If China does not take effective measures, it will have one of the highest numbers of AIDS infected people in the world" (Zeng Yi, an academic, June 2000)

Problem Areas in China

1.   Lack of research into spread of HIV/AIDS virus

2.   Lack of medical awareness of the virus

3.   Inadequate investment in prevention work

4.   Provincial secrecy and cover-ups

5.   Potential spread by migrant workers

6.   Substandard syringes and other medical equipment

7.   High cost of HIV tests

However, information coming out of China seems to suggest that the HIV infection rate is reaching crisis point. In a heart-breaking article by Jonathan Watts titled: "Hidden from the World, a village dies of AIDS while China refuses to face a growing crisis" – (Henan Province, the ground zero of an epidemic threatening villages), the Guardian Newspaper of 25 October 2003 comments:

"Chang Sun's wife is HIV positive. So is his mother. So is his aunt. So is his cousin and his cousin's wife. So is the woman next door and, probably, so is her husband. In fact, it is quite possible that almost every adult and many of the children in this small, remote village are infected.

And then, there are those who lie in the flat, brown vegetable fields, which are steadily filling with mossy green burial mounds.

Among them is Chang's father, who died of Aids last year, and his three-year-old daughter, who succumbed the year before that. His first wife is there too – she threw herself down the village well in 2000 after a doctor told her she was no longer worth treating because she had the virus.

Another plot will soon be needed. As we walk furtively to Chang's home under cover of darkness, the crackling of firewood in a neighbour's yard reminds him that a traditional wake is being held for the latest son to be lost to the disease, the 10th victim in the village this year.

"It is our custom for strong male adults to carry the coffin, but so many people are sick or dead that there aren't enough of us left," says the 35-year-old farmer. "So now it is the old people who are doing the burying."

This is Xiongqiao village in the Henan province, the ground zero of arguably the world's worst HIV/AIDS epidemic, with up to a million people infected in this single province through a vast, largely unregulated blood-selling operation.

The situation is already a catastrophe, but the risks are growing. The medical treatment is inadequate and the authorities are trying to cover up the truth with a lethal mix of censorship and police intimidation.

The Guardian has gained rare access to the village and has spoken to HIV-positive villagers who have been arrested and beaten for trying to draw attention to their plight; to health officials who have been harassed, sued and kept under surveillance for speaking out, and to local reporters who have been fired for trying to publish the truth.

It has also heard from Aids experts, charity organisations and foreign diplomats who have either been refused access to Henan or only allowed to enter under heavy restrictions.

Outside journalists fare little better: two cameramen from China's state-run television channel, CCTV, were kicked out this week.

The problem and response are side-effects of modern China's peculiar blend of profit-at-all-costs capitalism and hid-and-control communism. Even more than the Sars scare this year, the HIV crisis in Henan underlines the growing gulf between the urban rich and rural poor and the state's overarching emphasis on social stability at the expense of individual rights and free speech.

Impoverished

It was almost inevitable that the outbreak occurred in Henan. Here is the most populous and impoverished of China's provinces, life is cheaper than almost anywhere else in the world. The average Henan farmer survives on 46 pence per day.

When local health authorities were suddenly told to start making profits in the late 1980s, as part of the country's drive towards capitalism, Henan's officials turned to almost their only untapped resource: the blood of the province's 90 million population. Vans were converted into mini-clinics and driven out into the countryside. Ambitious peasants established themselves as "bloodheads" (brokers) to meet the demand among both buyers and sellers.

For an 800cc donation, villagers were paid 45 Renminbi (RMB, about £3.50), enough to feed a family for a week. Realising that they could get far more for milking their veins than for tending the land, they lined up day-in and day-out for years to make donations. By the peak – around 1995 – Henan had become the nation's blood farm.

"Almost everybody did it," said Chang's cousin, Ming.

"We would sell extra if there was a marriage ceremony coming up or if we wanted to build a house. The most I ever did was four donations in a single day."

The system has been adapted so that villagers could give such huge amounts of blood without suffering anaemia. After extracting plasma from each 800cc donation, the collectors would pump 400cc back into the arms of the donors. It is believed that people's blood often got mixed up in this way, spreading HIV to almost everyone involved.

Ming started to show symptoms of Aids in February and now spends most of his time lying on a bed held together by string, watching snowy black-and-white TV images on an old television set. Under a single naked light that illuminates the fading newsprint that serves as wallpaper, he says he has only lasted so long because the central government began providing free retroviral drugs this year.

After years of denial, the health ministry in Beijing has recently started to face up to the problem in Henan. Officials cautiously acknowledge that tens of thousands of people may have been infected. Although the government dodges the question of responsibility, steps are being taken to ease the suffering of victims.

As well as the free medicine, money has been provided for HIV clinics and plans are mooted for free education and tax breaks for the growing numbers of Aids orphans and widows in Henan. But villagers say the authorities are still covering up the enormous scale of the outbreak. Based on the proliferations of blood collection units in the mid 1990s, Aids activists estimate that more than a million people in Henan were contaminated.

"If you sold blood, there is a 90% chance of infection," said a local man. "But people don't want to know. My wife is now sick, but is afraid to take a test."

The disease is also spreading across generations. At a nursery school for orphans in Houyang, all the 38 children have at least one parent who is HIV positive, many of whom are likely to have passed on the disease during birth. Only three of the five-and six-year olds have been tested, but all three were positive.

The founder of the school, Chen Xiangyang, said one girl is now sick. "Her mother died of Aids and her father ran away after he tested positive. We don't tell the children even if they have the disease; we try to make them as happy as possible."

In remote villages like Xionqiao, which has no road and only one telephone, residents say they are being neglected because corrupt local officials want to play down their own accountability.

"The headman told us that he doesn't want us to get the reputation as an 'Aids village' but it is a fact that almost everyone here has the disease," said Chang. Other villagers said their claims for the benefits due to HIV sufferers have been turned down.

Tempers snapped in June, after four villagers died of Aids in less than a week and two residents were detained by police on their way to petition the provincial government for help. The arrests sparked China's most violent Aids-related confrontation. Almost 100 villagers overturned an official's car and marched on the village headman's office to protest against their lack of health care. The authorities' response was swift and bloody: two days after the demonstration, 600 baton-wielding police stormed the village, battering down doors, smashing windows and beating residents, including HIV-sufferers, children and Chang's 56-year-old mother, who says she still feels pain in the arm they broke.

Death and darkness fill Chang's house, which was built with the money he made from selling blood. The mood is set by the black-framed picture of his father who died last year, and in the funeral poems – "The wide land weeps for those we have loved and lost" – to his first wife and child which are pasted to the walls. It also seems to have taken liquid form in a murky bottle of traditional medicine that is all he and his mother have to ward off Aids.

Negative

Astonishingly, Chang tested negative for HIV. He does not believe the results, nor has he changed his lifestyle despite being remarried to an HIV-positive wife from a neighbouring and equally infected village.

"Everyone in my family has HIV. Why should I be different?" he says.

It is a view shared by many – not least because they cannot afford the 3Rmb price of a condom, equivalent to half a day's wages. Also to blame is a lack of Aids education in the villages by Henan officials who would rather ignore the problem than teach people how to deal with it.

The consequences for China will be devastating as many infected villagers are migrating to work in Beijing and other big cities. "It is now too late to stop the spread of the disease," said Gao Yaojie, the most outspoken advocate of a rethink of China's policy on Aids.

Overseas, Ms Gao has won awards for her efforts to raise the problems of Henan. In China, she has been denied a passport, had her phone bugged and been placed temporarily under house arrest. Numerous others who have tried to raise the problem have encountered similar problems. Last year, a local doctor – Wan Yanhai – was detained for allegedly passing out information about the scale of the epidemic. A journalist, who asked not to be named, said he had been fired by three different newspapers in Henan for trying to get the story published.

On the way from the city, a few hours drive from Xiongquiao, I asked a taxi driver if she was aware of any HIV cases in the province.

"No, no definitely not", she replied. "That is just wicked rumour mongering, we have no Aids here. You don't have to worry. Trust me. A taxi driver knows these things.""

3. Regional HIV/AIDS Statistics

The following table shows regional HIV/AIDS statistics:

UNAIDS/WHO HAIV/AIDS Regional Estimates as of end 2002 (AIDS Epidemic Update: December 2002)

Estimated Number living with HIV/AIDS during 2002	Adults & Children	Adults (15-49)	Children (<15)	% of HIV-positive adults who are women	Adult (15-49) prevalence rate
Sub-Saharan Africa	29,400,000	26,500,000	2,800,000	58%	8.8%
East Asia & Pacific	1,200,000	1,200,000	4,000	24%	0.1%
Australia/New Zealand	15,000	15,000	<200	7%	0.1%
South & South East Asia	6,000,000	5,800,000	240,000	36%	0.6%
Eastern Europe & Central Asia	1,200,000	1,200,000	16,000	27%	0.6%
Western Europe	570,000	560,000	5,000	25%	0.3%
North Africa & Middle East	550,000	510,000	40,000	55%	0.3%
North America	980,000	970,000	10,000	20%	0.6%
Caribbean	440,000	420,000	20,000	50%	2.4%
Latin America	1,500,000	1,500,000	45,000	30%	0.6%
TOTAL	**42,000,000**	**38,600,000**	**3,200,000**	**50%**	**1.2%**

Estimated number of new HIV infections during 2002	Adults & Children	Adults (15-49)	Children (<15)
Sub-Saharan Africa	3,500,000	2,700,000	720,000
East Asia & Pacific	270,000	270,000	3,000
Australia/New Zealand	500	500	<100
South & South East Asia	700,000	640,000	60,000
Eastern Europe & Central Asia	250,000	250,000	1,000
Western Europe	30,000	30,000	<500
North Africa & Middle East	83,000	70,000	13,000
North America	45,000	45,000	<500
Caribbean	60,000	50,000	7,000
Latin America	150,000	140,000	10,000
TOTAL	**5,000,000**	**4,200,000**	**800,000**

Estimated Deaths from HIV/AIDS during 2002	Adults & Children	Adults (15-49)	Children (<15)
Sub-Saharan Africa	2,4000,000	1,800,000	550,000
East Asia & Pacific	45,000	43,000	2,000
Australia/New Zealand	<100	<100	<100
South & South East Asia	440,000	400,000	43,000
Eastern Europe & Central Asia	25,000	25,000	<100
Western Europe	8,000	8,000	<100
North Africa & Middle East	37,000	30,000	6,800
North America	15,000	15,000	<100
Caribbean	42,000	35,000	7,000
Latin America	60,000	55,000	5,000
TOTAL	**3,100,000**	**2,500,000**	**610,000**

4. Global Country Specific HIV/AIDS Statistics

The following table shows country-specific statistics of people living with HIV in the world.

Country	Adults & Children	Adults (15-49)	Adult (15-49) rate (%)	Women (15-49)	Children (0-14)	Orphans (0-14) alive now	Deaths Adults & Children	Total (thousands)	Adults (15-49) (thousands)
Global Total	40,000,000	37,100,000	1.2	18,500,000	3,000,000	14,000,000	3,000,000	6,119,328	3,198,252
Sub-Saharan Africa	28,500,000	26,000,000	9.0	15,000,000	3,600,000	11,000,000	2,200,000	633,816	291,310
Angola	350,000	320,000	5.5	190,000	37,000	100,000	24,000	13,527	5,767
Benin	120,000	110.000	3.6	67,000	12,000	34,000	8,100	6,446	2,929
Botswana	330,000	300,000	38.8	170,000	28,000	69,000	26,000	1,554	762
Burkina Faso	440,000	380,000	6.5	220,000	61,000	270,000	44,000	11,856	5,046
Burundi	390,000	330,000	8.3	190,000	55,000	240,000	40,000	6,502	2,887
Cameroon	920,000	860,000	11.8	500,000	69,000	210,000	53,000	15,203	7,065
Central African Republic	250,000	220,000	12.9	130,000	25,000	110,000	22,000	3,782	1,722
Chad	150,000	130,000	3.6	76,000	18,000	72,000	14,000	8,135	3,570
Comoros	...	...	...	...	...	...	...	727	351
Congo	110,000	99,000	7.2	59,000	15,000	78,000	11,000	3,110	1,364
Cote d'Ivoire	770,000	690,000	9.7	400,000	84,000	420,000	75,000	16,349	7,854
Dem. Republic of Congo	1,300,000	1,100,000	4.9	670,000	170,000	930,000	120,000	52,522	22,073
Djibouti	...	...	...	...	...	...	...	644	284
Equatorial Guinea	5,900	5,000	3.4	3,000	420	...	370	470	211
Eritrea	55,000	49,000	2.8	30,000	4,000	24,000	350	3,816	1,760
Ethiopia	2,100,000	1,900,000	6.4	1,100,000	230,000	990,000	160,000	64,459	28,952
Gabon	...	...	...	...	...	...	...	1,262	552
Gambia	8,400	7,900	1.6	4,400	460	5,300	400	1,337	647
Ghana	360,000	330,000	3.0	170,000	34,000	200,000	28,000	19,734	9,700
Guinea	...	...	...	...	...	...	...	8,274	3,868
Guinea-Bissau	17,000	16,000	2.8	9,300	1,500	4,300	1,200	1,227	557
Kenya	2,500,000	2,300,000	15.0	1,400,000	220,000	890,000	190,000	31,293	15,333
Lesotho	360,000	330,000	31.0	180,000	27,000	73,000	25,000	2,057	984
Liberia	...	...	...	...	...	...	...	3,108	1,518
Madagascar	22,000	21,000	0.3	12,000	1,000	6,300	...	16,437	7,538
Malawi	850,000	780,000	15.0	440,000	65,000	470,000	80,000	11,572	5,118
Mali	110,000	100,000	1.7	54,000	13,000	70,000	11,000	11,677	5,096
Mauritania	...	...	...	...	...	...	...	2,747	1,268
Mauritius	700	700	0.1	350	<100	...	<100	1,171	667
Mozambique	1,100,000	1,000,000	13.0	630,000	80,000	420,000	60,000	18,644	8,511
Namibia	230,000	200,000	22.5	110,000	30,000	47,000	13,000	1,788	820
Niger	...	...	...	...	...	...	...	11,227	4,831
Nigeria	3,500,000	3,200,000	5.8	1,700,000	270,000	1,000,000	170,000	116,929	53,346
Rwanda	500,000	430,000	8.9	250,000	65,000	260,000	49,000	7,949	3,756
Senegal	27,000	24,000	0.5	14,000	2,900	15,000	2,500	9,662	4,521
Sierra Leone	170,000	150,000	7.0	90,000	16,000	42,000	11,000	4,587	2,093
Somalia	43,000	43,000	1.0	...	...	...	...	9,157	4,015
South Africa	5,000,000	4,700,000	20.1	2,700,000	250,000	660,000	360,000	43,792	23,66
Swaziland	170,000	150,000	33.4	89,000	14,000	35,000	12,000	938	450
Togo	150,000	130,000	6.0	76,000	15,000	63,000	12,000	4,657	2,152
Uganda	600,000	510,000	5.0	280,000	110,000	880,000	84,000	24,023	10,290
United Rep. Of Tanzania	1,500,000	1,300,000	7.8	750,000	170,000	810,000	140,000	35,965	16,701
Zambia	1,200,000	1,000,000	21.5	590,000	150,000	570,000	120,000	10,649	4,740
Zimbabwe	2,300,000	2,000,000	33.7	1,200,000	240,000	780,000	200,000	12,852	5,972
East Asia & Pacific	1,000,000	970,000	0.1	230,000	3,000	85,---	35,000	1,497,066	833,058
China	850,000	850,000	0.1	220,000	2,000	76,000	30,000	1,284,972	726,031
Dem. Peo. Rep. Of Korea	...	...	...	...	...	...	...	22,428	11,876
Fiji	300	300	0.1	<100	...	-	...	823	443
Hong Kong	2,600	2,600	0.1	660	<100	-	<100	6,961	4,134
Japan	12,000	12,000	<0.1	6,600	110	2,000	430	127,335	59,109
Mongolia	<100	<100	<0.1	...	...	-	...	2,559	1,416
Papua New Guinea	17,000	16,000	0.7	4,100	500	4,200	880	4,920	2,491
Republic of Korea	4,000	4,000	<0.1	960	<100	1,000	220	47,069	27,558

People living with HIV in different countries of the world (cont.)

Country	Adults & Children	Adults (15-49)	Adult (15-49) rate (%)	Women (15-49)	Children (0-14)	Orphans (0-14) alive now	Deaths Adults & Children	Total (thousands)	Adults (15-49) (thousands)
Australia	12,000	12,000	0.1	800	140	...	<100	19,338	9,933
New Zealand	1,200	1,200	0.1	180	<100	...	<100	3,808	1,911
South & South-East Asia	5,600,000	5,400,000	0.6	2,000,000	220,000	1,800,000	400,000	1,978,430	1,031,463
Afghanistan	...	...	...	...	...	...	...	22,474	10,435
Bangladesh	13,000	13,000	<0.1	3,100	310	2,100	650	140,369	72,340
Bhutan	<100	<100	<0.1	...	...	...	...	2,141	972
Brunei Darussalam	...	...	...	...	...	...	...	335	187
Cambodia	170.000	160,000	2.7	74,000	12,000	55,000	12,000	13,441	6,314
India	3,970,000	3,800,000	0.8	1,500,000	170,000	...	...	1,025,096	533,580
Indonesia	120,000	120,000	0.1	27,000	1,300	18,000	4,600	214,840	118.163
Iran (Islamic Republic of)	20,000	20,000	<0.1	5,000	<200	...	290	71,369	37,396
Lao People's Dem. Rep	1,400	1,300	<0.1	350	<100	...	<150	5,403	2,542
Malaysia	42,000	41,000	0.4	11,000	770	14,000	2,500	22,633	11,868
Maldives	<100	<100	0.1	...	...	...	...	300	141
Myanmar	...	...	...	...	...	...	...	48,364	25,855
Nepal	58,000	56,000	0.5	14,000	1,500	13,000	2,400	23,593	11,106
Pakistan	78,000	76,000	0.1	16,000	2,200	25,000	4,500	144,971	67,964
Philippines	9,400	9,400	<0.1	2,500	<10	4,100	720	77,131	39,600
Singapore	3,400	3,400	0.2	860	<100	...	140	4,108	2,324
Sri Lanka	4,800	4,700	<0.1	1,400	<100	2,000	250	19,104	10,695
Thailand	670,000	650,000	1.8	220,000	21,000	29,000	55,000	63,584	36,636
Viet Nam	130,000	130,000	0.3	35,000	2,500	22,000	6,600	79,175	43,343
Eastern Europe & Central Asia	1,000,000	1,000,000	0.5	260,000	15,000	<5000	23,000	393,245	209,038
Armenia	2,400	2,400	0.2	480	<100	...	<100	3,788	2,152
Azerbaijan	1,400	1,400	<0.1	280	...	...	<100	8,096	4,529
Belarus	15,000	15,000	0.3	3,700	...	...	1,000	10,147	5,397
Bosnia and Herzegovina	...	900*	<0.1*	...	...	...	...	4,067	2,292
Bulgaria	...	400*	<0.1*	...	...	...	...	7,867	3,915
Croatia	200	200	<0.1	<100	<10	...	<10	4,655	2,331
Czech Republic	500	500	<0.1	<100	<10	...	<10	10,260	5,233
Estonia	7,700	7,700	1.0	1,500	...	...	<100	1,377	702
Georgia	900	900	<0.1	180	...	...	<100	5,239	2,726
Hungary	2,800	2,800	0.1	300	<100	...	<100	9,917	5,001
Kazakhstan	6,000	6,000	0.1	1,200	<100	...	300	16,095	8,866
Kyrgyzstan	500	500	<0.1	<100	...	...	<100	4,986	2,627
Latvia	5,000	5,000	0.4	1,000	<100	...	<100	2,406	1,215
Lithuania	1,300	1,300	0.1	260	<100	...	<100	3,689	1,901
Poland	...	14,000*	0.1*	...	...	...	...	38,577	20,685
Republic of Moldova	5,500	5,500	0.2	1,200	-	...	300	4,285	2,339
Romania	6,500	2,500	<0.1	...	4,000	...	350	22,388	11,761
Russian Federation	700,000	700,000	0.9	180,000	...	...	9,000	144,664	78,166
Slovakia	<100	<100	<0.1	<100	...	...	<100	5,403	2,934
Tajikistan	200	200	<0.1	<100	...	...	<100	6,135	3,111
Turkmenistan	<100	<100	<0.1	<100	...	...	<100	4,835	2,508
Ukraine	250,000	250,000	1.0	76,000	...	...	11,000	49,112	25,251
Uzbekistan	740	740	<0.1	150	<100	...	<100	25,257	13,395
Western Europe	550,000	540,000	0.3	140,000	5,000	150,000	8,000	407,021	200,286
Albania	...	...	...	...	...	...	...	3,145	1,692
Austria	9,900	9,900	0.2	2,200	<100	...	<100	8,075	4,058
Belgium	8,500	8,100	0.2	2,900	330	...	<100	10,264	4,987
Denmark	3,800	3,800	0.2	770	<100	...	<100	5,333	2,519
Finland	1,200	1,200	<0.1	330	<100	...	<100	5,178	2,462
France	100,000	100,000	0.3	27,000	1,000	...	800	59,453	29,001
Germany	41,000	41,000	0.1	8,100	550	...	660	82.007	40,191
Greece	8,800	8,800	0.2	1,800	<100	...	<100	10,623	5,269
Iceland	220	220	0.2	<100	<100	...	<100	281	144
Ireland	2,400	2,200	0.1	660	190	...	<100	3,841	2,022
Italy	100,000	100,000	0.4	33,000	770	...	1,100	57,503	28,018
Luxembourg	...	360	0.2	...	...	...	<100	442	221
Malta	...	240	0.1	...	...	...	<100	392	193
Netherlands	17,000	17,000	0.2	3,300	160	...	110	15,930	7,997
Norway	1,800	1,800	0.1	400	<100	...	<100	4,488	2,155

People living with HIV in different countries of the world (cont.)

Country	Adults & Children	Adults (15-49)	Adult (15-49) rate (%)	Women (15-49)	Children (0-14)	Orphans (0-14) currently living	Deaths Adults & Children	Total (thousands)	Adults (15-49) (thousands)
Slovenia	280	280	<0.1	<100	<100	...	<100	1,985	1,047
Spain	130,000	130,000	0.5	26,000	1,300	...	2,300	39,921	20,794
Sweden	3,300	3,300	0.1	880	<100	...	<100	8,833	4,012
Switzerland	19,000	19,000	0.5	6,000	300	...	<100	7,170	3,437
TFYR Macedonia	<100	<100	<0.1	<100	<100	...	<100	2,044	1,079
United Kingdom	34,000	34,000	0.1	7,400	550	...	460	59,542	28,559
Yugoslavia	10,000	10,000	0.2	...	...	...	<100	10,538	5,341
North Africa & Middle East	500,000	460,000	0.3	250,000	35,000	65,000	30,000	349,142	180,506
Algeria	...	13,000*	0.1*	...	...	...	...	30,841	16,779
Bahrain	<1000	<1000	0.3	150	...	...	...	652	390
Cyprus	<1000	<1000	0.3	150	...	...	...	790	396
Egypt	8,000	8,000	<0.1	780	...	...	...	69,080	36,301
Iraq	<1000	<1000	<0.1	150	...	...	...	23,584	11,527
Israel	...	2,700	0.1	...	...	...	...	6,172	3,067
Jordan	<1000	<1000	<0.1	150	...	...	...	5,051	2,561
Kuwait	...	...	...	...	...	...	...	1,971	1,123
Lebanon	...	...	...	...	...	...	...	3,556	1,949
Libyan Arab Jamahiriya	7,000	7,000	0.2	1,100	...	...	...	5,408	2,952
Morocco	13,000	13,000	0.1	2,000	...	...	...	30,430	16,373
Oman	1,300	1,300	0.1	200	...	...	...	2,622	1,211
Qatar	...	...	...	...	...	...	...	575	350
Saudi Arabia	...	...	...	...	...	...	...	21,028	9,667
Sudan	450,000	410,000	2.6	230,000	30,000	62,000	23,000	31,809	15,496
Syrian Arab Republic	...	...	...	...	...	...	...	16,610	8,481
Tunisia	...	...	...	...	...	...	...	9,562	5,392
Turkey	...	3,700*	<0.1*	...	...	...	...	67,632	36,857
United Arab Emirates	...	...	...	...	...	...	...	2,654	1,533
Yemen	9,900	9,900	0.1	1,500	...	...	...	19,114	8,098
North America	950,000	940,000	0.6	190,000	10,000	320,000	15,000	316,941	161,413
Canada	55,000	55,000	0.3	14,000	<500	-	<500	31,015	16,164
United States of America	900,000	890,000	0.6	180,000	10,000	-	15,000	285,926	145,249
Caribbean	420,000	400,000	2.3	210,000	20,000	250,000	40,000	32,489	17,183
Bahamas	6,200	6,100	3.5	2,700	<100	2,900	610	308	170
Barbados	...	2,000*	1.2*	...	...	...	...	268	154
Cuba	3,200	3,200	<0.1	830	<100	1,000	120	11,237	6,121
Dominican Republic	130,000	120,000	2.5	61,000	4,700	33,000	7,800	8,507	4,561
Haiti	250,000	240,000	6.1	120,000	12,000	200,000	30,000	8,270	4,053
Jamaica	20,000	18,000	1.2	7,200	800	5,100	980	2,598	1,376
Trinidad and Tobago	17,000	17,000	2.5	5,600	300	3,600	1,200	1,300	748
Latin America	1,500,000	1,400,000	0.5	430,000	40,000	330,000	60,000	488,031	262,151
Argentina	130,000	130,000	0.7	30,000	3,000	25,000	1,800	37,488	18,741
Belize	2,500	2,200	2.0	1,000	180	950	300	231	119
Bolivia	4,600	4,500	0.1	1,200	160	1,000	290	8,516	4,131
Brazil	610,000	600,000	0.7	220,000	13,000	130,000	8,400	172,559	96,894
Chile	20,000	20,000	0.3	4,300	<500	4,100	220	15,402	8,121
Colombia	140,000	140,000	0.4	20,000	4,000	21,000	5,6000	42,803	23,003
Costa Rica	11,000	11,000	0.6	2,800	320	3,000	890	4,112	2,204
Ecuador	20,000	19,000	0.3	5,100	660	7,200	1,700	12,880	6,874
El Salvador	24,000	23,000	0.6	6,300	830	13,000	2,100	6,400	3,289
Guatemala	67,000	63,000	1.0	27,000	4,800	32,00	5,200	11,687	5,459
Guyana	18,000	17,000	2.7	8,500	800	4,200	1,300	763	432
Honduras	57,000	54,000	1.6	27,000	3,000	14,000	3,300	6,575	3,214
Mexico	150,000	150,000	0.3	32,000	3,600	27,000	4,200	100,368	54,019
Nicaragua	5,800	5,600	0.2	1,500	210	2,000	400	5,208	2,539
Panama	25,000	25,000	1.5	8,700	800	8,100	1,900	2,899	1,549
Paraguay	...	...	...	...	...	...	...	5,636	2,836
Peru	53,000	51,000	0.4	13,000	1,500	17,000	3,900	26,093	13,878
Suriname	3,700	3,600	1.2	1,800	190	1,700	330	419	238
Uruguay	6,300	6,200	0.3	1,400	100	3,100	<500	3,361	1,625

Source: UNAIDS, 2002

It is worth noting that these are official figures. It is generally accepted that the actual figures are a lot worse than the official ones

Conclusion

AIDS affects every continent on earth. Although some countries are coping with the disease better than others by the use of planning, education and health care provision, the disease is having a major effect world-wide, with some countries on the point of being devastated by the disease. Sadly, this trend looks likely to continue, at least in the short term, as many countries struggle to cope with the effects of HIV and AIDS on their citizens.

HIV/AIDS has indeed progressed from a global epidemic to a **global pandemic**. AIDS is now being called the worst pandemic experienced by humanity in 600 years, even compared with the **bubonic plague (the black death)** that killed 25 million people in Europe in the 17th Century.

Self-Assessment Questions

1. *How did you feel when you read the statistics in the article? Write down 5 key words that describe your feelings or emotions.*

2. *Based on the statistics given in this chapter, approximately how many people does the HIV virus infect every day?*

3. *What percentage of HIV infections takes place in Africa?*

4. *What is the most common way HIV is transmitted on the African continent?*

5. *Why do some heads of state fail to address the problem of HIV infection and AIDS in their countries and what is the consequence of this failure for the people who live in these countries?*

6. *What will be the implications of the reduction in average life expectancy, perhaps by as much as 10 –29 years, as looks likely in some African countries.*

7. *Why does it seem likely that Asia will be the next major region to suffer from an HIV/AIDS epidemic?*

8. *Where is the next wave of the pandemic expected?*

Chapter 6

The Origin of AIDS

Contents of this Chapter

1. Introduction

One of the most fiercely disputed areas of the study of HIV/AIDS is its origin. Understanding the origins of diseases have in the past, helped scientists to find cures for some of them.

AIDS was first identified among homosexuals in June 1981 in San Francisco and New York, USA. However, HIV was identified as the probable cause of AIDS in 1984, by Dr Robert Gallo of the Institute of Human Virology, Baltimore, USA.

There are many theories of the origin of the disease. HIV 1 and HIV 2 are said to have different origins, which will be explained in this chapter.

2. Origin of HIV 1

There are several theories of the possible origin of HIV 1. These are discussed below:

a) The Congo Theory

Scientists believe that HIV was first contracted by humans in the 1940s and 1950s from the African Green Monkeys (AGMs) in Belgian Congo, now the Democratic Republic of Congo (formerly Zaire), either through sexual contact (Bestiality) with the primate or contact with the primate's blood during the process of butchery of the animal for food. This is because some of these primates are now found to have been infected with a close variant of HIV known as **'Simian Immunodeficiency Virus' (SIV)** which is thought to have jumped the species barrier and mutated into HIV. A variant similar to SIV has also been found among some primates in Asia. This virus is known as **Simian type-D Retroviruses (SRV).**

It is worth noting that though some of these monkeys have SIV, it does not seem to cause immuno-deficiency in them. Immune-deficiency is said to occur when the primates cross-infect one another.

The belief under this theory is that though humans first contracted the disease from primates, it was brought to North America by a very well-travelled wayward Canadian airline steward **Gaëtan Dugas**, who was born in 1953 and died of AIDS in 1984. He is known as **'patient zero'**, the man who brought the disease to North America. This theory gained so much weight because it was found that many of those who were the first known persons to be infected with the virus had some form of sexual relationship with Mr Dugas.

However, later findings seem to conclude that Mr Dugas could not be the first to be contracted with HIV in the west, as HIV pre-dated the patient zero, as the following cases suggest:

i.   Tissue samples that were taken from a 15 year old American teenager named "Robert" who died in St Louis, Missouri in 1969 was reported to be HIV positive. However, subsequent tests in 1990 were said to be inconclusive.

ii.   In 1966, a well-travelled Norwegian sailor who had a history of sexually transmitted infections was found to have the symptoms of HIV/AIDS. His wife and daughter later had the same symptoms; and they all died of opportunistic infections. Their blood, which was frozen in 1971, was said to be HIV positive, when tested.

iii.   Also blood samples collected and frozen by a hospital in Zaire in the late 1950s from a patient was found to be HIV positive when it was tested in 1986.

iv.   Stored tissues of a sailor from Manchester, England who died in 1959 was reported to have tested HIV positive in 1990.

b) The Polio Vaccine Theory

Closely related to the above theory, is the **Polio Vaccine Theory**, which suggests that HIV originated from complications caused by an experimental Oral Polio Vaccine (OPV) called **'CHAT'** used on 1 million Africans in Rwanda, Burundi and Congo (all former colonies of Belgium) in the 1950s. This trial polio vaccine was made out of kidney cells of the African Green Monkeys (AGMs) and Macaques in Central Africa. It is said that about 500 primates were used for the experiment.

The vaccine was developed by **Dr Hilary Koprowski** of Wistar Institute in Philadelphia, USA, in collaboration with Belgian researchers in the then Belgian Congo.

However, an analysis of the vaccine in 2000 (the results of which was published in 2001), cast doubt on this theory, as there were no traces of HIV in it.

Nevertheless, there are very strong supporters of this theory. One of the most powerful works in this area is a book written by **Edward Hooper**, titled **The River: A Journey Back to the Source of HIV and AIDS** (Harmondsworth: Penguin; Boston: Little, Brown, 1999; revised edition, Penguin, 2000). In summarising this theory, **Dr Brian Martin** (an associate professor in Science, Technology and Society) from the University of Wollongong in Australia notes:

- *"The location coincides dramatically. The earliest known cases of AIDS occurred in Central Africa, in the same regions where Koprowski's polio vaccine was given to over a million people in 1957 – 1960.*

- *The timing coincides. There is no documented case of HIV infection or AIDS before 1959. Centuries of the slave trade and European exploitation of Africa exposed Africans and others to all diseases then known; it is implausible that HIV could have been present and spreading in Africa without being recognised.*

- *Polio vaccines are grown (cultured) on monkey kidneys which could have been contaminated by SIVs. Polio vaccines could not be screened for SIV contamination before 1985.*

- *Another monkey virus, SV-40 is known to have been passed to humans through polio vaccines. A specific pool of Koprowski's polio vaccine was later shown to have been contaminated by an unknown virus.*

- *In order for a virus to infect a different species, it is helpful to reduce the resistance of the new host's immune system. Koprowski's polio vaccine was given to many children less than one month old, before their immune systems were fully developed. Indeed, in one trial, infants were given 15 times the standard dose in order to ensure effective immunisation.*

If this theory is correct, it has serious ethical, health and policy implications. In particular, it points to the danger of interspecies transfer of material through vaccinations, organ transplants, etc., which could lead to insights about responding to AIDS and preventing new diseases.

However, there has been no sustained attempt to test the theory. This could be done, for example, by testing stocks of polio vaccine for the presence of SIV. An offer to undertake tests was made as early as 1991; only in 2000 were some samples tested, and then only US-made vaccine. Another possibility would be to test stored blood samples in Africa from before 1950. If HIV is found, this would undermine the theory.

Although the theory has not been properly examined, many people seem to believe it has been refuted. Hilary Koprowski published a letter in Science in 1992 attacking the theory. In 1993, Rolling Stone, which had published a widely publicised article by Tom Curtis about the theory, published an 'update', interpreted by Science as a retraction. The public record thus suggests that these contributions have been the final word.

Actually, this appearance of 'refutation' was due to the exercise of power, not scientific judgement. Science refused to publish a reply to Koprowski's letter by Curtis and, later, another reply by eminent biologist W.D. Hamilton. Nature has received substantial submissions about the theory from at least six scholars but has not published any of them. Rolling Stone's 'update' was the aftermath of a legal action for defamation by Koprowski against Rolling Stone and Curtis. Thus, it has been editorial prerogative and legal action that have given the impression that critics of the theory have been unanswered."

Brian Martin continues:

"Hooper recently interviewed several of those who used to work in the Medical Laboratory of Stanleyville, Belgian Congo, and a nearby Lindi Chimpanzee camp, in the late 1950s. Their testimonies reveal that CHAT polio vaccine was being prepared locally at the medical laboratory...at a time when the only tissue culture available in the lab was made from chimpanzee kidney cells. This is significant, because the common chimpanzee is the

carrier of (SIVcpz) which is the immediate ancestor of HIV-1, the virus responsible for the AIDS pandemic....

...Furthermore, there are remarkable correlations between the towns and villages where CHAT vaccine was fed in the late fifties and the first appearance of HIV-1 and AIDS in Africa. This does not prove that CHAT started AIDS. But at this point many will consider that the OPV theory has become the most plausible theory of origin. This new evidence also raises questions about the ways in which the scientific community has, until now, responded to an 'uncomfortable theory'. Hooper Concludes: "I believe that this new information about CHAT preparation in Belgian Congo in the 1950s is vitally important, and not only with regard to the OPV theory, and the question of how AIDS may have started. It also raises important ethical questions about the ways in which modern research is funded; the ways in which the scientific establishment and the major scientific journals respond to theories which they find threatening, or embarrassing; and the ways in which experimental trials have been, and are still being, conducted in the developing world."

In responding to rebuttal by those who were directly involved in the production of the vaccine, **Edward Hooper** comments:

"Paul Osterrieth, Stanley Plotkin and Hilary Koprowski (letters, 8 May), all of whom were intimately involved with the trials of the CHAT polio vaccine in Central Africa, continue to insist that this vaccine was never prepared in chimpanzee cells, and thus to deny any connection between the CHAT vaccination of about a million Africans in 1957-60 and the emergence of AIDS in the same towns and villages between ten and twenty years later.

Osterrieth dismisses the memories of African technicians by saying that one was a 'low-level employee', while the testimony of the other 'isn't of any value'. He adds that he has already denied these claims in the Philosophical Transactions of the Royal Society. In that article, he contradicted some of his own previous statements (concerning, for instance, to which American institutions he sent chimpanzee kidneys), while remaining tight-lipped about other crucial details. He insisted that CHAT vaccine was never handled in his virology department at the Laboratoire Médical de Stanleyville (LMS), and that it 'could not have been prepared' there. Numerous witnesses from North America, Europe and Africa (not just the two I cited) disagree with Osterrieth on these two points, and some state that he prepared the vaccine himself.

But in which cells? Plotkin says that baboon kidneys were used for tissue culture, but the LMS annual reports record only a relatively tiny quantity of cells cultured from (at most) two baboons in 1958. Plotkin claims that 'when chimpanzees were used' for any work, this was 'readily acknowledged'. In the annual reports, however, references to the CHAT testing programme and the vaccination trials are obscure and minimal, and there is no information as to what activities necessitated the use of more than four hundred chimpanzees between 1956 and 1960. Several witnesses recall that Osterrieth handled tissue, cells and sera from chimpanzees throughout this period.

Finally, Plotkin complains that most of what I claim to be early AIDS cases from Africa are unconfirmed. Nine of my 39 cases were confirmed serologically; the others were diagnosed as probable AIDS cases by experienced Africa-based physicians. For both the full series and the subset of confirmed cases, the statistical correlations with the CHAT vaccination sites are highly significant."

c) The Conspiracy Theories

i.   One of the conspiracy theories is that HIV is the result of a western scientific biological weapons experiment that went wrong, which mutated the HIV virus. The supporters of this theory have their reasons for believing this possible.

Concerning this theory of the origin of AIDS, **Alan Cantwell Jr, MD** wrote a paper titled: AIDS – A Doctor's Note on the Man-Made Theory:

> *"A decade before the first cases of AIDS, Dr Donald M. MacArthur, a spokesman for the U.S. Department of Defense, told a Congressional Hearing that a "super germ" could be developed as part of our experimental bio-warfare program. This genetically engineered germ would be very different from any previous microbe known to mankind. The agent would be a highly effective killing agent because the immune system would be powerless against this super-microbe (Testimony before a Subcommittee of the Committee on Appropriations, House of Representatives, Department of Defense Appropriations for 1970, dated July 1, 1969). A transcript of this meeting on "Synthetic Biological Agents" records the following comments of Dr. MacArthur:*

> 1. *All biological agents up to the present time are representatives of naturally occurring disease, and thus are known by scientists throughout the world. They are easily available to qualified scientists for research, either for offensive or defensive purposes.*

> 2. *Within the next 5 to 10 years, it would probably be possible to make a new infective microorganism which could differ in certain important aspects from any known disease-causing organisms. Most important of these is that it might be refractory to the immunological and therapeutic processes upon which we depend to maintain our relative freedom from infectious disease.*

> 3. *A research program to explore the feasibility of this could be completed in approximately 5 years at a total cost of $10 million.*

> 4. *It would be very difficult to establish such a program. Molecular biology is a relatively new science. There are not many competent scientists in the field, almost all are in university laboratories, and they are generally adequately supported from sources other than the Department of Defense. However, it was considered possible to initiate an adequate program through the National Academy of Sciences – National Research Council (NAS-NRC). The matter was discussed with the NAS-NRC, and tentative plans were made to initiate the program. However, decreasing funds in CB (chemical/biological) research, growing criticism of the CB program, and our reluctance to involve the NAS-NRC in such a controversial endeavor have led us to postpone it for the past two years. It is a highly controversial issue and there are many who believe such research should not be undertaken lest it lead to yet another method of massive killing of large populations…Should an enemy develop it, there is little doubt that it is an important area of potential military technological inferiority in which there is no adequate research program.*

> > *Was the AIDS virus, or other so-called "emerging viruses" such as Ebola and Marburg viruses, created in bio-warfare laboratories during the 1970s? During the 1970s, the U.S. Army's bio-warfare research program intensified, particularly in the area of DNA and gene splicing research. Renouncing germ warfare except for "medical defensive research,"*

President Richard Nixon in 1971 ordered that a major part of the Army's bio-warfare research be transferred over to the National Cancer Institute (where HIV would be discovered a decade later by Gallo). That same year, Nixon also initiated his famous "War on Cancer," and offensive bio-warfare research (particularly genetic engineering of viruses) continued under the umbrella of orthodox cancer research. Cancer virologists learned "to jump" animal cancer viruses from one species of animal to another. Chicken viruses were put into lamb kidney cells; baboon viruses were spliced into human cancer cells; the combinations were endless. In due process, deadly man-made viruses were developed, and new forms of cancer, immunodeficiency, and opportunistic infections were produced when these viruses were forced or adapted into laboratory animals and into human tissue cell culture.

As predicted by the bio-warfare experts, new cancer-causing monster viruses were created that had a deadly effect on the immune system. In one government-sponsored experiment reported in 1974, newborn chimpanzees were taken away from their mothers at birth and weaned on milk obtained from virus-infected cows. Some of the chimps sickened and died with two new diseases that had never been observed in chimps. The first was a parasitic pneumonia known as Pneumocystis Carinii pneumonia (later known as AIDS); the second was leukaemia."

ii.   Another conspiracy theory suggests that western scientists deliberately introduced the HIV virus into Africa as an attempt to reduce the population of Africa. However, the plan went wrong, so everyone else is affected in the world.

d) The Theocratic Theories

i.   Still others believe that, since it was first discovered among homosexuals, it is some form of Devine Retribution from God for the sins of humanity.

ii.   There are also those who believe that it is simply part of the fulfilment of the Devine Prophecy, as a sign of the nearness of the end of the world.

Whichever theory or belief a person chooses to prefer, the threat of HIV and AIDS affects everybody on earth, whether heterosexuals, homosexuals, bisexuals, children and even those who are celibate. Some are, however, at greater risk of being infected than others.

Nevertheless, the theory that **most scientists believe** in is the 'Congo Theory'. Writing about the "Congo theory" of the origin of AIDS, an article in The ECONOMIST of 7th February 1998 states:

*"Never throw anything away, you don't know when it might come in useful. In 1959 a man living in what was then the Belgian Congo (now the Democratic Republic of Congo) gave a blood sample to some American doctors who were studying human genetics. When they had finished with it, instead of dropping it in a rubbish bin the doctors put it in a freezer, where it hung around, half forgotten, until 1986. In that year it was examined, along with 1,212 similar samples, by André Nahmias of Emory University, in Atlanta. Dr Nahmias was looking for signs of human immuno-deficiency virus (HIV), the cause of the then newly recognised disease AIDS. The sample proved positive, showing that AIDS (or at least HIV) had long predated the so-called **"patient zero"**, an airline cabin attendant whose promiscuous peregrinations across North America helped the disease to get a good grip there before it was recognised by doctors.*

Surprisingly, considering the controversy that surrounds the origin of AIDS (popular conspiracy theories include the idea that it escaped from a military laboratory in the country of your choice or that it is part of a western racist plot to reduce the population of Africa, and there has even been a suggestion that it piggy-backed around on an early polio vaccine), that early sample has only just been dusted down for a further examination, to see what it has to say about where HIV actually came from. A group of researchers including Dr Nahmias and led by David Ho and Tuofu Zhu of the Aaron Diamond AIDS Research Centre in New York has fished out of the sample what remains of the virus after almost 40 years, and has analysed its genetic material to find out whereabouts it fits in the AIDS family tree.

The results, published this week in Nature, confirm the prevailing scientific consensus that HIV is a virus which has hopped over the "species barrier" and into mankind from another animal. But they suggest that the hop took place longer ago than had been suspected. They also suggest that, at least for the form of AIDS which is now spreading worldwide, this hop took place only once. In other words, there was a true "patient zero". He was not, however, the world's most notorious airline steward, but rather an anonymous African who somehow and in some manner that will probably remain forever unknown, tangled with a chimpanzee and came away with more than he bargained for".

The same article continues:

"Viruses are little more than packets of genetic material, usually wrapped in a protein coat. Generally, the genetic material involved is DNA - the molecule that also carries the genes in animals, plants and bacteria. HIV, however, is exceptional. It belongs to an aberrant class of virus known as the retroviruses, which package their genes in the form of DNA's sister molecule, RNA. Whether a virus's genes are made of DNA or RNA, however, a reading of the genetic "letters" of which they are composed (and which carry the information needed to build new viruses) allows a family tree to be constructed. The more similar the sequences of genetic letters in two viruses, the more recently they diverged from a common ancestor..."

3. Origin of HIV 2

While similar to HIV 1, the origin of HIV 2 is thought to be different.

HIV 2 is thought to have originated from Guinea Bissau in West Africa, by jumping the species (SIV) barrier from the grey back and white-collared monkey known as **Sooty Mangabey (SM).** The English word 'sooty' is as a result of its colour, and the name Mangabey is derived from the Madagascan port of Mangaby, as the monkey was originally thought to be from the island of Madagascar in South Eastern Africa. Sooty Mangabeys have very long tails and normally walk on four legs.

However, Sooty Mangabeys are actually native, primarily to Gabon, Cameroon and Guinea Bissau. Another variant of the monkey, the Red Capped Mangabey, can be found in Nigeria, Cameroon, Gabon and Equatorial Guinea.

The scientific name for Sooty Managabey is **Cerocebus Torquatus** which means when translated in Greek 'Tail Monkey'. While the scientific name for the subtype 'red capped sooty Mangabey' is **Cerocebus Torquatas Torquatus.**

Some now think that the virus' spread in West Africa may have been facilitated by Guinea Bissau's War of Independence from Portugal from 1962 – 1974, as people migrated from the war zone.

Conclusion

There is also research which suggests that HIV may have existed as early as the 1930s. Some even say it may have been around for as long as 100 years. It may just have been made popular by political instability, wars, increase in tourism/travel and poverty. Some now doubt if primates are the actual origin of HIV/AIDS. Even those who believe that the virus originated from primates, feel that the virus may have jumped the species barrier more than once, in many different ways.

However, the origin of the disease is increasingly becoming unimportant, as it affects persons from all races, sexes, ages and walks of life. Thus, the preoccupation should be how best to prevent and eventually cure the disease.

Furthermore, although HIV was first discovered among homosexuals, by far the most common mode of transmission is now heterosexual intercourse.

It is possible that we will never truly understand exactly how AIDS originated. It is certainly a disease, which is impacting in a most terrible way on the lives of tens of millions of people throughout the world. Perhaps it is appropriate that the main effort is now to concentrate on finding ways of preventing and curing the disease.

Self-Assessment Questions

1. *Having read the Congo Theory of the origin of AIDS, how likely is it that AIDS originated in the Belgium Congo? Give reasons for your answer and if you think that this theory is unlikely, suggest a more realistic alternative.*

2. *Who was named 'patient zero' and why was he so named?*

3. *What are the 2 main HIV viruses which have been identified and where are they predominantly found?*

4. *How plausible is the Polio Vaccine Theory of AIDS? Justify your answer.*

5. *To what extent do you sympathise with the conspiracy theories?*

6. *How, in your opinion, did HIV/AIDS originate?*

Chapter 7

Prevention of HIV

Contents of this Chapter

1. Introduction

Since there is currently no cure for AIDS, preventing infection with HIV in the first place will clearly be the key to preventing AIDS developing. Some of the best known methods of prevention are examined below

2. Awareness and Education

There is a common saying that "if you know your opponent very well, the battle is half-way won". Thus, an awareness of the disease is vital. In order to avoid people dying in ignorance, it is important to communicate a frank and unambiguous message when educating people about HIV. This is where governments as well as communities should join forces and draw up strategies to tackle the problem.

For example, it might be possible to use role models or those who have already become infected to promote awareness. These people could tell their own story in order to make people understand that it could easily happen to others too and to enlighten them about the risks attached to certain types of behaviour.

HIV/AIDS and Sexually Transmitted Infections (STIs) prevention education can also be incorporated into the educational curriculum of schools, colleges and universities, where these diseases and their prevention is taught.

3. Avoid Unnecessary Risk

People should avoid attitude or activities that will expose them to unnecessary risk of contracting HIV. Everyone is at risk (though some are at greater risk), not withstanding their age, sex, race, occupation and status. Thus, it is important not to be complacent about the epidemic.

4. Avoid Sexual Promiscuity

Closely related to (3) above is that people should avoid sexually promiscuous behaviour, as such behaviour carries a greater risk of contracting HIV that is transmitted via sexual intercourse. Remember that by far the biggest mode of HIV transmission in the world is through heterosexual intercourse.

Avoiding sexual promiscuity calls for restricting sexual partners to one if not zero.

5. Abstinence from Sexual Activities

The best way to prevent sexually transmitted HIV infection is to abstain from sex itself. In reality, however, evidence shows that the vast majority of people will continue to engage in some sort of sexual activities. Thus, strategies other than abstinence will have to be employed as well.

For some however, abstaining from pre-marital sex is not just about HIV prevention, but is about firm religious or moral convictions.

6. Practice Safer Sex

For those who choose to be sexually active, the most effective (and by far the most widely used method of preventing HIV infection) is the use of a condom by the man during sexual intercourse. This is commonly referred to as 'safer sex' or protected sex. Condoms, if properly used, prevent the man's semen from entering the woman's vagina and also prevent the woman's vaginal fluid from entering the man's penis.

As already seen, both semen and vaginal secretions are potential carriers of HIV. It is important to note, however, that condoms do not provide 100% protection. For instance, a condom may break or slip off the man's penis during intercourse. Nevertheless, it is by far the most effective prevention available against sexually transmitted HIV.

It is one thing to advise people to use condoms at any time they engage in sexual activities, but it is another to know how to use a condom properly in order to protect themselves.

According to UNAIDS (2003), the following is a guide on how a condom may be used to achieve effective prevention of HIV and other sexually transmitted infections:

- *Only open the package containing the condom when you are ready to use it. Otherwise, the condom will dry out. Be careful not to tear or damage the condom when you open the package. If it does get torn, throw it away and open a new package.*

- *Condoms come rolled up into a flat circle. They can only be unrolled onto an erect penis.*

- *Before the penis touches the other person, place the rolled-up condom, right side up, on the end of the penis.*

- *Hold the tip of the condom between your thumb and first finger to squeeze the air out of the tip. This leaves room for the semen to collect after ejaculation.*

- *Keep holding the top of the condom with one hand. With the other hand (or your partner's hand), unroll the condom all the way down the length of the erect penis to the pubic hair. If the man is uncircumcised, he should first pull back the foreskin before unrolling the condom.*

- *Always put the condom on before entering the partner.*

- *If the condom is not lubricated enough for you, you may choose to add a "water-based" lubricant, such as silicone, glycerine, or K-Y jelly. Even saliva works well for this. Lubricants made from oil (cooking oil or shortening, mineral or baby oil, petroleum jellies such as Vaseline, most lotions) should never be used because they can damage the condom.*

- *If you feel the condom slipping off during sex, hold it at the base to keep it in place during the rest of the sexual act. It would be safest for the man to pull his penis out and put on a new condom, following all the steps again.*

After sex, you need to take the condom off the right way.

- *Right after he ejaculates, whilst still inside his partner, he must hold onto the condom at the base, near the pubic hair, to be sure the condom does not slip off.*

- *Now, the man must pull out while the penis is still erect. If you wait too long, the penis will get smaller in size, and the ejaculate will spill out of the condom.*

- *When the penis is completely out, take off the condom and throw it away.*

If you are going to have sex again, use a new condom and start the whole process over again!

Even in cases where a couple are both infected with HIV, safer sex is still recommended, as they may cross-infect each other with different strains of the virus.

There are also now condoms for women.

7. Avoid Sharing Needles, Razors, Toothbrushes and Similar Items

Sharing syringes and needles, razor blades and toothbrushes with other people carries the risk of transmitting HIV because blood (which is a carrier of HIV) could be passed from one person to another by the use of such items.

Therefore, sharing these or similar items should always be avoided. This is a particularly important point to note in barber shops, where sharing of razors and trimmers is the norm when having hair cut. There are HIV disinfectant sprays and lubricants now available that every barber shop should apply on items after every individual hair cut, to avoid infecting others.

Furthermore, instruments used for circumcision on one person should never be used on another under any circumstances, to avoid possible transmission of the virus. Female circumcision as a practice should be completely discouraged, as it has no medical benefits. In fact the reverse is the case.

8. Blood, Tissue and Organ Screening

The best possible way to prevent HIV infection under this heading would be to avoid blood transfusion and body tissue or organ transplantation. Some may avoid it as a result of religious or personal beliefs. However, blood or organ transplantation during illness or accident continues to be a common and popular mode of treatment. Thus, an effective and efficient blood, tissue and organ screening programme should be in place to detect and eliminate HIV infected blood, tissue or organ. There have been such reported cases of infection in the United Kingdom in the past.

While modern screening equipment can be very effective, it may still not possible to be 100% accurate in identifying HIV infection in infected blood or organs.

9. Do Not Donate Infected Blood

Closely related to (8) above is that a person infected with HIV should not donate blood or body organs for the purpose of transfusion or transplantation. The dangers of such donation are obvious to see; namely the risk of infecting others. In particular, it is important to bear in mind that some of the groups most at risk of having HIV, such as drug addicts who share needles, may be quite eager to donate blood, so that they can get money to 'feed' their drug habit.

10. Avoiding Breast Feeding While Infected

As breast-feeding is one of the methods of transmitting the disease, an infected mother should avoid breast-feeding her child. Although it may be difficult in some cases to avoid breast-feeding, other ways of feeding the child should be used in order to prevent the child from being infected. Family members may be a source of help in this regard, for example if there is another woman in the family who is not infected with the HIV virus but can breast feed the child for the mother. Bottle feeding the baby is another method. The problem in so many developing countries is that parents cannot afford to buy milk to bottle feed the baby as a result of their grinding poverty.

11. Prevention During Pregnancy

This is a particularly difficult area to deal with, as 1 in every 6 children born to infected mothers can be expected to be infected by the virus. How can an infected pregnant woman then prevent the unborn child from being infected with HIV?

It is now possible to drastically reduce the likelihood of infecting an unborn child. There are certain drugs available that an infected pregnant woman can take to facilitate prevention.

Furthermore, it is also suspected that having the baby delivered by caesarean section is more likely to reduce the risk of infecting the baby than by natural methods, where there is likely to be more blood and hence the possibility of transmitting the disease that way.

In either case, it is advisable to consult a specialist medical practitioner for advice and medication.

12. Prevention During Kissing

Kissing is not a conventional mode of transmitting HIV. However, a person with sores or deep cuts in the mouth should avoid mouth-to-mouth kissing just to be on the safe side. People should avoid putting themselves at unnecessary risk at all times.

13. Avoid Sharing Sex Toys

Sex toys are equipment, instruments or items that some people use on themselves or on their sexual partners during sexual activities. There is the danger of transmitting HIV if an infected person's body fluids are on the sex toy and it was used on the other person.

It is advisable therefore, for people who use or intend to use sex toys not to share them with others at all.

14. Prevention and Prompt Treatment of other STDs

Other Sexually Transmitted Diseases (STDs) such as syphilis and chancroid, which produce genital sores or wounds, can increase the risk of transmitting HIV through sexual intercourse. Thus, preventing being infected with other STDs is vital. Where there is an STD infection, prompt consultation and treatment is necessary to reduce the risk of HIV infection. This is because sores caused by untreated or improperly treated sexually transmitted infections (STIs) can become an entry point for HIV.

Either abstinence or 'safer sex' (using condom during intercourse) is by far the safest known means of preventing STDs.

15. Other Harm-Reduction Methods

The prompt treatment and rehabilitation of hard drug addicts is also part of the prevention process, particularly in cases of HIV infection, as a result of sharing contaminated needles and syringes.

While not yet treated and rehabilitated, drug addicts may be given clean syringes and needles to avoid sharing them.

As part of the harm-reduction programme, condoms may be distributed free of charge to those who need them. Alternatively, people should be informed so that they are aware of where to always pick up a free condom.

It is understandable that some will find these methods unacceptable in their communities, as a result of religious or cultural convictions. Nevertheless, they have proved to be an effective means of HIV/AIDS prevention in many countries.

16. Readily Available Prevention Tools

There is no point in talking about prevention when the prevention tools are not available. Thus, HIV prevention tools such as condoms and awareness information should be readily available. Governments should play a major role in this area, because it is beyond the means of most ordinary individuals in many developing countries to obtain preventative measures on their own, as they are too poor to afford them.

17. Advice and Counselling Centres

It is advisable for governments to set up advice and counselling centres as part of their HIV prevention campaign. This advice and counselling role may be played by existing health centres, hospitals or organisations/departments specifically set up for this purpose. These centres should have close working relationship with community organisations, community heads and the people themselves. This is important so that the people are trusting enough to seek assistance if they need it. This is particularly the case when people are afraid of the stigma associated with HIV/AIDS.

These centres could also be used as training centres for HIV/AIDS and other STDs prevention and co-ordination programmes.

18. Empowerment of Women

Another important mechanism in the prevention of HIV/AIDS, particularly in the developing world is to devise strategies and initiatives where women are empowered in terms of employment, education, healthcare, business and sexual decisions. Economic empowerment of women will enhance sexual empowerment, so that they can decide when and who to have sex with, and not to be forced into unwanted sex as a result of economic and social deprivation.

19. Poverty Reduction Strategies

As there is a clear relationship between HIV/AIDS and poverty, governments should be dedicated and have in place effective strategies to create viable jobs and reduce poverty in their communities.

20. HIV Antibody Testing

Prevention should also include the provision of facilities for HIV testing, otherwise it would be difficult, if not impossible, to know who and how many people are infected by the disease. Thus, test centres should be established in various locations of the country.

Such testing facilities would be useful for both preventative, therapeutic and statistical purposes.

21. Prevention Budget

Every government or authority should allocate a budget for preventing and fighting HIV/AIDS. The importance of a sensibly allocated budget cannot be overemphasised.

22. Strategic Committee

There should be a strategic committee set up by governments at both central and local levels for the planning, co-ordinating and monitoring of HIV/AIDS infections and to examine the effectiveness of existing strategies, so that changes may be effected where necessary.

There should also be a carefully written HIV/AIDS Policy, which will serve as a guide to all, on how, where and when the prevention strategies will be implemented.

23. Obstacles to Preventing HIV

There are several obstacles in the way of preventing HIV, particularly in developing countries. One such obstacle is the belief in some communities that a super-natural force such as voodoo or witchcraft is the cause of their illness, rather than HIV/AIDS. As a result, they rely on the magical powers of witch doctors, rather than on prevention or treatment.

In an article titled "A Global Disaster" (2nd January 1999), the Economist Magazine describes some other obstacles to preventing HIV in developing countries:

"The best hope for halting the epidemic is a cheap vaccine. Efforts are under way, but a vaccine for a virus that mutates as rapidly as HIV will be hugely difficult and expensive to invent. For poor countries, the only practical course is to concentrate on prevention. But this, too, will be hard, for a plethora of reasons:

- *Sex is fun…many feel that condoms make it less so. Zimbabweans ask: "Would you eat a sweet with its wrapper on?"*

- *…and discussion of it often taboo. In Kenya, Christian and Islamic groups have publicly burned anti-AIDS leaflets and condoms, as a protest against what they see as the encouragement of promiscuity. A study in Thailand found that infected women were only a fifth as likely to have discussed sex openly with their partners as were uninfected women.*

- *Myths abound. Some young African women believe that without regular infusions of sperm, they will not grow up to be beautiful. Ugandan men use this myth to seduce schoolgirls. In much of southern Africa, HIV-infected men believe that they can rid themselves of the virus by passing it on to a virgin.*

- *Poverty. Those who cannot afford television find other ways of passing the evening. People cannot afford antibiotics, so the untreated sores from STDs provide easy openings for HIV.*

- *Migrant labour. Since wages are much higher in South Africa than in the surrounding region, outsiders flock in to find work. Migrant miners (including South Africans forced to live far from their homes) spend most of the year in single-sex dormitories surrounded by prostitutes. Living with a one-in-40 chance of being killed by a rockfall, they are inured to risk. When they go home, they often infect their wives.*

- *War. Refugees, whether from genocide in Rwanda or state persecution in Myanmar, spread HIV as they flee. Soldiers, with their regular pay and disdain for risk, are more likely than civilians to contract HIV from prostitutes. When they go to war, they infect others. In Congo, where no fewer than seven armies are embroiled, the government has accused Ugandan troops (which are helping the Congolese rebels) of deliberately spreading AIDS. Unlikely, but with estimated HIV prevalence in the seven armies ranging from 50% for the Angolans to an incredible 80% for the Zimbabweans, the effect is much the same.*

- *Sexism. In most poor countries, it is hard for a woman to ask her partner to use a condom. Wives who insist risk being beaten up. Rape is common, especially where wars rage. Forced sex is a particularly effective means of HIV transmission, because of the extra blood.*

- *Drinking. Asia and Africa make many excellent beers. They are also home to a lot of people for whom alcohol is the quickest escape from the stresses of acute poverty. Drunken lovers are less likely to remember to use condoms."*

Though there can be obstacles, evidence from many developing countries suggests that prevention and education continue to be the key and can be successful.

Conclusion

There are many ways that people can adapt their behaviour in order to prevent infection with HIV. Although some of these strategies do depend on the help of the government or medical experts, many preventative measures are simply common sense and can be used by anyone. However, the role of education is always vital; people cannot change their behaviour unless they realise the benefits of doing so and the risks associated with not doing so. In other words, if they are not taught the ways of preventing infection, then they are always going to be at greater risk of contracting it.

By far the most effective mode of preventing sexually transmitted HIV is using a condom during intercourse. Thus, the 'safer sex' campaign should be vigorously employed. Sex will not be 'fun' if engaging in it without using a condom means that it will lead to an early death.

Self-Assessment Questions

1. *What is the single best preventative measure that will reduce HIV infection?*

2. *What are the main ways that people can change their sexual behaviour to reduce the risk of being infected with HIV?*

3. *What medical procedures carry the most risk of HIV infection?*

4. *Why do you think poorer countries might find it particularly difficult to help their people reduce the risk of HIV infections?*

5. *What are some of the possible obstacles to preventing HIV infection?*

6. *What practical steps need to be followed when using a condom, in order to ensure effective prevention of HIV infection?*

Chapter 8

HIV and Tuberculosis

Contents of this Chapter

1. Introduction

One of the most common HIV/AIDS related opportunistic infections is tuberculosis (TB). It is the leading infectious killer of people living with HIV/AIDS, especially in the developing world. TB used to be known as the 'WHITE PLAGUE' or 'CONSUMPTION' in the early part of the 20th century.

TB is caused by the bacterium **MYCOBACTERIUM TUBERCULOSIS** which is an extremely infectious rod-shaped germ or micro-organism referred to as **BACILLUS** (plural BACILLI).

There is a particular concept that everyone studying tuberculosis should understand. This is that not everyone who has a tuberculosis infection is suffering from tuberculosis. It is said that 90% of those infected with Mycobacterium Tuberculosis may never develop active TB, as the body's immune system tames and suppresses the germs, which then lie dormant in the body.

2. Different Stages of Tuberculosis

There are 3 main stages of tuberculosis infection which are briefly explained below.

(a)   _Early Infection (Stage – 1)_

This is the first stage of TB infection which normally heals either without being noticed or might pass off as common cold or flu.

(b)   _Dormant TB (Stage – 2)_

The dormant TB stage also known as **"SLEEPING TB"** is when the bacilli germs remain dormant (although maybe widespread) in the body. Though present in the body, the germs may have no harmful effect on the infected person.

(c)   _Active TB (Stage – 3)_

Active TB, which is the third and final stage is when the dormant TB activates and "wakes up", causing sores in the lungs and possibly other parts of the body. It is at this stage that a person is referred to as having TB or suffering from TB.

3. Different Types of TB

Understanding tuberculosis is not as easy as some may expect. TB is a complex disease. Although about 80% of all infections relate to the TB of the lungs - known as pulmonary tuberculosis - TB can infect several other parts of the body (i.e. extra-pulmonary TB). It is worth noting however, that only Pulmonary tuberculosis is infectious.

a) Pulmonary Tuberculosis

As mentioned above, this is TB of the lungs which is the predominant types of tuberculosis. Even Pulmonary TB is by no means uniform, but diverged as explained below:

(i.)   Primary Tuberculosis Pneumonia

This is a very infectious pneumonia-based TB that comes with a high fever and productive cough. It is particularly predominant in young children, the elderly and HIV/AIDS patients.

(ii.)   Tuberculosis Pleurisy

This is tuberculosis that causes a rupture of the space (the pleural space) between the lung and the chest wall as the infection compresses the lung. Tuberculosis Pleurisy can cause shortness of breath and extreme chest pain that worsens when a deep breath is taken (pleurisy).

(iii.)   <u>Cavitary TB</u>

This is TB that causes the destruction of the lung by forming cavities or enlarged air spaces. The symptoms of cavitary TB may include weight loss, productive cough (sometimes with blood), weakness, night sweat and fever.

(iv.)   <u>Miliary TB</u>

Miliary TB can cause acute and chronic illness for patients who may appear to be dying slowly. As the name implies, this is tuberculosis in the form of many small lumps on the lung that look like millet seeds.

Other symptoms of Military TB include weight loss, night sweats and fever.

(v.)   <u>Laryngeal TB</u>

An extremely contagious form of pulmonary tuberculosis, is Laryngeal TB, which is TB of the Larynx or the vocal chord.

b) Extra-Pulmonary TB

As opposed to pulmonary TB, extra-pulmonary TB may infect many areas of the body other than the lungs. This is the type of TB that is peculiar primarily to people with a weak or compromised body immune system.

Extra-pulmonary TB itself is made-up of different strains of TB that are explained below.

(i)   <u>Lymph Node Disease</u>

Lymph is a colourless fluid containing white blood cells, drained from the tissues and conveyed through the body in the lymphatic system.

Lymph node means a small mass of tissue in the lymphatic system where lymph is purified and Lymphocytes are formed.

Lymph Node Disease, therefore, is TB that causes the lymph node to become enlarged. The disease may later spread to the skin.

<u>(ii) Tuberculosis Peritonitis</u>

This is TB that infects the outer linings of the intestines and the linings in the abdominal wall, which then produces increased fluid. This increase in fluid causes abdominal swollen and extreme pain.

Symptoms of TB Peritonitis include fever and illness.

<u>(iii) Tuberculosis Pericarditis</u>

Pericardium means the membrane surrounding the heart. Tuberculosis Pericarditis causes the space between the pericardium and the heart to be filled with fluid, preventing the heart from beating efficiently and restricting blood supply to the heart.

(iv) Osteal Tuberculosis

This is TB infection of the bones, but notably the spine which may fracture and cause deformation of the patient's back.

(v) Renal Tuberculosis

This type of tuberculosis can cause white blood cells in the urine. This may spread to the reproductive organs and may adversely affect the patient's ability to reproduce.

In men, renal tuberculosis can cause an inflammation of the epididymis; which is a convoluted duct behind the testis, along which sperm passes to the vas deferens.

(vi) Adrenal Tuberculosis

This is TB of the adrenal glands which can lead to the production of insufficient adrenalin in the body. Some of the symptoms are constant weakness and collapse.

(vii) TB Meningitis

This is TB of the nervous system. It is the TB that infects the membrane surrounding the brain and the spinal cord. TB meningitis can cause permanent impairment and possible death.

Symptoms include constant headache, sleepiness and frequent coma.

4. How TB is Transmitted

Tuberculosis is a very contagious air-borne disease, which can be transmitted by:

a)   Coughing

b)   Sneezing

c)   Spitting, or

d)   Talking

However, not everyone infected will necessarily get ill with TB, as the body immune system prevents the bacilli germs from progressing to active TB which, protected by a thick waxy coat, can be dormant for years. Only people who are ill with pulmonary tuberculosis are infectious.

5. *Symptoms of Tuberculosis*

Special skin tests and chest X-rays may show whether or not a person is infected with tuberculosis. There are however, some symptoms that indicate whether a person may have active TB. These include:

a)   Severe and irritating cough that hangs on, sometimes coughing out blood

b)   Chest pain

c)   Weight loss

d)   Pneumonia

e)   Breathlessness

f)   Loss of appetite

g)   Constant fevers

h)   Constant tiredness

i)   Night sweats

j)   Vomiting

k)   Dark urine

l)   Yellowish skin

m)   Stomach cramps

n)   Changes in eyesight

While not everyone experiencing any of these symptoms may be suffering from TB, it is important to note that these are some of the signs to watch out for, in people with active TB.

6. *Prevalence of Tuberculosis*

Tuberculosis infection is so prevalent in the world that in 1993, the World Health Organisation (WHO) declared it a global emergency.

According to WHO:

(a)   One-third of the world's population is currently infected with Mycobacterium tuberculosis;

(b)   Nearly one percent of the world's population is infected with TB each year;

(c)   Someone in the world is infected with TB every second;

(d)   5-10 percent of people who are infected with TB become sick or infections at some time during their life;

(e)   TB kills about 2 million people each year;

(f)   Around 8 million people become sick with TB each year;

(g)   Over 1.5 million TB cases per year occur in sub-Saharan Africa. This number is rising rapidly as a result of the HIV/AIDS epidemic;

(h)   Nearly 3 million TB cases per year occur in south-east Asia;

(i)   It is estimated that between 2000 and 2020, nearly 1 billion people will be newly infected, 200 million people will get sick, and 35 million will die from TB – if control is not further strengthened;

(j)   TB is the leading infectious killer of youth and adults;

(k)   TB is the leading killer of women;

(l)   TB is likely to create more orphans than any other infectious disease;

(m)   The level of TB in prisons all over the world has been reported to be up to 100 times higher than the civilian population;

(n)   Cases of TB in prisons may account for up to 25% of a country's burden of TB;

(o)   Transmission of Mycobacterium tuberculosis may also occur during long (i.e. more than 8 hours) commercial aircraft flights, from an infectious source (a passenger or crew member) to other passengers or crew members. The risk of infection is related to the proximity and the duration of exposure to the source patient. Decreased ventilation in crowded and confined environments is often a contributing risk factor;

(p)   As many as 50 percent of the world's refugees may be infected with TB. As they move, they may spread TB;

(q)   TB is also very prevalent among the homeless population in both industrialised and poor countries.

TB has indeed become a global epidemic in both developed and developing countries.

7. *Treatment and Control of TB*

Though complicated, TB can be effectively treated and controlled with various anti-TB medicine that is normally taken over 6 months.

The World Health Organisation's (WHO) recommended strategy for effective TB control is known as DOTS, meaning Directly Observed Treatment, Short-course. DOTS combines five elements:

(a)   Political commitment;

(b)   Microscopy services;

(c)   Anti-TB drug supplies;

(d)   Surveillance and monitoring system; and

(e)   Use of lightly efficacious regimes with direct observation of treatment.

Sputum smear testing is repeated after 2 months, to check progress, and again at the end of treatment. A recording and reporting system documents patient's progress throughout, and the final outcome of treatment.

According to WHO:

(a)   DOTS produces cure rates of up to 95 percent even in poorest countries;

(b)   DOTS prevents new infections by curing infectious patients;

(c)   DOTS prevents the development of Multi-Drug Resistant TB (MDR-TB) by ensuring the full course of treatment is followed;

(d)   A six-month supply of drugs for DOTS costs **US $11** per patient in some parts of the world. The World Bank has ranked the DOTS strategy as one of the "most cost-effective of all health interventions".

The DOTS strategy means that with the direct observation of treatment, the patient does not bear the sole responsibility of adhering to treatment. Healthcare workers, public health officials, governments and communities must all share the responsibility and provide a range of support services patients need to continue and finish treatment.

8. Drug Resistant TB

There is now the emergence of the frightening Drug Resistant TB that has complicated the whole treatment of tuberculosis.

Multi-Drug Resistant Tuberculosis (MDR-TB or DRT) as it is normally called, is caused by the improper, inconsistent and partial treatment and management of existing tuberculosis. This may be the case where TB patients fail to take their medication regularly and as prescribed, probably because they feel better, or when doctors prescribe the wrong combination of drugs.

The MDR-TB strain of tuberculosis is known to be resistant to the most important drugs in TB treatment namely **ISONIAZID** and **RIFAMPICIN.** Other common drugs used in treating TB are pyrazinamide and Ethambutol.

While there can be a successful treatment of MDR-TB, the cost of treatment is astronomically high as much as **US $250,000** per patient. As a result, MDR-TB is now an incurable disease in many developing countries, as people cannot afford the cost of such treatment.

9. Preventing TB

The only effective way of preventing being infected with active TB is:

a)   To have regular consultation and check-ups by a qualified doctor;

b)   To take any medication promptly and regularly as prescribed by a qualified doctor;

c)   To get enough rest

d)   To eat healthy food; and

e)   To avoid alcoholic drinks

f)   By vaccination (mostly BCG vaccination). BCG means **Bacillus Calmette Guerin**. It is said that the BCG vaccination has 80% protection rate for ten years.

10. Tuberculosis and HIV/AIDS

There is now conclusive proof that there exists a strong connection between HIV and Tuberculosis (TB), which makes HIV/AIDS prevention a lot more complicated. "AVERT" UK (1999), provided the following information concerning the relationship between HIV/AIDS and Tuberculosis:

"The interaction between the HIV epidemic and the Tuberculosis (TB) epidemic is lethal. TB adds to the burden of illness of people with HIV. The HIV epidemic spurs the spread of TB.

World-wide around 1 in 3 people are infected with the germ that can lead to tuberculosis. Prevalence is highest in conditions of poverty and overcrowding. In some of the developing world's poorest and most overcrowded cities, up to 80% of the adults carry the TB germ. Cities are also the epicentres of the epidemic of HIV, the virus that causes AIDS. In some cities in East Africa, as many as 25-35% of all adults are infected with HIV.

Millions of people infected with the TB germ who would otherwise have escaped active tuberculosis are now developing the disease because their immune system is under attack from HIV. Studies in Italy, Rwanda, Spain, the USA and Zaire found that people who were infected with the TB germ who were also infected with HIV were 30-50 times more likely to develop active tuberculosis than those without HIV.

Unlike HIV, the TB germ can spread through the air. So individuals with active tuberculosis can pass it on to those with whom they come into close contact. If left untreated for a year, one individual can typically infect 10 – 15 other people.

For these reasons, once HIV is introduced into a community where there are people infected with the TB germ, the population faces parallel epidemics of AIDS and TB. In the USA a long-standing annual decline in TB cases ended abruptly in 1985, at the peak of HIV spread. In Asia 14% of all TB cases will be attributable to HIV by the end of the 1990s. This figure was only 2% at the start of the decade. The growing wave of TB is not only a menace for those infected with HIV. Tuberculosis can spread through the air to HIV-negative people. It is the only major AIDS-related opportunistic infection to pose this kind of risk.

Africa, where HIV has spread widely since the late 1980s, already faces a disastrous dual epidemic. In some countries, TB cases have doubled or even tripled since 1985. Tuberculosis is the leading killer of HIV-positive Africans. More than 5 million of the 13 million Africans now alive with HIV are expected to develop TB, and over 4 million will die unnecessarily early deaths because of TB.

Almost all individuals with TB can live longer with proper treatment, and treatment with anti tuberculosis drugs is just as effective in people with HIV, as in those who are not infected. Controlling the dual epidemic requires a dual strategy-treatment TB and preventing new infections with HIV.

The TB germ, a bacterium called Mycobacterium tuberculosis, is highly prevalent in much of the developing world and in poor urban "pockets" of industrialised countries. In these communities, people typically become infected in childhood. But a healthy immune system usually keeps the infection in check. People can remain infected for life with dormant, uninfectious TB. Such people are called TB carriers.

In the past, most TB infected people remained healthy carriers. Only 5-10% ever developed active tuberculosis. Those few kept the TB epidemic going by transmitting the TB germ to their close contacts. TB germs can be spread through the air from patients with active pulmonary (lung) tuberculosis.

Today, as TB carriers increasingly become infected with HIV, many more are developing active tuberculosis because the virus is destroying their immune system. For these dually infected people, the risk of developing active tuberculosis is 30-50 fold higher than for people infected with TB alone. And, because Mycobacterium tuberculosis can spread through the air, the increase in active tuberculosis cases among dually infected people means:

- More transmission of the TB germ,
- More TB and carriers,
- More TB disease in the whole population.

As a consequence, the HIV/AIDS epidemic is reviving an old problem in developed countries and exacerbating an existing one in the developing world. Altogether, TB may claim as many as 30 million lives during the 1990s from among the HIV positive and HIV-negative populations.

As HIV slowly weakens the immune system, the individual gradually becomes unable to fight off "opportunistic infections" – infection with viruses, bacteria parasites and fungi that would normally pose little threat. Common opportunistic infections include fungal infections of the mouth and throat, intestinal infections, and pneumonia.

Tuberculosis, a major opportunistic infection, poses a particular threat to the well-being and survival of HIV-positive people. Only 35-50% of HIV positive people have pulmonary tuberculosis, detectable from just a sputum sample. The remainder develop "disseminated" tuberculosis, which can be diagnosed only with special laboratory facilities. Tuberculosis also progresses faster in HIV-infected people and is more likely to be fatal if undiagnosed or left untreated".

Conclusion

Although TB is not transmitted through sexual contact, it does have a very close relationship with HIV and the statistics show that the 2 diseases are often linked, so a person with HIV/AIDS is advised to undergo tuberculosis test for prompt treatment and vaccination.

Self-Assessment Questions

1. What is the name of the bacterium which causes TB?

2. Roughly how many people may be carriers of this bacterium without ever developing TB?

3. Name the 3 main stages of TB infection

4. What is the main part of the body affected by Pulmonary Tuberculosis?

5. List the main types of Pulmonary Tuberculosis.

6. Which areas of the body may be affected by Extra-Pulmonary TB?

7. List the main types of Extra-Pulmonary TB

8. What are the 4 main ways of transmitting TB?

9. Why can it be difficult to diagnose that someone has TB?

10. What does DOTS stand for?

11. Why is MDR-TB such a worrying form of TB?

12. Why is the link with HIV so strong? Explain your answer fully.

Chapter 9

Financial and Social Cost of HIV/AIDS

Contents of this Chapter

1. Introduction

The ever-increasing HIV infection rate (particularly in developing countries), has a profound associated cost to society. This cost is not only financial, but also includes social, emotional and psychological. Below is an examination of some of the associated financial and human costs of this terrible disease.

2. Changes in Population Demography

The increasing number of HIV infections in developing countries and the resulting increased death rate is expected to cause a major change in population demography of those countries.

As so many young people die of AIDS (possibly because they are the group most likely to be sexually active) some communities will be left with a population full of old people and children but short of young adults. Some developing countries in Sub-Saharan Africa are already experiencing this tilt in population demography.

3. Loss of Manpower

A direct consequence of (2) above is that in the long run, it will lead to a huge loss of manpower, which will be too catastrophic to imagine. Those who are strongest and fittest are the young adults and these are the people most at risk of catching the disease. Loss of manpower is increasingly becoming a reality in some countries directly as a result of the devastating effects that AIDS is having on those societies.

As already mentioned in an earlier chapter, elderly parents are burying their sons and daughters, workers are burying their bosses or colleagues and they are left to fill the gaps in the production process. This is leading to shortfall in overall productivity.

HIV/AIDS has now been declared as the worst pandemic that has afflicted mankind for 600 years.

4. Reallocation of Resources

The increasing rate of HIV infection is making some countries reallocate and divert some of their already scarce resources into HIV prevention strategies. These can run into hundreds of millions of pounds. This money may previously have been spent on other vital areas like healthcare, employment, poverty reduction and economic development.

5. An Impediment to Economic Development

The re-allocation of scarce resources into HIV prevention or treatment, coupled with the loss of manpower as a result of AIDS will, in the long run, certainly impede economic development in those countries or continents. This is a particularly worrying prospect in much of the African continent, where the already problematic state of economic development is in danger of being worsened by the AIDS epidemic.

6. Increased Poverty

Lack of economic development is a recipe for increased poverty, both of the nation and of the individual. This in turn will adversely affect the state of education, health, manpower and confidence of a nation.

7. Political Instability and Threat to National Security

A direct consequence of poverty is political instability, triggered by frustration, dissent, unrest, conflicts and wars, as people fight to protect the little they have. The consequence of all of this is even greater poverty and death. This is the case in so many conflict-torn countries in Africa, Asia and South America. Furthermore, such large numbers of these catastrophic deaths and the associated manpower loss through AIDS is clearly a threat to national security, as a country may find that it has insufficient young soldiers able to form an effective army or defence force.

8. Other Diseases and Pressures on Health Care

As already discussed in a previous chapter, AIDS attracts other diseases, as a person's body immune system is damaged by Human Immuno-Deficiency Virus. Thus, diseases such as tuberculosis are on the rise again in countries that have previously eliminated or drastically reduced its prevalence. The consequence of HIV/AIDS and the increase in other diseases caused by AIDS is that it puts enormous pressure on hospitals and health centres and also puts additional burden on health care finances, which may already be stretched to breaking point.

As a direct consequence of the AIDS epidemic, African leaders have agreed to spend **15% of their countries GDP** on healthcare.

9. Increase in Numbers of Orphaned Children

AIDS is also creating large numbers of orphans in many developing countries as their parents die of the disease. This is particularly becoming a major problem in sub-Saharan Africa where increasing numbers of children are growing up in orphanages. There are now over **13 million orphans** in the world in as a result of AIDS. This figure is expected to rise to 20 million by 2010

As well as the immediate effects as shown above, there are very real long-term problems caused to the fabric of society, as a whole generation grows up with no parental care, guidance and discipline.

10.Increase in Hunger and Famine

The HIV/AIDS epidemic is also creating famine in some countries in sub-Saharan Africa.

As the farmers in the community are killed by AIDS, the children they have left behind may be too young to have acquired, the farming, fishing or trading skills by being left orphaned. Thus, creating a food shortage in many regions of Africa.

11. Increased Care Needs

A consequence of HIV infection and the increase in orphans means that there will be a greater demand for social care and care professionals to cater both for those who are infected and the children left orphaned. This in turn will lead to an increased financial burden on society, as well as an increase in demand for social support, which some countries may simply not be able to provide.

12. Social Ostracisation and Discrimination

Being infected with HIV can lead to a great deal of discrimination. Even relatives and friends of an infected person are often victims of the discrimination. Discrimination may include social ostracisation, lack of employment opportunities, intimidation and violence. There have been several reported cases of lynching and murder of infected persons.

13. Loss of Confidence

A society so bruised by AIDS in terms of resources and manpower is likely to lose confidence in its ability to develop and progress. A great deal of work would need to be done to restore confidence and hope to the people. If not, it will turn out to be a wounded, bewildered, subdued and humiliated society.

14. Depression, Suicide, Assisted Suicide and Mercy Killing

By its very nature, HIV infection is likely to lead to an increase in depression and suicide among HIV positive persons. In some cases, it can even lead to assisted suicide by friends and relatives. This is illegal in the United Kingdom and most countries in the world.

Conclusion

Clearly the costs to society of HIV and AIDS are many and varied, whether economic, social, or psychological. As in so many areas, it is often those in the developing world who have the most to lose as they are the worst afflicted.

Self-Assessment Questions

1. *Of all the costs to society listed, which do you think is:*

   a) *The greatest financial cost?*

   b) *The greatest social cost?*

   c) *The greatest long-term cost?*

   d) *The greatest psychological cost?*

2. *Why is the cost of HIV/AIDS so often greater in the developing world than in the developed world? Give examples to illustrate your answer.*

Chapter 10

Managing and Living With HIV Infection

Contents of this Chapter

1. Introduction

The discussion so far has focused on the prevalence and prevention of HIV and AIDS. Sadly, some have already been infected by HIV and the infection rate continues to rise. Thus, this chapter seeks to explain ways of living and coping with HIV infection.

There is so much ignorance about the disease that there have been many reported cases of discrimination, persecution, social ostracisation and even lynching of infected persons in some communities. It is very important that such actions should be discouraged and prevented.

2. Effects of Infection

Reaction to a positive HIV test ranges from disbelief, shouting, crying, anger, loneliness, suicidal tendencies, to a feeling of failure and unfairness. It could be a depressing time indeed; a time when knowledge on how to manage and cope with the infection will prove to be very useful and quite possibly life-saving.

3. Consequences of Infection

One of the sad consequences and realities of being infected with HIV is that it could result in the development of AIDS and an early death.

Thus, carefully drawing up a strategy on how to live longer is necessary. Some of the tips on prolonging life will be examined below. Another very crucial point to bear in mind is to make sure that an infected person does not infect others deliberately or negligently.

The various prevention methods have been discussed in the chapter on preventing HIV. There are now known to be several cases where people deliberately infected others as means of revenge or as a reflection of the feeling that "if I am infected, I will also infect as many as possible". However, it is important to note that deliberately or negligently infecting others is both morally and ethically wrong, as well as being a criminal offence.

4. Why Proper Management of HIV Infection is Vital

Proper management of HIV will not only help the infected person to live a healthier life, but will also help in the prevention of the disease.

Proper management of HIV would involve:

a) Helping Infected Person come to terms

Helping the infected person come to terms with his illness so that he can accept his status of being HIV positive. Not coming to terms with his new status could lead to continuous anger, disbelief, frustration and feelings of revenge infection.

b) Complete change of behaviour

An infected person needs to have a complete behaviour change, particularly in respect of sexual matters and healthy living. He should also make sure that others are not infected by him.

c) Others accepting his status

It is important that those around him and the community as a whole accepts his status as being HIV positive. This will not only better enable an infected person to come to terms with his status, but will also enable him to change his sexual behaviour and lifestyle.

d) HIV as just another terminal illness

The feeling here is that an infected person will cope better in their communities if HIV was seen as just another terminal illness like:

- Cancer
- Motor neuron disease
- Alzheimer's disease
- Parkinson's disease

If this were to be the case, then there will be less stigma and discrimination against those infected with HIV.

e) Stigma and Discrimination

One of the biggest issues in HIV/AIDS is the stigma that is attached to being infected. Sadly, stigma and discrimination against infected persons, their family and friends is very common in some societies.

As a result, many infected persons will not reveal their status or present themselves for an HIV test, which is bad for the prevention and management of the disease.

f) Community-Wide Effort

Effective management of the disease should be a whole community effort, so as not to socially exclude the infected person. By doing that, the infected person will have a better quality of life and be better prepared to cope with the disease.

5. *What to do next*

When a person discovers that he or she is infected with HIV, it will be a time for an entire change of attitude and behaviour; a time to draw up strategies on how to cope, survive and to live longer. It will be a time to seek as much information as possible about the disease and where to find help. It is also a time to regain lost confidence and to stay strong.

6. *Telling Others*

Telling someone about the infection may become inevitable if help is sought. Such moral and medical support is absolutely vital to improve the quality of life and to prolong it. Others may find religious or spiritual comfort very useful.

It would however, be unwise to tell everyone about the infection because, as mentioned above, it could result in discrimination, persecution and violence directed at not only the infected person but also at friends or family members. This information has to be handled very carefully and sensibly. In tolerant and well-informed societies, going public about an infection could, in some cases, yield positive results, as it would serve as a warning to others of the seriousness of the problem and the need to prevent the infection in the first place. This is particularly true where the infected person is a celebrity.

Usually only very close relatives and other trusted persons such as a doctor may be told.

7. *Keeping Fit and Healthy*

One of the features of HIV infection is that as the infection progresses, the patient loses weight and their muscles become weaker. Thus, keeping fit and staying healthy would help to prevent or slow down the rate of this physical deterioration.

Regular exercise will enable the patient to build more muscle and eating sensible amounts of healthy food at regular intervals will help to prevent the loss of existing muscle.

The US Centre for Disease Control and Prevention (1998) provides some advice on how to stay healthy longer:

- *Make sure you have a doctor who knows how to treat HIV.*

- *Follow your doctor's instructions. Keep your appointments. Your doctor may prescribe medicine for you. Take the medicine just the way he or she tells you to, because taking only some of the medicine gives your HIV infection more chance to fight back. If you get sick from your medicine, call your doctor for advice; don't change how you take your medicine on your own or because of friends.*

- *Get immunizations (shots) to prevent infections such as pneumonia and flu. Your doctor will tell you when to get these shots.*

- *If you smoke or if you use drugs not prescribed by your doctor, quit.*

- *Exercise regularly to stay strong and fit.*

- *Get enough sleep and rest.*

- *Take time to relax. Many people find prayer and meditation, along with exercise and rest, helps them cope with the stress of having HIV infection or AIDS.*

- *Eat healthy foods. This will help keep you strong, keep your energy and weight up, and help your body protect itself.*

As the HIV burns up a lot of the body's energy, it is advisable that the patient eats regularly (without waiting to be hungry), food that contains high amounts of protein and calories.

It is always advisable, however, for HIV positive persons to consult a qualified doctor or nutritionist before embarking on a healthy diet plan. The particular diet plan itself is left for the doctor or nutritionist (specialised in HIV management) to decide, as diet plans may vary from individual to individual. However, it is worth mentioning here some of the recommended diet for people with HIV.

a)   Protein

As already seen in a previous chapter, one of the consequences of HIV/AIDS infection is that the patient may lose massive amounts of body weight. This is because of the loss of the body's protein caused by muscle wasting. Thus, regular intake of protein is necessary for body and muscle building and maintenance.

Protein-based food would include:

- Meat and fish
- Chicken
- Milk
- Beans
- Peanut butter
- Eggs

b)   Carbohydrates/energy foods

Regular intake of carbohydrate/energy based food is necessary for patients with HIV/AIDS to gain much needed energy and calories. This is to enable patients to be able to withstand their ever diminishing energy levels.

Carbohydrate foods include:

- Bread
- Cereals
- Rice
- Potatoes
- Pasta
- Noodles
- Wheat
- Corn
- Sugar
- Syrups

c)   Calcium

Regular calcium intake is also essential for HIV patients, in order to maintain healthy bones, regular heartbeat and proper blood flow in the body.

Calcium-based foods include:

- Fish/Sea food
- Yoghurt
- Milk
- Cheese
- Most other dairy products

d)   Fat

The proper maintenance of body fat is essential for the effective management of HIV. However, excessive or saturated fat can cause problems such as high cholesterol levels, prostate cancer and heart attacks. Thus, a selective fat-based diet is recommended. This would include:

- Oily Fish
- Peanut oil
- Nuts
- White meat/poultry
- Olive oil

The following are very high sources of fat so may only be taken in limited quantities:

- Full fat milk
- Butter
- Fried foods

e)   Fruit and Vegetables

Another important food group that should form part of a healthy diet for HIV management is fruit and vegetables. These are great sources of different varieties of vitamins and minerals that an HIV infected body needs. Thus, it is advisable to have a regular intake of different types of fruit and vegetables.

f)   Fluid

It is good to have a regular and plentiful intake of water, fruit juices and other non-alcoholic beverages (preferably with a high proportion of water). This will ensure that the body has enough fluid to operate properly. However, HIV patients should **avoid alcoholic beverages**.

Staying fit and healthy is paramount if a patient wants to continue to prolong his or her life.

8. When an Infected Person Decides to Have Children

This is a particularly sensitive issue where a person, even though he or she is infected with HIV, decides to have children. As already seen in the chapter on how the disease is transmitted, an infected mother can transmit HIV to the child during pregnancy or at birth. However, there are now anti-retroviral drugs available to infected pregnant mothers where, if they are taken regularly as prescribed, could prevent the unborn child from being infected.

On the other hand, for an infected man who wants a child, a technique known as **"sperm washing"** may be used. This is where, in a medically controlled situation, the HIV is identified in the patient's semen and removed. The now HIV-free sperm is then transplanted into the woman by means of artificial insemination. This is however, a relatively new technique so may not be 100% successful. Therefore, patients should always make an informed decision about any action they take. Always seek specialist advice before engaging in any of the methods mentioned above.

9. *Helping others*

Another very important way to live with HIV infection is to help other infected people to manage and cope with their illness, or to help uninfected persons prevent themselves from being infected, for instance, by education. This will bring happiness and satisfaction and could reduce the stress and frustration associated with HIV infection.

10. *An infected Person need not die of AIDS.*

In developed societies, although HIV infections continue to rise, people do not have to die of AIDS. This is because of the improvements in HIV treatment that now exist and the fact that there are now effective anti-retroviral drugs available which, when taken regularly as prescribed, may prevent the disease from progressing to AIDS.

A major problem, however, is that many people in developing countries cannot afford these drugs as they are very expensive.

However, as mentioned in previous chapter, prices of HIV drugs are coming down after the court case in South Africa in April 2001 and they may one day be accessible to all those who want them. That will be good news indeed for many hundreds of thousands of people.

In the mean time however, government support is necessary as the cost is still beyond the means of the vast majority of the people in the world who live in grinding poverty.

These drugs, coupled with keeping fit and eating healthily, can continue to prolong and improve the life of an infected person.

Nevertheless, the best "treatment" for HIV continues to be prevention itself, even when a cure for AIDS is found.

11. Some of the Most Common Antiretroviral drugs available

The following table shows some of the most common antiretroviral drugs which are currently available.

Brand Name	Generic Name	Firm Name
Retrovir Capsules	Zidovudine, AZT	Glaxo SmithKline
Retrovir Syrup	Zidovudine, AZT	Glaxo SmithKline
Retrovir Injection	Zidovudine, AZT	Glaxo SmithKline
Videx	Didanosine, ddl	Bristol Myers-Squibb
Hivid	Zalcitabine, ddC	Hoffmann-La Roche
Zerit	Stavudine, d4T	Bristol Myers-Squibb
Epivir	Lamivudine, 3TC	Glaxo SmithKline
Invirase	Saquinavir	Hoffman-La Roche
Norvir	Ritonavir	Abbott Laboratories
Crixivan	Indinavir	Merck & Co., Inc
Viramune	Nevirapine	Boehringer Ingelheim Pharmaceuticals, Inc
Viracept	Nelfinavir	Agouron Pharmaceuticals
Rescriptor	Delavirdine	Pharmacia & Upjohn
Combivir	Zidovudine and lamivudine	Glaxo SmithKline
Fortovase	Saquinavir	Hoffman-La Roche
Sustiva	Efavirenz	DuPont Pharmaceuticals
Ziagen	Abacavir	Glaxo SmithKline
Agenerase	Amprenavir	Glaxo SmithKline
Norvir (soft gelatine capsule)	Ritonavir	Abbott Laboratories
Videx EC (enteric coated capsule)	Didanosine	Bristol-Myers Squibb
Kaletra (oral capsule and solution)	Lopinavir and ritonavir	Abbott Laboratories
Trizivir	Abacavir, zidovudine and lamivudine	Glaxo SmithKline
Viread	Tenofovir disoproxil fumarate	Gilead Sciences, Inc

Source: US Food and Drug Administration (2002)

The fact that HIV is so varied and has a ferocious ability to mutate means that a single drug alone is not, at the moment, capable of containing the progression of HIV infection. Rather a cocktail of different combinations of anti-retroviral drugs is necessary to properly attack the virus and keep it under control.

Warning:

Patients are strongly advised to always consult doctors who are specialists in HIV treatment, before any of these anti-retroviral drugs are used.

12. Drug Resistant HIV

There are now reported cases of the emergence of multi-drug resistant HIV. Viruses may mutate into drug resistance when patients fail to follow strictly the drug combination or dosage prescribed by their doctor.

Not only is HIV now resistant to some of the anti-retroviral drugs available, but there have also been several documented cases where the drug resistant HIV has been transmitted directly to a person who was previously uninfected with HIV.

The emergence of this multi-drug resistant HIV has brought a dangerous new twist in the management and treatment of HIV.

It is therefore, strongly advisable for patients to follow strictly the drug combinations and dosage prescribed by their doctor.

It is also clear that it would be unwise even for two HIV infected persons to engage in unprotected sex, as they may cross-infect each other with different strains of HIV; and there is now the possibility that one of these strains could be the multi-drug resistant strain.

13. Side Effects of Anti-retroviral Drugs

While regularly taking anti-retroviral drugs is necessary for HIV/AIDS patients to have an improved quality of living and to prolong life, they are not without problems.

Some of the main side effects experienced by people taking such drugs over a long period are:

- Fatigue
- Nausea/dizziness
- Headache
- Vomiting
- Upset stomach
- Diarrhoea
- Fat growths/lumps
- Mood swings
- Prominent veins
- Liver and kidney problems
- Enlarged breasts

- Anaemia
- Painful toes and fingers

Considering the possibility of these side effects, patients are strongly advised to have regular contact with their doctor for the proper management of the disease.

14. A Problem for the Whole Community

By its nature, HIV/AIDS is a problem not just for the infected person, but also for family members and the community at large. Community awareness and participation is therefore very important in the managing and living with the disease.

An infected person is more likely to survive in an understanding, supportive and caring community environment.

Conclusion

The way that people react to the news that they are infected with HIV can vary from person to person. However, it is important to bear in mind that there are ways of living and coping with HIV, and in particular, to be aware that there are some very real and practical steps that can be taken to improve the quality of life of the infected person. Happily, such steps can sometimes prevent AIDS developing in the future, so it is important to educate people about the benefits of maintaining a positive attitude in the face of what many people believe is an automatic death sentence.

Self-Assessment Questions

1. What is the major possible effect of having an HIV infection?

2. Why is proper management of HIV infection important?

3. What are the most sensible first steps a person should take when he or she finds out that they are infected with HIV?

4. How would a person decide who to tell about the infection?

5. What simple, common sense things can an infected person do to stay healthy?

6. What are the risks associated with an infected person having children and to what extent could they be overcome?

7. What are some of the possible consequences of the new strains of drug-resistant HIV?

8. Why is it important that people are aware of the potential side effects of the anti-retroviral drugs before they start to take them?

Chapter 11

HIV Testing and Immunology Silence

Contents of this Chapter

1. Introduction

One of the most important means by which HIV can be prevented is for those who are already infected to refrain from infecting others. However, for this to be effective, infected people need to *know* that they are actually infected, rather than relying on guesswork, hearsay and perception. This is where HIV testing becomes so important for the management, treatment and prevention of the spread of HIV/AIDS.

It is advisable that anyone embarking on an HIV test should undergo counselling prior to and after the test. The chapter on HIV and counselling deals extensively with this subject matter.

2. Advantages of HIV Testing

There are many advantages for HIV testing. Some of these are listed below:

a) As already mentioned above, testing is useful for the prevention of the spread of HIV infection, as the infected person can take more care not to infect others.

b) A negative test result will bring peace of mind, so reduce unnecessary worry, stress and uncertainty. This is particularly the case with people in high risk categories.

c) A positive result would lead to early treatment and management of the disease, so preventing or prolonging HIV progressing to AIDS.

d) A positive result could also lead to family members (and the community as a whole) making efforts to educate others about the disease and its prevention. It will also enable the community to provide some sort of support network for infected persons.

e) A positive result would also influence an infected person to change his/her future plans, for example:

- Having children.

- Engaging in a particular type of career.

- Embarking on particular business transactions, projects, investments or activities.

- Knowing that he/she is HIV positive will enable people to make more realistic decisions.

3. Possible Disadvantages of HIV Testing

Despite the many important benefits of HIV testing, there can be problems, some of which are:

a) A positive test can lead to discrimination, stigmatisation and possible ostracisation of both the infected persons and their family members or friends.

b) There is also the constant worry and stress of being tested positive.

c) As a result of the adverse consequences of a positive test, some infected persons are known to have suffered anxiety and depression, in some cases, leading to suicide.

d) In many developing countries, testing positive will not result in effective treatment and management of the disease, as governments may be too poor to provide such treatment free of charge.

e) Even a negative test result could lead to potential discrimination and stigmatisation of all kinds.

Overcoming some of these problems will require proper education and enlightenment of society as a whole, particularly as to the nature of the disease and dispelling myths associated with it.

4. Different Kinds of HIV Testing

There are different kinds of HIV testing, as explained below:

a) Involuntary Testing

This is generally not an acceptable way of HIV testing, as it breaches the fundamental human rights of the person tested. Involuntary testing means that a person is forced to undergo an HIV test against his or her will. Involuntary testing may be forced upon a person by:

- Governments

- Schools/colleges

- Immigration services (for potential immigrants)

- Parents

- Teachers

- Community groups

While involuntary testing should continue to be discouraged, it has been an accepted practice by many immigration services of several countries to subject potential immigrants to medical examination before allowing them entry into the country. The medical examination may include not only an HIV test but a test for several other diseases, such as tuberculosis, Hepatitis and SARS.

There may, however, be other **exceptional circumstances** where involuntary testing could be tolerated by law. This may be where a person who is infected or suspected to be infected is deliberately infecting or trying to infect others with the virus.

These exceptions are partially suggested in both English and European Law, as shown below:

Under English Law

Section 38 Public Health (Controls of Disease) Act 1984 [as amended by Section 5 Public Health (infectious diseases) Regulation 1988] allows for the detention in hospital of an inmate of that hospital suffering from HIV/AIDS, if he is likely to spread the disease if he leaves the hospital.

Under European Law

Article 5(1) (e) of the European Convention on Human Rights allows for the lawful detention of persons for the prevention of the spread of infectious diseases.

The assumption here is that, while being detained, a forced HIV testing might be possible, though undesirable.

b) Confidential Testing

This type of testing is normally done by a doctor who is known to (or will eventually be known to) the person being tested. Test results are normally kept confidential so that information will not be divulged to a third party.

Some of the main benefits of confidential testing are:

i)   Confidentiality is maintained.

ii)   A written test result is provided, which could be used as an evidence of a person's HIV status for various purposes.

iii)   Quicker access to medical care, where test is positive.

iv)   A pregnant woman who is at risk of infection may have to get tested through her doctor, in order to have proper medical advice and care.

v)   Some countries immigration services require written HIV test results from potential immigrants.

vi)   Counselling is provided prior to and after the test.

However, there may be limits to this confidentiality where the test result is positive. This is because a test centre may, in some cases, be able to tell parents, schools, insurance companies, or an employer of the patient without necessarily breaking the law.

Nevertheless, patients confidentiality should always be maintained by doctors and other professionals. The chapter on "Access to and Disclosure of Medical Records" deals with the subject matter of confidentiality.

Maintenance of confidentiality is vital in order for people to come forward for tests. The opposite is that many will shy away from testing if they know that confidentiality will be disrespected. This will clearly be counter-productive to any HIV/AIDS prevention initiatives.

c) Anonymous Testing

This type of testing is where doctors and medical professionals at the test centre are not known to the person being tested. Patients are not even required to give their name, address, or any personal detail. Rather a random reference number is given to patients. In this way, the test result is known only to the person tested, and complete confidentiality is maintained. Normally, counselling and advice services are also given to patients.

However, where the test result is positive, the patient will just have to inform other persons such as parents, relatives or a doctor who specialises in the treatment and management of HIV/AIDS.

d) Self-Help Home Sample HIV Testing

As part of the anonymous testing regime, another kind of HIV testing that is gaining popularity is a self-help home sample testing kit. This is where an HIV test kit is bought from a chemist or pharmacy and a few drops of blood are deposited on a test card. This is mailed to the HIV test laboratory or centre. The person then calls the laboratory a few days or weeks later (quoting the special reference number) and is told the result over the telephone.

However, like the anonymous testing above, patients may have to tell others where the test was positive.

The problem with this type of testing is that patients may not get the benefit of face-to-face counselling.

e) DIY Instant HIV Test Kits

Still another form of anonymous testing is a Do-It-Yourself (DIY) instant HIV test kits. The idea of this type of test is that by following the instructions, a person can carry out the test by himself in his own home, with instant results. This test is not recommended, as it may be unreliable and can be inaccurate. This is because some patients may not follow test instructions accurately. Furthermore, like other anonymous testing, it lacks the face-to-face counselling and the emotional support required.

5. The HIV Antibody Testing

An HIV test is generally intended to identify antibodies in a person's blood and other bodily fluids. Antibodies are special chemicals produced by the body in response to an infection.

Thus, if antibodies to HIV are found in a person's blood, it means that the person has been infected with HIV.

6. Immunology Silence

Generally speaking, HIV antibodies take 3 months to develop in the blood. In very rare cases they may take up to 6 months to develop.

Thus, a test that is carried out earlier than 3 months after a person's exposure to HIV, may not detect antibodies, even though the person is infected. They may therefore, unknowingly continue to transmit the disease to others. This false test result is known as a **false negative.**

Therefore, it is always advisable for such persons to undergo repeat testing after 3 months. Some would even recommend that another test be done after 6 months, just to be sure. It is worth nothing however, that the reliability of the test result will depend on whether the person subjected himself to further exposures to HIV within this **3 month "window period".** This window period of not testing positive (though infected) is referred to as **SEROCONVERSION.**

If there was no further exposure and the test was negative of antibodies even after 6 months of the original exposure, the person is not infected with HIV. An appreciation of the window period is essential for the prevention and control of HIV, as persons infected with HIV may not Seroconvert (test positive) for HIV antibodies during this time.

It is also important to reiterate the point that the symptoms of AIDS itself may not be detected for years, by just looking at a person. However, an HIV antibody test done within 3-6 months of exposure should detect whether or not a person is infected with HIV. An antibody test will however, not reveal the level and extent of the damage the virus has caused the immune system, and how close is it to developing AIDS. Another test known as a **viral load test** is required for this information and information relating to the quantity of the virus that is present in the patient.

7. A False Positive Test

While the body's immune system can be silent (**false negative**), even though a person is infected with HIV, it is also possible for an HIV antibody test to produce a positive result even though the person is not infected with HIV. The circumstances where such a false positive result may occur include:

a) The existence of other viral infections

b) Prior immunisations

c) Test error at test centre, or

d) Women who have had multiple pregnancies may have antibodies similar to HIV.

8. Methods of HIV Antibody Testing

There are 3 main methods used in HIV antibody testing namely:

a)   ELISA Method

Enzyme-Linked Immunosorbent Assay (ELISA), also referred to as Enzyme Immunoassay (EIA) is the most common and fundamental method of testing HIV infection. ELISA HIV testing is not a test to detect the virus itself, rather, it is a test to detect HIV fighting antibodies in the blood. It is the fastest and easiest method of HIV antibody testing. The first HIV test that a person undergoes is usually an ELISA test.

The test involves using a needle to collect a small amount of blood from the arm of the person. Though it takes about 3 to 5 hours to get a result, it might take up to 3 weeks or more, if the sample was sent to another laboratory for analysis. There are also now ELISA tests that uses **the urine and saliva** (oral fluid test known as **Orasure**) of the person.

ELISA is a very sensitive test. It is known to be about 99.5% sensitive, in that it can detect even very small amounts of antibody. Thus, false negatives are rare. ELISA is normally the method used in screening donated blood.

Where an ELISA test is positive, a second test known as "Western Blot" is carried out to confirm the validity of the ELISA test result.

b)   Western Blot Testing

Western Blot (WB) HIV testing is a secondary test, in that it is only done where an ELISA test is positive. Thus, it is a more specific test than ELISA. Western Blot is purely a test to confirm the validity of a positive ELISA test result. Like an ELISA test, it also uses the blood sample.

Western Blot is a more difficult test to perform and interpret. Therefore, it requires high technical skills from those administering the test. A western blot test can be either:

i)   Positive;

ii)   Negative; or

iii)   Indeterminate (i.e. neither positive nor negative)

An indeterminate test result could mean that the patient may have just started to seroconvert at the time the test was done. If this is the case, the test should be repeated in 1 to 2 months later.

However, a false-positive test result is very rare with a Western Blot test as it is able to differential HIV antibodies from other non-HIV antibodies that may react to an ELISA test.

WB is generally more expensive and takes longer to get a result from than ELISA testing.

c)   IFA Test

A newer alternative method of secondary testing is Indirect Immunofluoresence Assay (IFA), which is used as an alternative to a Western Blot Test. Like the WB test, IFA uses blood samples to confirm and validate a positive ELISA test result.

The risk of an IFA test to produce an indeterminate result is, on the whole, much lower than a Western Blot Test. It is, however, generally much more expensive than WB test.

d)   Rapid Murex-SUDS Test

A much newer and quicker primary HIV antibody test, similar to ELISA is now in existence. It is a very rapid test known as Murex-SUDS **(Single Use Diagnostic System).** Results are available in 10-40 minutes. However, where blood samples are sent to a separate laboratory for analysis, it may take up to 1-2 weeks for the result. It is a much more expensive method than ELISA. Where a SUDS test is positive, it has to be validated by either a Western blot or IFA tests. Generally, the sensitivity of SUDS is similar to that of ELISA.

9. Viral-Load Testing

All the testing methods described above are antibody test methods, which do not actually reveal either the virus itself or the quantity of the virus that is present in the patient. What it does reveal, however, is that there is evidence of HIV-fighting antibodies present in the patient's blood. The conclusion therefore, is that if these are present, then the patient must be infected with HIV.

It is worth recalling that an HIV antibody test may give a false negative result if the test was done within the 3 months "window period".

The Viral Load Testing on the other hand, seeks to measure the amount of the HIV-RNA that is present in the patient's blood. Knowledge of this is important as it can identify the stage of the infection, which could aid decision-making relating to the type of treatment and management regime that is required.

Some of the **advantages of a viral load test** are that:

a)   it detects the progression of the disease.

b)   it enables doctors to determine when to start treatment.

c)   it enables doctors to determine the level of treatment required.

d)   it enables doctors to monitor the treatment itself.

e)   it enables doctors to determine when to change treatment.

f)   it facilitates better management of the disease in general.

There are **2 main methods of viral testing**, both of which measure the level of the patient's HIV-RNA in the blood.

The 2 methods of viral load testing are:

a)   bDNA test; and

b)   PCR test

However, further discussion of these tests is beyond the scope of this book.

10. Other Test Methods

There are also home-based self-help tests available that have already been discussed above.

Conclusion

HIV testing is extremely vital for the prevention, management and treatment of HIV/AIDS. However, for HIV testing to be attractive, patients have to be convinced that confidentiality will be maintained.

Self-Assessment Questions

1. *What is the role of HIV testing?*

2. *What are the advantages and disadvantages of HIV testing?*

3. *Describe the different kinds of tests that are available.*

4. *What is HIV antibody testing?*

5. *What do you understand by false positive and false negative tests?*

6. *Explain the different methods used in HIV antibody testing.*

7. *Explain Viral Load testing.*

Chapter 12

HIV/AIDS Counselling Techniques

Contents of this Chapter

1. What is Counselling?

Counselling is the act of giving advice, or assisting and guiding a person to resolve difficulties by a trained and experienced person.

However, this chapter will concentrate on counselling in relation to HIV and AIDS. With the ever increasing rate of HIV infections worldwide and the resulting death rate from AIDS, the importance of counselling cannot be over emphasised.

Some of the previous chapters have already dealt with some form of counselling, but it is still worth considering an introduction to counselling in relation to HIV/AIDS.

A person who is a specialist in counselling is known as a Counsellor.

2. *Who should be a Counsellor?*

Being a counsellor in any field is a very challenging and daunting task that requires a great deal of knowledge, skill and experience. Thus, some of the qualities expected of the counsellor are:

(a)   Listening skills

(b)   problem solving skills

(c)   interview skills

(d)   ability to maintain confidentiality

(e)   inter-personal skills and diplomacy

In their book "Learning to Counsel" (Cromwell Press) 1997, Jan Sutton and William Stewart state that the qualities and skills of a counsellor should include the following:

(a)   providing the core conditions for effective counselling to take place namely:

-     genuineness
-     non-possessive warmth
-     unconditional positive regard

(b)   acceptance

(c)   demonstrating empathy

(d)   remaining impartial and suspending judgement

(e)   getting on the client's wavelength

(f)   listening actively and responding appropriately

(g)   being able to enter the client's frame of reference

(h)   offering support

(i)   keeping pace with the client

(j)   expressing understanding of the client's feelings

(k)   keeping the interview moving forward

(l)   maintaining objectivity when planning action

(m)   using silences constructively: waiting for a reply

(n)   reading between the lines: listening to what the client is feeling but not actually communicating

(o)   saying "goodbye" constructively

(p)   using the skills of:

- primary level empathy
- active listening
- attending
- paraphrasing content
- reflecting feelings
- open questions
- summarising
- focusing
- being concrete
- challenging and confronting the client
- advanced level empathy
- immediacy
- disclosing self

Thus, counsellors should always demonstrate professionalism in their work.

3. Counselling in relation to HIV/AIDS

As we have seen, counselling in general, and in particular relating to HIV/AIDS requires a great deal of professionalism.

The main objectives of HIV/AIDS counselling are:

(a)   to prevent HIV transmission, through changes in behaviour and life style,

(b)   to provide better care for those infected and to enable them and their families to manage and cope with the infection.

(c)   to educate people about the realities of HIV/AIDS infection.

(d)   To demystify the disease.

However, for an effective counselling service to be provided, The Joint United Nations Programme on HIV/AIDS [UNAIDS – (Technical Update, 1997)], states that a number of things are needed, including:

(a)   careful selection of trainers who will be able to provide counselling services.

(b)   training that includes supervised placement after initial training, and follow-up training after a period of work experience,

(c)   retention of trained counsellors, by providing them with sufficient space and reasonable working hours; sufficient administrative and professional support and also support from their colleagues,

(d)   the creation of appropriate settings for counselling, avoiding an environment which prevents clients from freely expressing personal concerns; confidentiality for clients; and ensuring that informed consent is always given and counselling offered before an HIV test;

(e)   referral systems that link counselling services with medical clinics and with a range of other services – such as social support, legal services and supportive care available through religious communities – usually provided by non-governmental organisations (NGOs).

It is important therefore, that management provide full support in these areas if effective counselling is to be achieved.

It is also absolutely vital that counsellors have a full and thorough understanding of HIV/AIDS, its prevention and the possible consequences of infection, namely;

(a)   The nature of the disease.

(b)   Public perception of HIV/AIDS.

(c)   The fact that being HIV positive could lead to death by AIDS.

(d)   The social consequences like stigma, discrimination, ostracisation, isolation and depression.

(e)   The effects on friends, family members and the community at large.

(f)   Understanding of terminal illness, bereavement and mourning customs.

Indeed HIV/AIDS counsellors should be persons of high experience and skills; persons who:

(a)   Are willing to listen and provide advice and support.

(b)   Will be non judgmental about the client's sex history. For instance, whether the client is:

- a prostitute

- a homosexual/bisexual

- transvestite

- a transsexual

- an intravenous drug user

- an alcoholic

- a person with numerous sex partners

- a person who does not see the need to use condoms

- ex-offenders

A judgmental attitude will prevent clients from providing vital information required for proper and effective advice. Basically, counsellors should not impose their personal beliefs and values on clients.

While support, care, guidance and advice should be provided, counsellors should encourage the client and his/her family to make their own decisions.

HIV/AIDS counsellors may therefore be:

- doctors
- psychiatrists
- midwives
- nurses
- health educationists
- psychologists
- other health professionals
- social workers
- probation officers
- dieticians/nutritionists
- drug rehabilitation officers
- humanitarian personnel
- religious personnel
- community leaders
- role models

It is advisable to have a control and feedback system to evaluate the effectiveness of counsellors, in order to improve service provision.

4. Who Needs Counselling?

Considering the devastating impact that HIV/AIDS is having on humanity, everyone should have knowledge of its prevention. However, not everyone requires the type of counselling that is discussed in this chapter.

Those who require HIV/AIDS counselling are people who are at a greater risk of being infected or transmitting HIV. This category of persons would include:

(a) intravenous drug users and their partners,

(b) those who have multiple sex partners,

(c) those who engage in unprotected sex,

(d) pregnant women who are HIV positive,

(e) Prostitutes and their partners,

(f) Those who have recently been treated by a doctor or other medical practitioner who is now known to have HIV/AIDS

(g) Those who have had blood transfusion or organ transplantation and are worried about HIV infection.

(h) Anybody who engages in certain sexual practices or other activities that exposes them to the risk of HIV/AIDS infection.

(i) HIV positive women who are breast feeding their babies.

(j) HIV positive men/women who want to have a baby.

(k)   Those who are worried as to whether or not they are infected.

(l)   Those found to be HIV positive and their families,

(m)   Rape victims.

5. Counselling Before an HIV Test

Pre-HIV test counselling is a vital part in HIV/AIDS prevention, management and education.

In its Fact Sheet 7 (Counselling and HIV/AIDS 2002), the World Health Organisation (WHO) states that:

"the aim of pre-test counselling is to provide information to the individual about the technical aspects of testing the various implications of being diagnosed as either HIV positive or negative".

Pre-test counselling should focus on two main topics:

(a)   the person's personal history of risk behaviours, or having been exposed to HIV, and

(b)   assessment of the person's understanding of HIV/AIDS (including methods of transmission) and the person's previous experiences in crises situations.

Information given should be up to date and given in a manner that is easy to understand. Pre-marital testing of couples and testing of blood donors is different from testing those suspected of having HIV/AIDS. However, both groups require sensitivity. Testing should be discussed as a positive act that is linked to changes in risk behaviour, coping and increasing the quality of life.

According to the WHO, the components of a proper pre-test counselling would include the following elements:

*"**Assessment of risk***

Assessing the likelihood that the person has been exposed to HIV requires considering the following:

Frequency and type of sexual practices, in particular, high risk practices such as vaginal and anal intercourse without a condom, or unprotected sex with prostitutes;

Whether the person was/is part of a group with high risk prevalence for HIV infection (intravenous drug users, male and female prostitutes and their clients, prisoners, refugees, migrant workers, homosexual and bisexual men, and health care workers where the use of Universal Precautions is erratic or incomplete.

Whether the individual has received a blood transfusion, organ transplant, or blood or body products. Note that in some developing countries, testing of blood for HIV might not occur.

Has the person been exposed to non-sterile invasive procedures, such as tattooing, scarification, female and male circumcision?

Assessment of understanding

The following questions should be asked in assessing the need for HIV testing:

Why is the test being requested?

What are the behaviour patterns of symptoms of concern?

What does the person know about the test and its uses?

What are the person's beliefs and knowledge about HIV transmission and its relationship to at risk behaviours?

Who could provide emotional and social support (e.g. family, friends, etc)?

Has the person sought VCT before, if so, when, from whom, for what reason and what was the result?

Has the person considered what to do or how he/she would react if the result if positive, or if it is negative?

Preparation for pre test counselling

Effective pre test counselling will prepare the person for the test by:

Discussing confidentiality and informed consent for the HIV test including providing an understanding of the policies governing consent.

Explaining the implications of knowing one is or is not infected.

Exploring the implications for marriage, pregnancy, finances, work, and stigma.

Facilitating discussion about ways to cope with knowing one's HIV status (For example, has the person considered what to do or how she/he would react if the test is positive, or if the test is negative?).

Promoting discussion on sexuality and sexual practices.

Promoting discussion on relationships, with emphasis on the benefits of shared confidentiality between the person and his/her loved ones.

Promoting discussion on sexual and drug related risk behaviours, as appropriate.

Exploring emotional coping mechanisms and the availability of social support.

Explaining how to prevent HIV transmission.

Correcting myths, misinformation and misunderstanding related to HIV/AIDS."

Pre-test counselling can be very beneficial and some of the benefits include:

a)   Greater awareness of HIV/AIDS and its education.

b)   Enabling clients to change behaviour and lifestyle patterns.

c)   Enabling clients to accept HIV/AIDS status if the test turns out to be positive.

d)   Better preparation of clients to manage HIV where the test turns out to be positive.

e)   Enabling clients to reduce the risk of infecting others.

f)   Enabling clients to be better able to cope with the pressures and consequences of being tested positive.

g)   Giving clients hope and the will to continue to live.

h)   It enables friends and family members to better understand HIV/AIDS so that they can give the client the needed support during these difficult times.

Basically, pre-test counselling will better prepare clients emotionally for the worst. It is suggested that a trained and experienced HIV positive person might also be used as a counsellor. This might be a source of encouragement and prevention for others.

6. Counselling After a Negative HIV Test

It is essential that post-HIV/AIDS test counselling is also provided for clients. This counselling is necessary whether or not the client has tested positive. The meeting should be to ascertain how the client feels about the test results and also to ascertain to what extent the client still remembers the pre-test counselling information and advice that was provided. Where it seems to the counsellor that the client has forgotten some of the information, advice should be repeated and the counsellor should make sure that it is understood.

Although the test is negative, clients should be encouraged to come back for another HIV test within 3 months and regularly thereafter. They should also be made to understand that they continue to be at risk of infecting themselves and others if they do not change their behaviour and lifestyle.

7. Counselling after a Positive HIV/AIDS Test

In cases where the test was positive, a lot more would need to be done.

Some of the consequences of a positive test have already been discussed in previous chapters, however, one obvious consequence is the possibility of death. It is therefore, absolutely essential that such a positive result is given with extreme care. It is suggested that where possible, the result is given by the same counsellor who conducted the pre-test counselling, as this is likely to create a more comfortable environment and an atmosphere of continuity.

Being HIV positive means a complete life-style change for the client.

The information and advice provided for the client should include:

a)   availability of health care services,

b)   doctors who are specialists in HIV/AIDS treatment and management,

c)   counselling facilities close to the client's home,

d)   information on some of the most common infections associated with HIV/AIDS,

e)   any other help and services that may be available,

f)   hope that an HIV infection is not an automatic death sentence,

g)   how best not to infect other people,

h)   how to cope with the pressures and consequences.

Counselling at this stage should be a continuous and long-term service. The client should be encouraged to involve trusted family members in future counselling sessions as they will also be affected by the consequences and impact of being infected with HIV/AIDS. While the counselling should be continuous, the client should without delay, be referred to a doctor that specialises in the treatment and management of HIV/AIDS. To start early in both treatment and management is essential for clients to have a healthier life.

Some HIV positive persons find great deal of comfort, joy and peace of mind by educating others on how to avoid being infected.

Others may find comfort from engaging in religious or charitable activities.

8. Counselling at AIDS Stage

This is counselling at the stage where HIV has progressed to AIDS. This is the terminal stage of the disease where counselling will involve some extra consideration such as:

a)   discussion of the drafting of a will,

b)   discussions about the state of physical disability,

c)   discussion about death and dying,

d)   discussions about disappointment, anger, guilt, regret, shame and expectation,

e)   making peace with friends and family; probably also requesting for forgiveness for past events and misunderstandings,

f)   who will be at the bedside at death,

g)   funeral arrangements concerning how, when and where,

h)   encouraging the client to encourage friends, family and others to always take precautionary measures not to be infected by HIV/AIDS, thus enabling clients to die with some comfort that their advice may save others,

i)   the opportunity to say goodbye to friends and relatives.

9. Counselling the Counsellors/Carers

Counselling in HIV/AIDS and caring for people with HIV/AIDS are not only humanitarian, but also very challenging and difficult. Thus, counsellors and carers may in the long run experience physical and emotional burnout (become run down) for several reasons, namely:

a)   the constant encounter with the full impact of human suffering,

b)   the emotional tie/relationship they have built up with the client,

c)   the guilt for their inability to completely help the client from his/her illness,

d)   emotional and physical fatigue,

e)   the uncaring world (governments and community) around them,

f)   the frustration as a result of lack of support and motivation,

g)   lack of resources and essential services,

h)   government bickering as to how best to fight HIV/AIDS,

i)   the general hopelessness around them,

j)   the expectation of some patients that the counsellor or carer may assist in finding a cure for the disease,

k)   where patients want counsellors and carers to assist them (patients) to die (euthanasia),

l)   the whole atmosphere of sadness around them,

m)   worries and fears of divine retribution for their inability to relieve the patients of their illness.

Therefore, counsellors and carers also need periodic counselling in order to be in a good and balanced frame of mind. Such counselling may include:

a)   applauding them for the fantastic and humanitarian work that they are doing,

b)   motivating them to continue the amazing work that they do,

c)   assuring them that they are in no way at fault for not being able to help beyond their abilities,

d)   expressing management's full and continuous support for their work,

e)   actually providing both emotional and material (resources) support,

f)   giving them breaks and short holidays to recuperate from the emotional and physical drain,

g)   providing periodic training in the form of workshops and short courses on how to cope and be efficient,

h)   the fact that there is the hope that HIV/AIDS could be cured in the future,

i)   increasing the status of the HIV/AIDS counsellor,

j)   encouraging regular physical exercise.

Red Cross counsellors experienced similar emotional burn out when dealing with the family members of the victims of the atrocities committed during the 1995 Yugoslavian war in Bosnia-Herzegovina. According to Amanda William, a press officer of the Red Cross:

> *"It is pioneering work and the effects will not be known for a long time. As for the impact on delegates (counsellors), Bieren de Haan says,"*

> *'They will probably never be the same people again. It is normal in some ways to be hurt by an experience like this, but it is a very important human lesson.'"*

Counselling is indeed very challenging work.

10. Counselling Children

It is important that children should not be exempted from the counselling services provided for clients and other family members. This is particularly important where a parent(s) is tested HIV positive or has progressed to the AIDS stage of the disease as children will also face (in the community or at school) some of the consequences of a parent being tested positive, namely:

a) guilt,

b) sadness and anger,

c) isolation and discrimination,

d) shame and humiliation,

e) death and dying of a parent,

f) stress,

g) low self-esteem.

It is important to reassure children that they are in no way at fault for their parent(s) being infected. It may be that the child is also infected. In such cases, he/she should be provided with the counselling that has already been discussed. However, it has to be conducted with a person who fully understands children and how to interact with them; using simple words and examples that they will understand. They should be told the truth about HIV/AIDS, the possible consequences of being infected and its management regime.

Children might find joy and comfort by educating other children about HIV/AIDS and its prevention as examples in South Africa shows.

11. Strategies to Introduce and Support Counselling Services

Despite the many benefits of counselling in HIV/AIDS prevention and its management, many governments and organisations have no strategy to provide effective counselling services. It could be that they have not fully appreciated the importance of counselling or they have no trained and experienced personnel to be counsellors, or they have not enough resources to provide counselling services.

The World Health Organisation (fact sheet 7) provides the following strategies to introduce and support counselling services:

"Convince the decision makers of the need and value of counselling services by quoting evidence of effective services in other communities, as evidenced by reports from a small evaluation project in your area.

Select counsellors and counselling trainees appropriately. These people should have warm and caring personalities, be good listeners, be respected by others, and be motivated and resilient.

Provide training workshops followed by supervised practice and ongoing training for the counsellors.

Provide instrumental and psychological support to the counsellors.

Be sensitive to the location and time of services. The time of services should address accessibility for women, men, youths and couples. In addition, the sites where services are provided could be expanded to include maternal and child health clinics, hospital out patient clinics, community based programs, and STD and TB clinics. These locations could help reduce the stigma attached to an exclusive HIV or STD clinic.

Have adequate supply of condoms (with information on use).

Approach sex workers, street workers, and intravenous drug users in the places where they live and work.

Introduce educational campaigns that increase awareness of counselling services.

Provide counsellors with adequate referral services. This includes referrals to other counsellors, support services, treatment management, laboratory testing, ante natal care/breast feeding/family planning services, and orphan care.

Set up clear counselling standards and protocols."

It is hoped that many more will come to realise the important role that counselling plays in the effective prevention and management of HIV/AIDS.

Conclusion

Although the provision of counselling cannot physically cure a person infected with HIV/AIDS, it can make a huge difference in terms of morale; especially regarding their future well being. Counselling should also be seen as an opportunity to promote education and prevention amongst those who are not yet infected, but who may be at risk if they do not change their behaviour.

Self-Assessment Questions

1.   In your opinion, why is it important to have people who are prepared to offer counselling?

2.   What are the 4 main objectives when providing counselling?

3.   Why is the sort of counselling given to people who test positive for HIV so different from that given to those who are HIV negative?

4.   Why do counsellors themselves need counselling?

5.   What is the WHO recommendation in terms of strategies to introduce and support counselling services?

6.   Who should be an HIV/AIDS counsellor?

Chapter 13

How to Educate People About HIV Prevention

Contents of this Chapter

1. Introduction

Effectively preventing HIV requires an enormous amount of education of the people; it is a time to change people's minds, attitudes and sexual behaviour which may require a great deal of skill and public relations expertise. As there is still no cure for the disease, education and prevention will continue to be the key.

Some of the main points to remember when educating people are discussed below.

2. Government Involvement and Support

Successful education requires total and unambiguous government support and involvement, as governments are best equipped to deal with a large scale education programme in terms of resources and finance. In addition to government, appropriate non-governmental organisations (NGOs), charities and indeed the entire population should be involved in the fight against HIV and AIDS.

3. Convincing People that the Disease Exists

One key issue that needs to be dealt with is convincing people that the disease actually exists. This is important because some people do not believe that HIV and AIDS exists. Rather, they are willing to believe that their illness was caused by witchcraft, voodoo or other supernatural forces. Others believe that it was some other disease rather than AIDS that kills their loved ones.

Thus, convincing people that the disease really exists will go a long way in helping to prevent it.

4. Awareness

Similar to (3) above is that once people are convinced of the existence of the disease, ideally everybody should be made to have full understanding of it and its effects; in other words ensuring that people are aware of the catastrophic effects of AIDS and how to prevent it. Information about the disease and its prevention should be made readily available in literature that is easily accessible to everyone. Such information should be appropriately translated into relevant local languages where possible, so that everyone is given the opportunity to be informed about the disease.

5. A sincere and realistic message

It is important that any educational message should be presented in a sincere, realistic and simple way. The truth about the disease should be told so that people can make an informed decision about their behaviour rather than dying through ignorance and half-truths. As such, simple words and phrases, rather than technical jargon should be used. Some simply call it the **"safer sex"** campaign.

In addition, educators should not impose their views on the people they are educating. They should reason with them and act as service providers rather than lording over them.

6. Community Involvement

Communities, towns or villages should be encouraged to form organisations or forums through which the educational campaign is spread to everyone in that community. This will ensure that no one is left, out as HIV/AIDS is a problem for the entire community.

7. At Schools and Colleges

A perfect opportunity to educate young people about the disease is at schools, collages and universities. This means that from a young age, people are informed of the realities and implication of HIV/AIDS and other Sexually Transmitted Diseases and how to prevent being infected.

Some governments in sub-Saharan Africa are already thinking of incorporating HIV/AIDS education in their school/colleges curriculum; an example that should be emulated by other governments.

8. Advice and Test Centres

There should be in place different regional HIV advice centres which people could contact or visit for information and advice about the disease and HIV anti-body testing. Local hospitals, clinics, health centres and teaching hospitals may be used as advice centres. Staff of such centres should be made to realise that the confidentiality of the client should continue to be maintained, as HIV testing is a very sensitive matter.

9. Recruiting Campaigners and Educators

Sufficient capable and genuine people should be recruited as educators and campaigners to carry the message of HIV/AIDS and its prevention to all the corners of the country taken into consideration people who understands local languages and customs.

10. Training the Campaigners

Educating people in general (but particularly HIV/AIDS) can be a very challenging and daunting task. As a result, the educators/campaigners themselves should be properly trained in not only HIV/AIDS prevention, but also in public relations, marketing and interpersonal skills.

The educators/campaigners appointed should be people who are capable of convincing others about the facts of the disease and its prevention.

The catastrophe or possible catastrophe caused by HIV/AIDS is such that a half-hearted approach to tackling the problem is bound to fail. Thus, governments should have the courage to use full force and resources to fight it, as the possible consequences for failure are so grave.

Such educators/campaigners may be referred to as an **"HIV/AIDS hit squad" or "AIDS Busters"** whose job it will be to educate people about the disease.

It is estimated that the average country would require **about 6,000 - 10,000 of such trained persons** to carry the campaign to all the corners of the country. Larger countries will require even larger numbers. Whatever the cost involved in the training, the cost of funding these campaigners would be far less than the ultimate consequences of an AIDS pandemic; an unimaginable wide-spread death and a population that would be bewildered, wounded and totally subdued.

It is also estimated that the poorer nations would require a total of **US $9.2 billion** a year to tackle AIDS, half of which would be needed for Sub-Saharan Africa alone.

The campaigners may work closely with the community organisations.

11. Using Consultants

Because of the specialist and diverse nature of HIV/AIDS education, the use of consultants (especially at the early stages of the prevention campaign) may be necessary. This may be in terms of strategy and training of the educators/campaigners not only in HIV/AIDS prevention but also in areas such as public relations, marketing, quality control, decision-making, management and human rights, that conventional medical doctors or practitioners may be ill-equipped to provide effectively.

The College of Venereal Disease Prevention provides extensive consultancy services in this area. Some governments have already shown interest.

12. Regional Planning Committees

Apart from field workers or educators, there should also be regional planning committee in every province, state or region of the country. The committee's duty should include the planning and co-ordinating and monitoring the HIV/AIDS educational and awareness campaign in their state or province.

The committee should be made up of capable and trusted people who are experts in different areas of knowledge. This will facilitate uniformity, consistency and effectiveness. The committees should also supervise and control the work of the campaigners and educators.

These committees should be accountable to the strategic planning committee.

13. Strategic Planning Committee

This was briefly mentioned in the previous chapter but it is worth mentioning again. At the pivotal point of this education process, there should be a strategic planning committee at central or federal government level, which should include experts, consultants, managers, and community representatives whose tasks will include planning, logistics, coordination, policy formulation and monitoring and control of the regional planning committee.

There should also be a research and intelligence unit within the committee, which gathers information and monitors the effectiveness of the education and prevention campaign and the prevalence of HIV. This information will facilitate effective planning and strategy in the future.

The strategic planning committee should be answerable to the Prime Minister or President via the Minister of Health.

14. Budget

Again this has been mentioned in a previous chapter, but it is worth mentioning again.

There is a considerable cost involved in the process of educating people. Thus, a realistic and substantial HIV prevention budget should be allocated to meet the costs before any educational campaign commences. Some international organisations and governments may be willing to help poorer countries meet this cost.

15. Control

There should also be in place a control system to regularly check the effectiveness of the strategic planning committee, which will in turn check the effectiveness of the regional planning committees. This will facilitate greater accountability in the system.

The fact that corruption is endemic in some countries means that unless there is effective control and accountability, the whole campaign could fail and turn out to be an exercise to enrich a corrupt few who have no interest at all in public welfare, but only in their personal interest.

16. Learning from Success Stories

Although HIV and AIDS have cast gloom and despair all over the world, there has been success stories that other countries can learn from.

The **"safer sex"** campaign in developed countries has resulted in a drastic reduction in HIV infections, as people became enlightened about the disease and its catastrophic effects.

However, success stories are not confined to developed countries. Some developing countries are also witnessing various degrees of success that should be of interest to policy makers and governments. Some of these success stories were discussed by THE ECONOMIST magazine of 2nd January 1999, under the heading, "A Global Disaster":

"...But three success stories show that the hurdles to prevention are not impossibly high.

*First, **Thailand**. One secret of Thailand's success has been timely, accurate information gathering. HIV was first detected in Thailand in the mid-1980s, among male homosexuals. The health ministry immediately began to monitor other high-risk groups, particularly the country's many heroin addicts and prostitutes. In the first half of 1988, HIV prevalence among drug users tested at one Bangkok hospital leapt from 1% to 30%. Shortly afterwards, infections soared among prostitutes.*

The response was swift. A survey of Thai sexual behaviour was conducted. The results, which showed men indulging in a phenomenal amount of unprotected commercial sex, were publicised. Thais were warned that a major epidemic would strike if their habits did not change. A "100% condom use" campaign persuaded prostitutes to insist on protection 90% of the time with non-regular customers.

By the mid-1990s, the government was spending $80m a year on AIDS education and palliative care. In 1990-93, the proportion of adult men reporting non-marital sex was halved, from 28% to 15%; for women, it fell from 1.7% to 0.4%. Brothel visits slumped. Only 10% of men reported seeing a prostitute in 1993, down from 22% in 1990. Among army conscripts in northern Thailand, a group both highly sexed and well-monitored, the proportion admitting to paying for sex fell from 57% in 1991 to 24% in 1995. The proportion claiming to have used condoms at their last commercial entanglement rose from 61% in 1991 to 93% in 1995.

People lie about sex, so reported good behaviour does not necessarily mean actual good behaviour. But tumbling infections suggests that not everyone was fibbing. The number of sexually transmitted diseases reported from government clinics fell from over 400,000 in 1986 to under 50,000 in 1995. Among northern conscripts, HIV prevalence fell by half between 1993 and 1995, from over 7% to under 3.5%.

Most striking was the government's success in persuading people that they were at risk long before they started to see acquaintances die from AIDS. There was no attempt to play down the spread of HIV to avoid scaring off tourists, as happened in Kenya. Thais were repeatedly warned of the dangers, told how to avoid them, and left to make their own choices. Most decided that a long life was preferable to a fast one.

*Second, **Uganda**. Thailand shows what is possible in a well-educated, fairly prosperous country. Uganda shows that there is hope even for countries that are poor and barely literate. President Yoweri Museveni recognised the threat shortly after becoming president in 1986, and deluged the country with anti-AIDS warnings.*

The key to Uganda's success is twofold. First, Mr Museveni made every government department take the problem seriously, and implement its own plan to fight the virus. Accurate surveys of sexual behaviour were done for only $20,000-30,000 each. Second, he recognised that his government could only do a limited amount, so he gave free rein to scores of non-governmental organisations (NGOs), usually foreign-financed, to do whatever it took to educate people about risky sex.

The Straight Talk Foundation, for example, goes beyond simple warnings about AIDS and deals with the confusing complexities of sex. Its staff run role-playing exercises in Uganda's schools to teach adolescents how to deal with romantic situations. Its newsletter, distributed free, covers everything from nocturnal emissions to what to do if raped. Visiting AIDS workers from South Africa and Zimbabwe asked the foundation's director, Catharine Watson, how she won government permission to hand out such explicit material, and were astonished to hear that she had not felt the need to ask.

The climate of free debate has led Ugandans to delay their sexual activity, to have fewer partners, and to use more condoms. Between 1991 and 1996, HIV prevalence among women in urban ante-natal clinics fell by half, from roughly 30% to 15%.

Third, **Senegal***. If Uganda shows how a poor country can reverse the track of an epidemic, Senegal shows how to stop it from taking off in the first place. This West African country was fortunate to be several thousand miles from HIV's origin. In the mid-1980s, when other parts of Africa were already blighted, Senegal was still relatively AIDS-free. In concert with non-governmental organisations and the press and broadcasters, the government set up a national programme to keep it that way.*

In Sengal's brothels, which had been regulated since the early 1970s, condom use was firmly encouraged. The country's blood supply was screened early and effectively. Vigorous education resulted in 95% of Senegalese adults knowing how to avoid the virus. Condom sales soared from 800,000 in 1988 to 7m in 1997. Senegalese levels of infection have remained stable and low for a decade - at around 1.2% among pregnant women.

Contrast these three with South Africa. On December 1st, World AIDS Day, President Nelson Mandela told the people of KwaZulu-Natal that HIV would devastate their communities if not checked. The speech was remarkable not for its quality - Mr Mandela is always able to move audiences, but for its rarity. Unlike Mr Museveni, South Africa's leader seldom uses his authority to encourage safer sex. It is a tragic omission. Whereas the potholed streets of Kampala are lined with signs promoting fidelity and condoms, this correspondent has, in eight months in South Africa, seen only two anti-AIDS posters, both in the UN's AIDS office in Pretoria".

Conclusion

There are clearly obstacles in the way of fully educating people about the risks of HIV. Some people will be fortunate to live in countries where there are many seeking to educate them about this terrible disease, but so many more people do not have access to even the most basic information. Until this happens it seems likely that many more millions of people will continue to be infected by HIV and possibly AIDS, leading to their untimely early death.

Self-Assessment Questions

1. *Why do you think that so many people refuse to even recognise that AIDS exists?*

2. *Although the cost of educating people about HIV/AIDS might be high, explain how the cost could be justified.*

3. *Why are stories about the successful HIV/AIDS education programmes so important?*

4. *Why should there be transparent accountability in the process of educating people about the disease?*

5. *Explain how best you can educate people about HIV/AIDS.*

Chapter 14

HIV/AIDS and the Workplace

Contents of this Chapter

1. Introduction

The prevention and management of HIV/AIDS at the workplace is increasingly becoming an important issue. According to the International Labour Organisation (ILO), of approximately 42 million people that were infected with HIV, at least 26 million were workers aged between 15 and 49. The ILO continues:

> "This has implications for the size and structure of the populations, for family and social cohesion, and for the livelihoods of individuals and the economies of the nations...
>
> ...The effects are felt by enterprises and national economies as well as workers and their families. The epidemic strikes at the most vulnerable groups in society including the poorest of the poor, women and children, exacerbating existing problems of inadequate social protection, gender inequalities, and child labour"

The epidemic affects the world of work in many ways, namely:

- Discrimination against people with HIV threatens fundamental principles and rights at work, and undermines efforts for prevention and care.

- The disease cuts the supply of labour and reduces income for many workers.

- Valuable skills and experience are being lost.

- Productivity is falling in enterprises and in agriculture, and labour costs are rising.

- Investment is being undermined and tax revenue cut just as countries face more pressure on public.

- The double burden on women gets heavier as they have to earn a livelihood and provide care to sick family members and neighbours.

2. Risk of HIV infection at Work

The possibility of HIV being transmitted at the workplace is now a great concern to many employers and their staff. Therefore, many employers are now devising means to minimise the risk. According to the World Health Organisation (WHO), the chance of contracting HIV at the workplace is estimated to be **0.3%.** Others approximate the risk at **0.4%.**

However, people in certain professions have greater risk of infection than others.

According to the ILO, **the following workers may have greater risk** of being infected with HIV at their workplace.

- Hospital, healthcare and paramedical personnel;

- Dental personnel;

- Police

- Firefighters;

- Rescue workers;

- Custodians;

- Correctional officers;

- Ground-keepers;

- Mental health institution workers;

- Laboratory workers;

- Mortuary attendants

It is also possible for these workers to transmit HIV to their patients or clients.

3. Sources of HIV infection at Work

The World Health Organisation (WHO) states that the primary sources of HIV infection at the workplace are as follows:

To Patients

- Through contaminated instruments that are re-used without adequate disinfection and sterilisation;

- Through transfusion of HIV infected blood, skin grafts, organ transplants;

- Through HIV-infected donated semen;

- Through contact with blood or other body fluids from an HIV-infected health care worker.

To Health Care Workers

- *Skin piercing with a needle or any other sharp instrument which has been contaminated with blood or other body fluids from an HIV infected person;*

- *Exposure of broken skin, open cuts or wounds to blood or other body fluids from an HIV infected person;*

- *Splashes from infected blood or body fluids onto the mucous membranes (mouth or eyes).*

4. Prevention of HIV at the Workplace

The World Health Organisation provides the following recommendation on HIV prevention at the workplace:

a) Creating a safe work environment

- education of employees about occupation risks (fact sheet 9), methods of prevention of HIV and other infectious diseases (fact sheet 12), and procedures for reporting exposure;

- provision of protective equipment such as gloves, goggles, plastic aprons, gowns, and other protective devices;

- provision of appropriate disinfectants to clean up spills of blood and other body fluids;

- increasing the accessibility of puncture resistant "sharps" containers;

- maintaining appropriate staffing levels;

- ensuring that Universal Precautions are implemented, monitored and evaluated;

- providing post-exposure counselling (fact sheet 7), treatment, follow-up and care;

- implementing measures that reduce and prevent stress, isolation and burnout;

- controlling shift lengths and providing supervision of inexperienced staff;

- addressing the healthcare, compensation and financial needs of HIV positive health care workers;

- providing flexible work allocation for HIV positive personnel and continuing their employment for as long as possible. Their participation will be dependant upon their condition, job demands, and the need to protect them from other infections such as tuberculosis;

- providing dispute settlement mechanisms for HIV infected personnel;

- wearing heavy-duty gloves when disposing of "sharps";

- assessing protective and other equipment for risk and safety;

- adopting safe techniques and procedures, such as disposing of needles without recapping, or recapping using the single-handed method, using sterile nasal catheters and other resuscitation equipment, using a separate delivery pack for each delivery, and not using episiotomy scissors to cut the umbilical cord;

- making appropriate disinfectants and cleaning materials available;

- sterilising equipment properly;

- eliminating unnecessary injections, episiotomies, and laboratory tests; avoiding, or covering, breaks in the skin, especially the hands.

b) Universal Precautions

Universal Precautions are simple standards of infection control practices to be used in the care of all patients, at all times, to reduce the risk of transmission of blood borne infections. They include:

- Careful handling and disposal of "sharps";

- Hand washing with soap and water before an after all procedures; use of protective barriers such as gloves, gowns, aprons, masks, goggles for direct contact with blood and other body fluids;

- Safe disposal of waste contaminated with blood or body fluids;

- Proper disinfection of instruments and other contaminated equipment;

- Proper handling of soiled linen

5. Safe Decontamination of Equipment

The following table helps in selecting the method for decontamination.

Level of Risk	Items	Decontamination Method
High Risk	Instruments which penetrate the skin/body	Sterilisation, or single use of disposables
Moderate Risk	Instruments which come in contact with non-intact skin or mucous membrane	Sterilisation, boiling, or chemical disinfection
Low Risk	Equipment, which comes in contact with intact skin	Thorough washing with soap and hot water

Source: World Health Organisation – 2003

6. ILO Guidelines to Address HIV Epidemic at the Workplace

These are comprehensive guidelines provided by the International Labour Organisation (ILO) to combat the HIV/AIDS epidemic at the workplace.

A. Objective of the code

The objective of this code is to provide a set of guidelines to address the HIV/AIDS epidemic in the world of work and within the framework of the promotion of decent work. The guidelines cover the following key areas of action:

a)   prevention of HIV/AIDS

b)   management and mitigation of the impact of HIV/AIDS on the world of work

c)   care and support of workers infected and affected by HIV/AIDS

d)   elimination of stigma and discrimination on the basis of real or perceived HIV status

B. Use of the code

This code should be used to:

a)   develop concrete responses at enterprise, community, regional, sectoral, national and international levels

b)   promote processes of dialogue, consultations, negotiations and all forms of co-operation between governments, employers and workers and their representatives, occupational health personnel, specialists in HIV/AIDS issues, and all relevant stakeholders (which may include community-based and non-governmental organisations (NGOs)

c)   give effect to its contents in consultation with the social partners

- in national laws, policies and programmes of actions
- in workplace/enterprise agreements and
- in workplace policies and plans of action

C. Scope and terms used in the code

This code applies to:

a)   all employers and workers (including applicants for work) in the public and private sectors, and

b)   all aspects of work, formal and informal

D. Key principles

a) Recognition of HIV/AIDS as a workplace issue

HIV/AIDS is a workplace issue, and should be treated like any other serious illness/condition in the workplace. This is necessary not only because it affects the workforce, but also because the workplace, being part of the local community, has a role to play in the wider struggles to limit the spread and effects of the epidemic.

b) Non-discrimination

In the spirit of decent work and respect for the human rights and dignity of persons infected or affected by HIV/AIDS, there should be no discrimination against workers on the basis of real or perceived HIV status. Discrimination and stigmatisation of people living with HIV/AIDS inhibits efforts aimed at promoting HIV/AIDS prevention.

c) Gender equality

The gender dimensions of HIV/AIDS should be recognised. Women are more likely to become infected and are more often adversely affected by the HIV/AIDS epidemic than men due to biological, socio-cultural and economic reasons. The greater the gender discrimination in societies and the lower the position of women, the more negatively they are affected by HIV. Therefore, more equal gender relations and the empowerment of women are vital to successfully prevent the spread of HIV infection and enable women to cope with HIV/AIDS.

d) Health work environment

The work environment should be healthy and safe, so far as is practicable, for all concerned parties, in order to prevent transmission of HIV, in accordance with the provisions of the Occupational Safety and Health Convention, 1981 (No. 155)

A health work environment facilitates optimal physical and mental health in relation to work and adaptation of work to the capabilities of workers in light of their state of physical and mental health.

e) Social dialogue

The successful implementation of an HIV/AIDS policy and programme requires cooperation and trust between employers, workers and their representatives and government, where appropriate, with the active involvement of workers infected and affected by HIV/AIDS.

f) Screening for purposes of exclusion from employment or work processes

HIV/AIDS screening should not be required of job applicants or persons in employment

g) Confidentiality

There is no justification for asking job applicants or workers to disclose HIV related personal information. Nor should co-workers be obliged to reveal such personal information about fellow workers. Access to personal data relating to a worker's HIV status should be bound by the rules of confidentiality consistent with the ILO's code of practice on the protection of workers' personal data, 1997.

h) Continuation of employment relationship

HIV infection is not a cause for termination of employment. As with many other conditions, persons with HIV-related illnesses should be able to work for as long as medically fit in available, appropriate work.

j) Prevention

HIV infection is preventable. Prevention of all means of transmission can be achieved through a variety of strategies which are appropriately targeted to national conditions and which are culturally sensitive.

Prevention can be furthered through changes in behaviour, knowledge, treatment and the creation of a non-discriminatory environment.

The social partners are in a unique position to promote prevention efforts particularly in relation to changing attitudes and behaviours through the provision of information and education, and in addressing socio-economic factors.

k) Care and support

Solidarity, care and support should guide the response to HIV/AIDS in the *world of work. All workers, including workers with HIV, are entitled to affordable health services. There should be no discrimination against them and their dependants in access to and receipt of benefits from statutory social security programmes and occupational schemes.*

E. General rights and responsibilities

a) Governments and their competent authorities

- *Coherence,* Governments should ensure coherence in national HIV/AIDS strategy and programmes, recognising the importance of including the world of work in national plans, for example by ensuring that the composition of national AIDS councils includes representatives of employers, workers, people living with HIV/AIDS and of ministries responsible for labour and social matters.

- *Multi-sectoral participation*. The competent authorities should mobilise and support broad partnerships for protection and prevention, including public agencies, the private sector, workers' and employers' organisations, and all relevant stakeholders so that the greatest number of partners in the world of work are involved.

- *Coordination*, Governments should facilitate and coordinate all interventions at the national level that provide an enabling environment for world of work interventions and capitalise on the presence of the social partners and all relevant stakeholders. Coordination should build on measures and support services already in place.

- *Prevention and health promotion*. The competent authorities should instigate and work in partnership with other social partners to promote awareness and prevention programmes, particularly in the workplace.

- *Clinical guidelines*. In countries where employers assume a primary responsibility for providing direct health-care services to workers, governments should offer guidelines to assist employers in the care and clinical management of HIV/AIDS. These guidelines should take account of existing services.

- *Social protection*. Governments should ensure that benefits under national laws and regulations apply to workers with HIV/AIDS no less favourably than to workers with other serious illnesses. In designing and implementing social security programmes, governments should take into account the progressive and intermittent nature of the disease and tailor schemes accordingly for example by making benefits available as and when needed and by the expeditious treatment of claims.

- *Research*. In order to achieve coherence with national AIDS plans, to mobilise the social partners, to evaluate the costs of the epidemic on workplaces, for the social security system and for the economy, and to facilitate planning to mitigate its socio-economic impact, the competent authorities should encourage, support, carry out and publish the findings of demographic projections, incidence and prevalence studies and case studies of best practice. Governments should endeavour to provide the institutional and regulatory framework to achieve this. The research should include gender-sensitive analyses that make use of research and data from employers and their organisations and workers' organisations. Data collection should, to the extent possible, be sector-specific and disaggregated by sex, race, sexual orientation, age, employment and occupational status and be done in a culturally sensitive manner. Where possible, permanent impact assessment mechanisms should exist.

- *Financial Resourcing*. Governments, where possible, in consultation with the social partners and other stakeholders, should estimate the financial implications of HIV/AIDS and seek to mobilize funding locally and internationally for their national AIDS strategic plans including, where relevant, for their social security systems.

- *Legislation*. In order to eliminate workplace discrimination and ensure workplace prevention and social protection, governments, in consultation with the social partners and experts in the field of HIV/AIDS, should provide the relevant regulatory framework and, where necessary, revise labour laws and other legislation.

- *Conditionalities for government support*. When governments provide start-up funding and incentives for national and international enterprises, they should require recipients to adhere to national laws and encourage recipients to adhere to this code, and policies or codes that give effect to the provisions of this code.

- *Enforcement.* The competent authorities should supply technical information and advice to employers and workers concerning the most effective way of complying with legislation and regulations applicable to HIV/AIDS and the world of work. They should strengthen enforcement structures and procedures, such as factory/labour inspectorates and labour courts and tribunals.

- *Workers in informal activities (also known as informal sector).* Governments should extend and adapt their HIV/AIDS prevention programmes to such workers including income generation and social protection. Governments should also design and develop new approaches using local communities where appropriate.

- *Mitigation.* Governments should promote care and support through public health-care programmes, social security systems and/or other relevant government initiatives. Governments should also strive to ensure access to treatment and, where appropriate, to work in partnership with employers and workers' organisations.

- *Children and young persons.* In programmes to eliminate child labour, governments should ensure that attention is paid to the impact of the epidemic on children and young persons whose parent or parents are ill or have died as a result of HIV/AIDS.

- *Regional and international collaboration.* Governments should promote and support collaboration at regional and international levels, and through intergovernmental agencies and all relevant stakeholders, so as to focus international attention on HIV/AIDS and on the related needs of the world of work.

- *International assistance.* Governments should enlist international assistance where appropriate in support of national programmes. They should encourage initiatives aimed at supporting international campaigns to reduce the cost of, and improve access to, antiretroviral drugs.

- *Vulnerability.* Governments should take measures to identify groups of workers who are vulnerable to infection, and adopt strategies to overcome the factors that make these workers susceptible. Governments should also endeavour to ensure that appropriate prevention programmes are in place for these workers.

b) Employers and their organisations

- *Workplace policy.* Employers should consult with workers and their representatives to develop and implement an appropriate policy for their workplace, designed to prevent the spread of the infection and protect all workers from discrimination related to HIV/AIDS.

- *National, sectoral and workplace/enterprise agreements.* Employers should adhere to national law and practice in relation to negotiating terms and conditions of employment about HIV/AIDS issues with workers and their representatives, and endeavour to include provisions on HIV/AIDS protection and prevention in national, sectoral and workplace/enterprise agreements.

- *Education and training.* Employers and their organisations, in consultation with workers and their representatives, should initiate and support programmes at their workplaces to inform, educate and train workers about HIV/AIDS prevention, care and support and the enterprise's policy on HIV/AIDS, including measures to reduce discrimination against people infected or affected by HIV/AIDS and specific staff benefits and entitlements.

- *Economic impact.* Employers, workers and their organisations, should work together to develop appropriate strategies to assess and appropriately respond to the economic impact of HIV/AIDS on their particular workplace and sector.

- *Economic impact.* Employers, workers and their organisations, should work together to develop appropriate strategies to assess and appropriately respond to the economic impact of HIV/AIDS on their particular workplace and sector.

- *Personal policies.* Employers should not engage in nor permit any personnel policy or practice that discriminates against workers infected with or affected by HIV/AIDS. In particular, employers should:

  - Not require HIV/AIDS screening or testing, unless otherwise specified in section 8 of this code;

  - Ensure that work is performed free of discrimination or stigmatisation based on perceived or real HIV status;

  - Encourage persons with HIV and AIDS-related illnesses to work as long as medically fit for appropriate work.

- *Grievance and disciplinary procedures.* Employers should have procedures that can be used by workers and their representatives for work-related grievances. These procedures should specify under what circumstances disciplinary proceedings can be commenced against any employee who discriminates on the grounds of real or perceived HIV status or who violates the workplace policy on HIV/AIDS.

- *Confidentiality.* HIV/AIDS-related information regarding workers should be kept strictly confidential and kept only on medical files, whereby access to information complies with the Occupational Health Services Recommendation, 1985 (No. 171), and national laws and practices. Access to such information should be strictly limited to medical personnel and such information may only be disclosed if legally required or with the consent of the person concerned.

- *Risk reduction and management.* Employers should ensure a safe and healthy working environment, including the application of Universal Precautions and measures such as the provision and maintenance of protective equipment and first aid. To support behavioural change by individuals, employers should also make available, where appropriate, male and female condoms, counselling, care, support and referral services. Where size and cost considerations make this difficult, employers and/or their organisations should seek support from government and other relevant institutions.

- *Workplaces where workers come into regular contact with human blood and body fluids.* In such workplaces, employers need to take additional measures to ensure that all workers are trained in Universal Precautions, that they are knowledgeable about procedures to be followed in the event of an occupational incident and that Universal Precautions, are always observed. Facilities should be provided for these measures.

- *Reasonable accommodation.* Employers, in consultation with the workers and their representatives, should take measures to reasonably accommodate the worker(s) with AIDS-related illnesses. These could include rearrangement of working time, special equipment, opportunities for rest breaks, time off for medical appointments, flexible sick leave, part-time work and return to work arrangements.

- *Advocacy.* In the spirit of good corporate citizenship, employers and their organisations should, where appropriate, encourage follow employers to contribute to the prevention and management of HIV/AIDS in the workplace, and encourage governments to take all necessary action to stop the spread of HIV/AIDS and mitigate its effects. Other partnerships can support this process such as joint business/trade union councils on HIV/AIDS.

- *Support for confidential voluntary HIV counselling and testing.* Employers, workers and their representatives should encourage support for, and access to, confidential voluntary counselling and testing that is provided by qualified health services.

- *Workers in informal activities* (also known as informal sector). Employers of workers in informal activities should investigate and, where appropriate, develop prevention and care programmes for these workers.

- *International partnerships.* Employers and their organisations should contribute, where appropriate, to international partnerships in the fight against HIV/AIDS.

c) Workers and their organisations

- *Workplace policy.* Workers and their representatives should consult with their employers on the implementation of an appropriate policy for their workplace, designed to prevent the spread of the infection and protect all workers from discrimination related to HIV/AIDS.

- *National, sectoral and workplace/enterprise agreements.* Workers and their organisations should adhere to national law and practice when negotiating terms and conditions of employment relating to HIV/AIDS issues, and endeavour to include provisions on HIV/AIDS protection and prevention in national, sectoral and workplace/enterprise agreements.

- *Information and education.* Workers and their organisations should use existing union structures and other structures and facilities to provide information on HIV/AIDS in the workplace, and develop educational materials and activities appropriate for workers and their families, including regularly updated information on workers rights and benefits.

- *Economic impact.* Workers and their organisations should work together with employers to develop appropriate strategies to assess and appropriately respond to the economic impact of HIV/AIDS in their particular workplace and sector.

- *Advocacy.* Workers and their organisations should work with employers, their organisations and governments to raise awareness of HIV/AIDS prevention and management.

- *Personnel policies.* Workers and their representatives should support and encourage employers in creating and implementing personnel policy and practices that do not discriminate against workers with HIV/AIDS.

- *Monitoring of compliance.* Workers' representatives have the right to take up issues at their workplaces through grievance and disciplinary procedures and/or should report all discrimination on the basis of HIV/AIDS to the appropriate legal authorities.

- *Training.* Workers' organisations should develop and carry out training courses for their representatives on workplace issues raised by the epidemic, on appropriate responses, and on the general needs of people living with HIV/AIDS and their carers.

- *Risk reduction and management.* Workers and their organisations should advocate for, and co-operate with, employers to maintain a safe and healthy working environment, including the correct application and maintenance of protective equipment and first aid. Workers and their organisations should assess the vulnerability of the working environment and promote tailored programmes for workers as appropriate.

- *Confidentiality.* Workers have the right to access their own personal and medical files. Workers' organisation should not have access to personnel data relating to a worker's HIV status. In all cases, when carrying out trade union responsibilities and functions, the rules of confidentiality and the requirement for the concerned person's consent set out in the Occupational Health Services Recommendation, 1985 (No. 171) should apply.

- *Workers in informal activities (also known as informal sector).* Workers and their organisations should extend their activities to these workers in partnership with all other relevant stakeholders, where appropriate, and support new initiatives which help both prevent the spread of HIV/AIDS and mitigate its impact.

- *Vulnerability.* Workers and their organisations should ensure that factors that increase the risk of infection for certain groups of workers are addressed in consultation with employers.

- *Support for confidential voluntary IIIV counselling and testing.* Workers and their organisations should work with employers to encourage and support access to confidential voluntary counselling and testing.

- *International partnerships.* Workers' organisations should build solidarity across national borders by using sectoral, regional and international groupings to highlight HIV/AIDS and the world of work, and to include it in workers' rights campaigns.

F. Prevention through information and education

Workplace information and education programmes are essential to combat the spread of the epidemic and to foster greater tolerance for workers with HIV/AIDS. Effective education can contribute to the capacity of workers to protect themselves against HIV infection. It can significantly reduce HIV-related anxiety and stigmatisation, minimise disruption in the workplace, and bring about attitudinal and behavioural change. Programmes should be developed through consultations between governments, employers and workers and their representatives to ensure support at the highest levels and the fullest participation of all concerned. Information and education should be provided in a variety of forms, not relying exclusively on the written work and including distance learning where necessary. Programmes should be targeted and tailored to the age, gender, sexual orientation, sectoral characteristics and behavioural risk factors of the workforce and its cultural context. They should be delivered by trusted and respected individuals. Peer education has been found to be particularly effective, as has the involvement of people living with HIV/AIDS in the design and implementation of programmes.

a) Information and awareness-raising campaigns

Information programmes should, where possible, be linked to broader HIV/AIDS campaigns within the local community, sector, region or country. The programmes should be based on correct and up-to-date information about how HIV is and is not transmitted, dispel the myths surrounding HIV/AIDS, how HIV can be prevented, medical aspects of the disease, the impact of AIDS on individuals, and the possibilities for care, support and treatment.

As far as is practicable, information programmes, courses and campaigns should be integrated into existing education and human resource policies and programmes as well as occupational safety and health and anti-discrimination strategies.

b) Educational programmes

Educational strategies should be based on consultation between employers and workers, and their representatives and, where appropriate, government and other relevant stakeholders with expertise in HIV/AIDS education, counselling and care. The methods should be as interactive and participatory as possible.

Consideration should be given to educational programmes taking place during paid working hours and developing educational materials to be used by workers outside workplaces. Where courses are offered, attendance should be considered as part of work obligations.

Where practical and appropriate, programmes should:

- Include activities to help individuals assess the risks that face them personally (both as individuals and as members of a group) and reduce these risks through decision-making, negotiation and communication skills, as well as educational, preventative and counselling programmes;

- Give special emphasis to high-risk behaviour and other risk factors such as occupational mobility that expose certain groups of workers to increased risk of HIV infection;

- Provide information about transmission of HIV through drug injection and information about how to reduce the risk of such transmission;

- Enhance dialogue among governments and employers' and workers' organisations from neighbouring countries and at regional level;

- Promote HIV/AIDS awareness in vocational training programmes carried out by governments and enterprises, in collaboration with workers' organisations;

- Promote campaigns targeted at young workers and women;

- Give special emphasis to the vulnerability of women to HIV and prevention strategies that can lessen this vulnerability (see section 6.3);

- Emphasise that HIV cannot be contracted through casual contact, and that people who are HIV-positive do not need to be avoided or stigmatised, but rather should be supported and accommodated in the workplace;

- Explain the debilitating effects of the virus and the need for all workers to be empathetic and non-discriminatory towards workers with HIV/AIDS;

- Give workers the opportunity to express and discuss their reactions and emotions caused by HIV/AIDS;

- Instruct workers (especially health-care workers) on the use of Universal Precautions and inform them of procedures to be followed in case of exposure;

- Provide education about the prevention and management of STIs and tuberculosis, not only because of the associated risk of HIV infection but also because these conditions are treatable, thus improving the workers' general health and immunity;

- Promote hygiene and proper nutrition;

- Promote safer sex practices, including instructions on the use of male and female condoms;

- Encourage peer education and informal education activities;

- Be regularly monitored, evaluated, reviewed and revised where necessary.

c) Gender-specific programmes

- All programmes should be gender-sensitive, as well as sensitive to race and sexual orientation. This includes targeting both women and men explicitly, or addressing either women or men in separate programmes, in recognition of the different types and degrees of risk for men and women workers.

- Information for women needs to alert them to, and explain their higher risk of, infection, in particular the special vulnerability of young women.

- Education should help both women and men to understand and act upon the unequal power relations between them in employment and personal situations; harassment and violence should be addressed specifically.

- Programmes should help women to understand their rights, both within the workplace and outside it, and empower them to protect themselves.

- Education for men should include awareness-raising, risk assessment and strategies to promote men's responsibilities regarding HIV/AIDS prevention.

- Appropriately targeted prevention programmes should be developed for homosexually active men in consultation with these workers and their representatives

d) Linkage to health promotion programmes

Educational programmes should be linked, where feasible, to health promotion programmes dealing with issues such as substance abuse, stress and reproductive health at the workplace. Existing work councils or health and safety committees provide an entry point to HIV/AIDS awareness campaigns and educational programmes. This linkage should highlight the increased risk of infection in the use of contaminated needles in intravenous drug-injection. It should also highlight that intoxication due to alcohol and drugs could lead to behaviour which increases the risk of HIV infection.

e) Practical measures to support behavioural change

- Workers should be provided with sensitive, accurate and up-to-date education about risk reduction strategies, and, where appropriate, male and female condoms should be made available.

- Early and effective STI and tuberculosis diagnosis, treatment and management, as well as a sterile needle and syringe-exchange programmes, should also be made available where appropriate, or information provided on where they can be obtained.

- For women workers in financial need, education should include strategies to supplement low incomes, for example, by supplying information on income-generating activities, tax relief and wage support.

f) Community outreach programmes

Employers, workers and their representatives should encourage and promote information and education programmes on prevention and management of HIV/AIDS within the local community, especially in schools. Participation in outreach programmes should be encouraged in order to provide an opportunity for people to express their views and enhance the welfare of workers with

HIV/AIDS by reducing their isolation and ostracism. Such programmes should be run in partnership with appropriate national or local bodies.

G. Training

Training should be targeted at, and adapted to, the different groups being trained; managers, supervisors and personnel officers, workers and their representatives, trainers of trainers (both male and female), peer educators, occupational health and safety officers, and factory/labour inspectors. Innovative approaches should be sought to defray costs. For example, enterprises can seek external support from national AIDS programmes or other relevant stakeholders by borrowing instructors or having their own trained. Training materials can vary enormously, according to available resources. They can be adapted to local customs and to the different circumstances of women and men. Trainers should also be trained to deal with prejudices against minorities, especially in relation to ethnic origin or sexual orientation. They should draw on case studies and available good practice materials. The best trainers are often staff themselves and peer education is therefore recommended at all levels. It should become part of a workplace's annual training plan, which should be developed in consultation with workers' representatives.

a) Training for managers, supervisors and personnel officers

In addition to participating in information and education programmes that are directed at all workers, supervisory and managerial personnel should receive training to:

- Enable them to explain and respond to questions about the workplaces' HIV/AIDS policy;

- Be well informed about HIV/AIDS so as to help other workers overcome misconceptions about the spread of HIV/AIDS at the workplace;

- Explain reasonable accommodation options to workers with HIV/AIDS so as to enable them to continue to work as long as possible;

- Identify and manage workplace behaviour, conduct or practices which discriminate against or alienate workers with HIV/AIDS;

- Enable them to advise about the health services and social benefits which are available;

b) Training for peer educators

- Peer educators should receive specialise training so as to:

- Be sufficiently knowledgeable about the content and methods of HIV/AIDS prevention so that they can deliver, in whole or in part, the information and education programme to the workforce;

- Be sensitive to race, sexual orientation, gender and culture in developing and delivering their training;

- Link into and draw from other existing workplace policies, such as those on sexual harassment or for persons with disabilities in the workplace;

- Enable their co-workers to identify factors in their lives that lead to increased risk of infection;

- Be able to counsel workers living with HIV/AIDS about coping with their condition and its implications

c) Training for workers' representatives

- Workers' representatives should, during paid working hours, receive training so as to:

- Enable them to explain and respond to questions about the workplace HIV/AIDS policy.

- Enable them to train other workers in trainer education programmes;

- Identify individual workplace behaviour, conduct or practices which discriminate or alienate workers with HIV/AIDS, in order to effectively combat such conduct;

- Help and represent workers with AIDS-related illnesses to access reasonable accommodation when so requested;

- Be able to counsel workers to identify and reduce risk factors in their personal lives;

- Be well instructed about HIV/AIDS in order to inform workers about the spread of HIV/AIDS;

- Ensure that any information that they acquire about workers with HIV/AIDS in the course of performing their representative functions is kept confidential;

d) Training for health and safety officers

In addition to becoming familiar with the information and education programmes that are directed at all workers, health and safety officers should receive specialised training in order to:

- Be sufficiently knowledgeable about the content and methods of HIV/AIDS prevention so that they can deliver information and education programmes to workers;

- Be able to assess the working environment and identify working methods or conditions which could be changed or improved in order to lessen the vulnerability of workers with HIV/AIDS

- Verify whether the employer provides and maintains a healthy and safe working environment and processes for the workers, including safe first-aid procedures;

- Ensure that HIV/AIDS-related information, if any, is maintained under conditions of strict confidentiality as with other medical data pertinent to workers and disclosed only in accordance with the ILO's code of practice on the protection of workers' personal data;

- Be able to counsel workers to identify and reduce risk factors in their personal lives;

- Be able to refer workers to in-house medical services or those outside the workplace which can effectively respond to their needs.

e) Training for factory/labour inspectors

The competent authority should ensure that factory and labour inspectors have sufficient means at their disposal to fulfil their supervisory, enforcement and advisory functions, in particular regarding HIV/AIDS prevention in enterprises. To achieve this, they should receive specialised training on HIV/AIDS prevention and protection strategies at the workplace. This training should include:

- Information on relevant international labour standards, especially the Discrimination (Employment and Occupation) Convention, 1958 (No. 111) and national laws and regulations;

- How to provide awareness about HIV/AIDS to workers and management;

- How to incorporate HIV/AIDS topics into their regular occupational safety and health briefings and workplace training;

- How to assist workers to access available benefits (such as how to complete benefit forms) and to exercise other legal rights

- How to identify violations, or the lack of implementation of workers' rights in respect of HIV status;

- Skills to collect and analyse data relating to HIV/AIDS in workplaces when this is for epidemiological or social impact studies and in conformity with this code.

f) Training for workers who come into contact with human blood and other body fluids

All workers should receive training about infection control procedures in the context of workplace accidents and first aid. The programmes should provide training:

- In the provision of first aid;

- About Universal Precautions to reduce the risk of exposure to human blood and other body fluids

- In the use of protective equipment;

- In the correct procedures to be followed in the event of exposure to human blood or body fluids;

- Rights to compensation in the event of an occupational incident;

And emphasise that the taking of precautions is not necessarily related to the perceived or actual HIV status of individuals

H. Testing

Testing for HIV should not be carried out at the workplace except as specified in this code. It is unnecessary and imperils the human rights and dignity of workers: test results may be revealed and misused, and the informed consent of workers may not always be fully free or based on an appreciation of all the facts and implications of testing. Even outside the workplace, confidential testing for HIV should be the consequence of voluntary informed consent and performed by suitably qualified personnel only, in conditions of the strictest confidentiality.

a) Prohibition in recruitment and employment

HIV testing should not be required at the time of recruitment or as a condition of continued employment. Any routine medical testing, such as testing for fitness carried out prior to the commencement of employment or on a regular basis for workers, should not include mandatory HIV testing.

b) Prohibition for insurance purposes

- HIV testing should not be required as a condition of eligibility for national social security schemes, general insurance policies, occupational schemes and health insurance.

- Insurance companies should not require HIV testing before agreeing to provide coverage for a given workplace. They may base their cost and revenue estimates and their actuarial calculations on available epidemiological data for the general population.

- Employers should not facilitate any testing for insurance purposes and all information that they already have should remain confidential.

c) Epidemiological surveillance

Anonymous, unlinked surveillance or epidemiological HIV testing in the workplace may occur provided it is undertaken in accordance with the ethical principles of scientific research, professional ethics and the protection of individual rights and confidentiality. Where such research is done, workers and employers should be consulted and informed that it is occurring. The information obtained may not be used to discriminate against individuals or groups of persons. Testing will not be considered anonymous if there is a reasonable possibility that a person's HIV status can be deduced from the results.

d) Voluntary testing

There may be situations where workers wish at their own initiative to be tested including as part of voluntary testing programmes. Voluntary testing should normally be carried out by the community health services and not at the workplace. Where adequate medical services exist, voluntary testing may be undertaken at the request and with the written informed consent of a worker, with advice from the workers' representative if so requested. It should be performed by suitably qualified personnel with adherence to strict confidentiality and disclosure requirements. Gender-sensitive pre and post-test counselling, which facilitates an understanding of the nature and purpose of the nature and purpose of the HIV tests, the advantages and disadvantages of the tests and the effect of the result upon the worker, should form an essential part of any testing procedure.

e) Tests and treatment after occupational exposure

- Where there is a risk of exposure to human blood, body fluids or tissues, the workplace should have procedures in place to manage the risk of such exposure and occupational incidents.

- Following risk of exposure to potentially infected material (human blood, body fluids, tissue) at the workplace, the worker should be immediately counselled to cope with the incident, about the medical consequences, the desirability of testing for HIV and the availability of post-exposure prophylaxis, and referred to appropriate medical facilities. Following the conclusion of a risk assessment, further guidance as to the workers' legal rights, including eligibility and required procedures for workers' compensation, should be given.

1. Care and Support

Solidarity, care and support are critical elements that should guide a workplace in responding to HIV/AIDS. Mechanisms should be created to encourage openness, acceptance and support for those workers who disclose their HIV status, and ensure that they are not discriminated against nor stigmatised. To mitigate the impact of the HIV/AIDS epidemic in the workplace, workplaces should endeavour to provide counselling and other forms of social support to workers infected and affected by HIV/AIDS. Where health-care services exist at the workplace, appropriate treatment should be provided. Where these services are not possible, workers should be informed about the location of available outside services. Linkages such as this have the advantage of reaching beyond the workers to cover their families, in particular their children. Partnership between governments, employers, workers and their organisations and other relevant stakeholders also ensures effective delivery of services and saves costs.

a) Parity with other serious illnesses

- HIV infection and clinical AIDS should be managed in the workplace no less favourably than any other serious illness or condition.

- Workers with HIV/AIDS should be treated no less favourably than workers with other serious illnesses in terms of benefits, workers' compensation and reasonable accommodation.

- As long as workers are medically fit for appropriate employment, they should enjoy normal job security and opportunities for transfer and advancement.

b) Counselling

- Employers should encourage workers with HIV/AIDS to use expertise and assistance outside the enterprise for counselling or, where available, its own occupational safety and health unit or other workplace programme, if specialised and confidential counselling is offered.

- To give effect to this, employers should consider the following actions

- Identify professionals, self-help groups and services within the local community or region which specialise in HIV/AIDS-related counselling and the treatment of HIV/AIDS;

- Identify community-based organisations, both of a medical and non-medical character, that may be useful to workers with HIV/AIDS;

- Suggest that the worker contact his or her doctor or qualified health-care providers for initial assessment and treatment if not already being treated, or help the worker locate a qualified health-care provider if he or she does not have one

- Employers should provide workers with HIV/AIDS with reasonable time off for counselling and treatment in conformity with minimum national requirements

- Counselling support should be made accessible at no cost to the workers and adapted to the different needs and circumstances of women and men. It may be appropriate to liaise with government, workers and their organisations and other relevant stakeholders in establishing and providing such support.

- Workers' representatives should, if requested, assist a worker with HIV/AIDS to obtain professional counselling.

- Counselling services should inform all workers of their rights and benefits in relation to statutory social security programmes and occupational schemes and any life-skills programmes which may help workers cope with HIV/AIDS.

- In the event of occupational exposure to HIV, employers should provide workers with reasonable paid time off for counselling purposes.

c) Occupational and other health services

- Some employers may be in a position to assist their workers with access to antiretroviral drugs. Where health services exist at the workplace these should offer, in cooperation with government and all other stakeholders, the broadest range of health services possible to prevent and manage HIV/AIDS and assist workers living with HIV/AIDS.

- These services could include the provision of antiretroviral drugs, treatment for the relief of HIV-related symptoms, nutritional counselling and supplements, stress reduction and treatment for the more common opportunistic infections including STIs and tuberculosis.

d) Linkages with self-help and community-based groups

Where appropriate, employers, workers' organisations and occupational health personnel should facilitate the establishment of self-help groups within the enterprise or the referral of workers affected by HIV/AIDS to self-help groups and support organisations in the local community.

e) Benefits

- Governments, in consultation with the social partners, should ensure that benefits under national laws and regulations apply to workers with HIV/AIDS no less favourably than to workers with other serious illnesses. They should also explore the sustainability of new benefits specifically addressing the progressive and intermittent nature of HIV/AIDS.

- Employers and employers' and workers' organisations should pursue with governments the adaptation of existing benefit mechanisms to the needs of workers with HIV/AIDS, including wage subsidy schemes.

f) Social security coverage

- Governments, employers and workers' organisations should take all steps necessary to ensure that workers with HIV/AIDS and their families are not excluded from the full protection and benefits of social security programmes and occupational schemes. This should also apply to workers and their families from occupational and social groups perceived to be at risk of HIV/AIDS.

- These programmes and schemes should provide similar benefits for workers with HIV/AIDS as those for workers with other serious illnesses.

g) Privacy and confidentiality

- Governments, private insurance companies and employers should ensure that information relating to counselling, care, treatment and receipt of benefits is kept confidential, as with medical data pertinent to workers, and accessed only in accordance with the Occupational Health Services Recommendation, 1985 (No. 171).

- Third parties, such as trustees and administrators of social security programmes and occupational schemes, should keep all HIV/AIDS-related information confidential, as with medical data pertinent to workers, in accordance with the ILO's code of practice on the protection of workers' personal data.

h) Employee and family assistance programmes

- In the light of the nature of the epidemic, employee assistance programmes may need to be established or extended appropriately to include a range of services for workers as members of families, and to support their family members. This should be done in consultation with workers and their representatives, and can be done in consultation with workers and their representatives, and can be done in collaboration with government and other relevant stakeholders in accordance with resources and needs.

- Such programmes should recognise that women normally undertake the major part of caring for those with AIDS-related illnesses. They should also recognise the particular needs of pregnant women. They should respond to the needs of children who have lose one or both parents to AIDS, and who may then drop out of school, be forced to work, and become increasingly vulnerable to sexual exploitation. The programmes may be in-house, or enterprises could support such programmes collectively or contract out for such services from an independent enterprise.

- The family assistance programme may include:

  - Compassionate leave;

  - Invitations to participate in information and education programmes;

  - Referrals to support groups, including self-help groups;

  - Assistance to families of workers to obtain alternative employment for the worker or family members provided that the work does not interfere with schooling;

  - Specific measures, such as support for formal education, vocational training and apprenticeships, to meet the needs of children and young persons who have lost one or both parents to AIDS;

  - Coordination with all relevant stakeholders and community-based organisations including the schools attended by the workers' children;

  - Direct or indirect financial assistance;

  - Managing financial issues relating to sickness and the needs of dependants;

  - Legal information, advice and assistance;

  - Assistance in relation to understanding the legal processes of illness and death such as managing financial issues relating to sickness, preparation of wills and succession plans;

  - Helping families to deal with social security programmes and occupational schemes;

  - Provision of advanced payments due to the worker;

  - Directing families to the relevant legal and health authorities or providing a list of recommended authorities.

Conclusion

It is clear from the discussion in this chapter that every employer and employee should put in every possible effort to achieve proper management, control and prevention of HIV/AIDS at the workplace.

Self-Assessment Questions

1.   *Why is proper prevention and management of HIV/AIDS at the Workplace necessary?*

2.   *What are the risks of contracting HIV at the Workplace?*

3.   *What are some of the possible sources of HIV infection at the Workplace?*

4.   *How can HIV infection be prevented at the workplace?*

5.   *How useful, in your opinion, is the ILO Code of Guidance on HIV/AIDS at the Workplace?*

6.   *Are there any other ways you can personally improve HIV/AIDS Prevention and Management at the Workplace?*

Chapter 15

HIV Vaccines And Microbicides

Contents of this Chapter

1. Introduction

This chapter is intended to introduce readers to the concept of vaccines and the possibility of an effective HIV vaccine and microbicide in the global fight against HIV/AIDS, especially now that it has graduated to the level of a pandemic.

2. *The Nature of Vaccines*

According to Black's Medical Dictionary (1999), the name vaccine:

> *"applied generally to a substance of the nature of dead or attenuated living infectious material introduced into the body with the object of increasing its [the body] power to resist or get rid of a disease".*

Thus, vaccines are used to boost the body's immune system and also used to boost the body's ability to fight diseases. Vaccines can therefore, be used for both preventative and therapeutic purposes.

3. *HIV Vaccines*

HIV vaccines are now seen as one of the most ideal methods of fighting the HIV/AIDS pandemic. With tens of millions of people already dead, and tens of millions destined to die of AIDS, vaccines will be the key to both the prevention and treatment of HIV/AIDS. Despite the potentially huge benefits of them, there are not currently any vaccines available for the fight against these terrible diseases.

The ideal HIV vaccine should be:

a)   100% effective,
b)   safe, and
c)   affordable

Some suggest that an oral vaccine would be more desirable.

As already mentioned, HIV vaccines will serve two primary purposes, preventative and therapeutic.

a) Preventative HIV Vaccines

As the name implies, these are HIV vaccines that will boost the helper cells (see chapter 2) so that people are immune from being infected by HIV. Since the vast majority of people in the world are not yet infected, the potential benefits of such a preventative vaccine are enormous. Many lives will be saved by an effective preventative vaccine.

Another preventative vaccine approach talked about is to develop a vaccine that can block the spikes (gp120) of HIV, so that the virus will be incapable of latching itself to CD4 (see chapter 2).

b) Therapeutic HIV Vaccines

A preventative vaccine will not be a consolation to those who have already been infected with HIV, as it could only prevent uninfected people from being infected. A therapeutic vaccine will therefore, be the solution for people who are already infected. This may be achieved by a vaccine that not only boosts the CD4+ - T cells, but also increases the number, spread and effectiveness of CD8 + (killer cells - see chapter 2), in order to destroy the virus, even when the person is infected. This will basically mean a cure for HIV/AIDS.

It will be a great day when a therapeutic vaccine is developed. However, it is a preventative vaccine that is in greatest need at the moment, as the vast majority of people are not yet infected.

c) Live Attenuated Virus Vaccine

Another vaccine approach that is advocated by an American scientist Dr Desrosiers, is the use of live attenuated HIV virus. Dr Ronald Desrosiers developed a trial vaccine that was 100% successful, when it was use to experiment on monkeys in 1993. Dr Desrosiers removed a gene from the SIV virus, the monkey equivalent of HIV. He then kept the virus live, but made it safe as a vaccine and it was given to monkeys. The monkeys were then injected with live SIV and the vaccine worked. The approach is that by using a live attenuated virus vaccine, the entire body defence mechanism is awakened and stimulated to fight the virus that has been introduced to the body.

This vaccine approach is not unique, as it is the same approach that was used in smallpox, yellow fever, polio, rubella, measles and mumps vaccines.

However, Dr Desrosiers' vaccine approach was rejected, because it was considered too risky and dangerous in the fight against HIV. While this approach worked very well in fighting other diseases, the fear is that HIV, being the fastest mutating virus humans have ever seen, may one day turn the virus against the body and might create an even more lethal brand of HIV. Some scientists feel that these uncertainties, combined with the limited knowledge that experts have about the virus, makes it too risky to be used on humans.

Nevertheless, other scientists feel that the live attenuated vaccine approach may have been the best opportunity for an effective HIV vaccine, as it has been the most effective trial vaccine so far.

4. Different Stages of HIV Vaccine Development

The vaccine development process is a very slow and long one that can take 10 to 20 years or even more. This process would normally involve the following stages:

a) Conceptual and Research

This is the stage when the basic concept and science of the vaccine is considered and research undertaken to see its feasibility.

b) Pre-Development

Once the feasibility of the science is ascertained, the next stage will be research on the development and the trials on creatures (other than human).

c) Clinical (Human) Trials Stage

If these tests on primates or other creatures were successful, then further research is undertaken and human trials are arranged. It could take as long as 8 to 15 years from the first stage of the human trial to the distribution stage of the vaccine.

There are 3 stages of human trials as explained below.

i) <u>Phase 1 Trials</u>

This is the first phase of human trials, which is normally conducted on between 10 to 80 volunteers who are low risk persons that are not infected with HIV.

The objective under a phase 1 trial is to assess the safety of the vaccine, including possible side effects. It also looks at the dosage, administration and the immune system's response to the vaccine.

Trials at this phase may take 8-12 months or more to complete.

ii) <u>Phase 11 Trials.</u>

To ensure safety and validate the results obtained under the Phase 1 trials, the phase 2 trials are conducted on much larger groups of about 50 to 500 volunteers that comprise persons of both low risk and high risk.

Phase 2 trials also look at safety and immune response, but over a much longer trial period. Thus, trials under this phase may take between 18-24 months.

A successful phase 2 trial will then move on to phase 3, which is the final phase.

iii) <u>Phase 111 Trials</u>

These are much more precise efficacy trials, which seek to verify the level of effectiveness of the vaccine in preventing HIV infection. As many as 5,000 to 16,000 high risk volunteers may be used for these trials.

The vaccine will be compared against other vaccines and against a placebo, to see the incidence of HIV infection amongst people given the vaccine and those that are given a placebo. Trials at this phase can take a minimum of 3 years.

d) Application for Licence

If the phase 111 efficacy trials are successful, then the vaccine manufacturers can apply for a license.

e) Manufacture and Distribution

Once a license is granted, then arrangements are made for the manufacture and effective distribution of the vaccine.

5. HIV Vaccine Research Funding

Apart from the fact that the vaccine development process takes a long time, there has not been enough willpower on the part of many pharmaceutical companies and governments to fund research into the development of HIV vaccine.

This is due in part to the feeling that the expected return on investment on HIV vaccine is not attractive enough, considering the fact that the people in most need of an HIV vaccine are from developing countries, with little financial standing. This may be why the majority of on-going vaccine trials are targetted towards fighting against HIV strains or subtypes that are prevalent in developed countries.

6. HIV Vaccines on Trial

There are many HIV vaccines that are now on trial. However, the vaccine development process is a long and slow one that takes many years to complete. The table below shows trial HIV vaccines and the phases they have reached.

Phase 1, 1/11 and 11 Safety, Dosing and Immunogenicity Trials

Principal research partners	Vaccine approach	Ongoing trials
IAVI; University of Oxford; UK Medical Research Council; University of Nairobi; Kenya AIDS Vaccine Initiative; Imperial College of Science, Technology and Medicine; Cobra Therapeutics Ltd; IDT GmbH	**DNA-MVA** Constructed from HIV subtype A HIV genes in naked DNA + HIV genes in modified vacinia Ankara (MVA), a pox virus	Phase 1/11: UK; Phase 1: Kenya
Merck & Co Inc; HIV Vaccine Trials Network (HVTN), Vical, Inc.	**DNA-adeno** Constructed from HIV subtype B HIV genes in naked DNA + HIV genes in adeno (common cold) virus	Phase 1: US
GlaxoSmithKline plc, HIV Vaccine Trials Network	**gp120, nef-tat** Constructed from HIV subtype B Gp 120 protein plus nef-tat fusion protein	Phase 1: US
Vaccine Research Center, US National Institutes of Health; Vical Inc.	**DNA** Constructed from HIV subtype B HIV genes in naked DNA	Phase 1: US
Agence Nationale de Recherche sur le VIH/SIDA (France), Biovector Therapeutics SA	**Lipopeptides** Constructed from HIV subtype B	Phase 1: France

Phase 111 Efficacy Trials

Principal Research Partners	Vaccine Approach	Ongoing Trials
VaxGen Inc; HIV Vaccine Trials Network (HVTN), Bangkok	**AIDSVAX**	Phase 111: US, Canada, Netherlands, Thailand
Metropolitan Authority	B & E	Data from North America and Europe
	gp 120 protein	
Aventis Pasteur SA, VaxGen Inc; US National Institutes of Health, Thailand Ministry of Public Health	**ALVAC-AIDSVAX** Constructed from HIV subtype B & E HIV genes in canarypox virus (ALVAC) + Gp120 protein (AIDSVAX)	Phase 111: Thailand, Earlier trial finishing in Brazil, Haiti, Trinidad and Tobago, US

Source: International AIDS Vaccine Initiative - 2003

7. *Failure of VaxGen*

VaxGen became the first and only company whose vaccine trials got the third and final stage. In early 2003, VaxGen announced that it had completed the stage 3, efficacy trials. However, these particular vaccines are designed to fight against HIV 1 subtype B and E (refer to chapter on different types of HIV), that are prevalent in North America, Puerto Rico, Japan, Australia, Western Europe, Central African Republic, Thailand and Southeast Asia. The vast majority of sub-Saharan Africa, where HIV/AIDS is much more prevalent would not have benefited from it. However, the belief is that once this is successful, then the development of vaccines for the other strains of HIV would be a lot easier.

In November 2003, VaxGen announced that the **vaccine failed**. The most promising HIV vaccine failed the test of efficacy. This created a huge setback in the quest for an effective HIV vaccine.

8. *HIV Subtypes, Strains and Vaccine*

As HIV is a very varied and fast mutating virus with different subtypes and strains, the worry amongst many is how to design a vaccine(s) that is effective against all the variants of the virus.

The varied nature of HIV poses a great deal of challenge to vaccine researchers.

9 . How soon is a Vaccine expected?

Producing a vaccine is a slow process, as it has to be scrutinized meticulously, as it passes through the different phases and trial stages. As mentioned above, the most promising HIV trial vaccine failed, thus, turning the clock backwards.

Therefore, an effective HIV vaccine is not expected until 2011 to 2016.

10. The Role of Ethics

Ethics play a major role in the trial and manufacture of HIV (indeed any) vaccines. The appropriate ethic committees have to be satisfied that the vaccine is not only effective and safe, but is also in agreement with important ethical issues, before approval is granted.

All of this prolongs the process of vaccine development for human use.

11. Introduction to Microbicides

Another possible source of HIV prevention, other than vaccines, is Microbicides. According to the National AIDS Trust, UK (2002):

> "A microbicide is a product, which when used (internally or rectally) can prevent HIV transmission as well as offer protection against a variety of STI's. It can take many different forms as a gel, cream or suppository that could be active in the body for several hours".

> Microbicides are not to be confused with spermicides, which prevent contraception, although it is possible that a microbicide could also act as a contraceptive".

While there is on-going research on the microbicides, it will take several years for them to be available for use.

It is important to realise that a microbicide will only be useful in the prevention of sexually transmitted HIV and STDs as it can be used as a liquid barrier. It may also be used to boost the immune system by killing HIV.

According to UNAIDS technical update (April 1998) titled: "Microbicides for HIV Prevention", the ideal microbicide should have the following characteristics:

- Effective against HIV and other STDs (when used either before or after intercourse)

- Active as soon as it is inserted, and for a long time

- Safe

- Inexpensive

- Available without prescription

- Colourless

- Odourless

- Tasteless

- Invisible

- Easy to Store

- Pleasure enhancing

- It may have or lack contraceptive properties

a) How Important are Microbicides?

Microbicides, if they can be developed, are regarded as very important to the prevention of HIV/AIDS.

The World Health Organisation (2003) States that:

> "It is important to support the development of microbicides because:

- Despite the knowledge of successful HIV prevention strategies – condom use, reduction in the number of sexual partners, diagnosis and treatment of STI's – HIV continues to spread at an alarming rate especially among women in developing countries;

- Without a preventative HIV vaccine, microbicides offer an alternative to condoms and are the most feasible method of primary prevention of HIV;

- Currently available HIV prevention techniques are often not feasible for women who live in resource poor settings. The availability of microbicides would greatly empower women to protect themselves and their partners. Unlike male and female condoms, microbicides are a potential preventative option that women can easily control and do not require the co-operation, consent or even knowledge of the partner.

b) Microbicides and Women

It is believed that an effective microbicide will be good for all, but particularly for women in the prevention of HIV and other STDs. Not only will it enable women to have a greater control in preventing themselves from infection, but microbicides can also serve as a vaginal lubricant during sexual intercourse.

c) When do we expect a Microbicide?

Considering the lengthy trial process that it has to pass through (as seen under vaccines), it is expected that the first microbicide is expected to be available between 2007 and 2010. This is still a long way off considering the state of emergency required in the prevention of HIV/AIDS, particularly in developing countries.

Therefore, huge investment in the research and development of microbicides is needed urgently to tackle this emergency.

So far, there are three stage 3 trials of microbicides.

Conclusion

There is no doubt that finding an effective vaccine and microbicide against HIV/AIDS will be one of the biggest breakthroughs against these vicious diseases that are gradually incapacitating humanity.

Self-Assessment Questions

1.   *What are Vaccines?*

2.   *What is the nature of HIV vaccines?*

3.   *Explain the different stages of HIV vaccine development?*

4.   *Why is vaccine development such a slow process?*

5.   *What are microbicides and how useful will they be in the fight against HIV?*

6.   *Considering the present stages of their development, how soon are we likely to have an effective vaccine and microbicide against HIV?*

Chapter 16

HIV and Criminal Law

Contents of this Chapter

A – Criminal Law

1. Introduction

A Criminal Offence is regarded as an "Offence Against the State" or "Entire Society". It would make sense to critically appraise the word 'regarded', in that an offence regarded as criminal in one country may not be regarded as criminal offence in another. Indeed, even in the same country, there can be variation in the law in different regions, as is the case in England and Scotland. Generally, bigamy is a criminal offence in the whole of the United Kingdom and conviction of the offence would normally carry a prison sentence and a criminal record. The same however, is not true in some other countries, where a man could not commit bigamy, as those societies allow polygamous marriages.

Conversely, while adultery is regarded as a Criminal Offence in some countries, which may even be punishable by death, it is not an offence at all in the United Kingdom; but only a ground for divorce.

Examples of Criminal Offences in the UK would include:-

a)	Homicide (Murder & Manslaughter)

b)	Treason

c)	Rape

d)	Assault and Battery

e)	Theft

f)	Fraud

g)	Dangerous driving

h)	Bigamy

i)	Burglary

j)	Criminal damage

k)	Incitement to violence

l)	Stalking

m)	Domestic Violence

n)	Grievous Bodily Harm (GBH)

A Civil wrong (known as **TORT**) on the other hand is regarded as a wrong against individual(s) as opposed to a criminal offence, which is regarded as offence against the state. The primary objective of the Civil Trial is compensation, rather than jail - no one goes to jail for a civil offence, nor will they get a criminal record. It may however, affect the credit record of the person concerned if it was a case of unpaid credit and the amount remained unpaid.

Some examples of civil wrongs would include:

a)   Breach of contract

b)   Private nuisance

c)   Defamation (i.e. slander and libel)

d)   Unpaid Debt

e)   Trespass to land (though aggravated trespass is a criminal offence)

f)   Negligence (though there is criminal negligence)

2. The following table illustrates some of the differences between Civil Wrongs & Criminal Offences.

Civil Wrongs	Criminal Offences
1. Cases tried in Civil Courts	1. Cases tried in Criminal Courts
2. Regarded as Wrongs Against Individual(s)	2. Regarded as Offences Against the State
3. The primary objective is to compensate the innocent party	3. The primary objective is to punish the guilty party.
4. The terminology used is 'sue' - which is done by either by the parties themselves or by their lawyers	4. Terminology here is to 'prosecute'. This is done by the Crown Prosecution Service (CPS). The head of the CPS is the Director of Public Prosecutions (DPP). In certain circumstances, however, other organisations such as Local Authorities may also bring a prosecution against offenders.
5. The verdict is 'liable' or 'not liable'	5. The verdict here is 'guilty' or 'not guilty'.
6. In the UK, the people involved are addressed as say BROWN Vs STEVEN. That is, Brown bringing the case against Steven.	6. Here, it is R Vs STEVEN. 'R' meaning REGINA which is the Latin name for Queen. Criminal cases are normally brought in the name of the Crown. It would still be 'R' if it was a King which means REX.
7. The person bringing the case is the PLAINTIFF while the other party is the DEFENDANT	7. The person bring the case (which is the state) is the PROSECUTION while the other party is the ACCUSED or the DEFENDANT.
8. The evidence and the burden of proof ON THE BALANCE OF PROBABILITIES. The plaintiff only needs to prove on the balance of probability that the defendant is liable.	8. Here a more stringent proof by the Prosecution is required namely to prove BEYOND THE REASONABLE DOUBT that the defendant is guilty.

9. Unless on legal aid, both parties meet their legal cost. The loser will have to pay the winner (costs and compensation)

9. The State also provides the defence for the accused so bears all costs unless the accused wants his own defence lawyers.

NOTE: Some cases are presented in a format similar to this:

R v SSHD ex parte STEVEN (1999)

These are cases of judicial review that are normally brought at the high course. Judicial review is the means by which an executive decision or a public body is challenged in the United Kingdom. An example is where a person challenges the decision of the Secretary of State for Home Department (SSHD) as is in this case. What this means is that Steven is petitioning the Crown to query her servant, (The Secretary of State) on the ground that the SSHD is acting or has acted beyond the powers conferred on him by legislation and by the Crown.

It can be seen from the above, that it would normally be more difficult to find a person guilty (especially in the Crown Court - jury trial) in a Criminal Court, than to find the person liable in a Civil Court, because of the more stringent demands on the prosecution in criminal law namely to "prove beyond the reasonable doubt'.

A good example is the well publicised 1996 case of Mr O. J. Simpson - an ex-American football player who was accused of killing both his wife (Nicole Brown Simpson) and her friend (Ron Goldman) in Los Angeles, California, USA. The case was read like this "THE PEOPLE OF CALIFORNIA vs O.J. SIMPSON".

He was found 'not guilty' by a Criminal Court in California, because the Prosecution could not prove 'Beyond the Reasonable Doubt' that he was the killer. If he was found guilty, he would have gone to jail for life.

However, the families of Nicole and Ron disagreed with the verdict and then went to a Civil Court. Remember, this was not a retrial (as many people in the public thought) but was a totally different trial by a totally different route - namely the civil route. The two families felt that it would be easier to find him liable in a civil court, as the evidence and burden of proof is not as high as in the Criminal Court. They needed only to prove on the 'Balance of Probabilities' that he was the killer. Their objective was to make him compensate the innocent i.e.:- to take from him all money and property that he had made over the years.

In 1997, O.J. Simpson was found 'liable' by the Civil Court and he was told to pay the estate of the deceased over Twenty Million US Dollars ($20,000,000).

Remember that this route does not lead to a jail sentence and there is no guarantee at all that he would be found guilty if he was sent back to a Criminal court (though such will not happen), as the burden of proof will continue to be higher and more stringent than the civil court.

3. The Nature of Criminal Liability

We have already seen some of the characteristics of civil wrongs and criminal offences. However, it is worth examining further the nature of criminal liability.

For someone to be found guilty under criminal law some basic requirements must exist. These are explained briefly below:

1) Actus Reus

    Actus Reus is that there must have been an act or action by the accused for him to be liable under criminal law. Action could take the form of assault, shooting, hitting, destroying, kicking, stabbing, etc.

    Actus reus would have to be proved by the prosecution. You can see why it would be very difficult if not impossible to prove that a victim was killed by witchcraft as actus reus would be missing. However, if a poison was used in killing the person, then the poisoning itself is the actus reus.

    In some of the circumstances however, actus reus could take the form of an omission rather than an action. This could occur where the accused had a duty to act but failed or refused to do so. Such a duty may arise from contract, legislation or at common law. One example of a duty arising from legislation is contained under the Children and Young Persons Act 1933 where it is a criminal offence for wilfully neglecting a child. For instance, not providing food for the child or not obtaining proper medical treatment for the child when necessary.

    However, no offence is committed for failing a moral duty. Example is where passers-by failed or refused to rescue a person drowning.

2) Mens rea

    Mens rea means 'mind or intention'. It could also be described as 'malice aforethought'. This is that even where actus reus has been proven, an accused may still not be liable under criminal law where there was no intention on his part to cause the act that he has been accused of.

    Thus, a person who threw a stone into the sky which fell down and kill a man would not be guilty of murder (as he had no intention to kill) but likely to be guilty of involuntary manslaughter, as he had been negligent. The same will be the case where A accidentally broke B's arm while defending himself from an attack by B.

3) Causation

    Another important requirement is criminal liability is the concept of causation. This basically means what is the actual cause of injury, death, etc. Which means that even where there is actus reus, a person is not guilty of murder if his act is not the cause of death. A brief example will illustrate this point.

    A and B are friends who are angry with J. On seeing J, A slapped him and B kicked J on the head so hard that J died. The question is, are both A and B guilty of murder? The question basically is "who caused the death of J?"

    Though there was actus reus on the part of both A and B, it was B that caused the death of J. However, A is likely to be guilty of assault or causing actual bodily harm depending on any injuries as a result of the slap. B on the other hand, might argue that even though he kicked J on the head, he had no intention to kill him. So if this defence of "lack of mens rea" was successful, then B is likely to be convicted of manslaughter rather than murder.

4)   <u>Negligence</u>

As seen above, even where mens rea has not been proven an accused person may still be convicted if he was criminally negligent.

However, for the criminal negligence to be successful, the prosecution must prove that:

1)   The accused owed the victim a duty of care; and

2)   That duty was broken; and

3)   As a result the victim suffered harm, injury or loss

Without these requirements being proven, the prosecution is unlikely to be successful.

There is an exception to these general rules in that there are circumstances where a claim for negligence may still succeed even though negligence cannot be proved. For instance, a patient who came out of a hospital operating theatre and found a needle in his chest may still succeed, though he cannot prove negligence on the part of the surgeon. Here the principle of **"Res ipsa loquitur"** can be applied which means "the evidence speaks for itself".

Apart from Criminal Negligence it is important to note that negligence as a whole is a civil wrong, so is dealt with under the law of tort.

4. The Crown Prosecution Service

The Crown Prosecution Service (CPS), headed by the Director of Public Prosecutions (DPP), is the body responsible for prosecuting people accused of committing criminal offences. The CPS equivalent in the United States is known as the District Attorney's office; and the DPP is known as the District Attorney. However, for the CPS to bring criminal proceedings against a person, two fundamental requirements must be met. These are:

1)   <u>Is the evidence available likely to lead to conviction?</u>

The answer to this question must be yes before the CPS proceeds with prosecuting so as not to waste public funds (tax-payers' money). This is why the CPS was severely criticised when its prosecution against the Maxwell Brothers (which cost the taxpayers £10 million) did not lead to a conviction.

The criticism focussed on the question of why the CPS spent £10 million of public funds when it did not have enough evidence to convict.

This is a particularly important point to remember as there have been circumstances when it is clear that a serious crime has been committed yet nobody was prosecuted, as evidence was not forthcoming. Besides, a person convicted without enough evidence is likely to be successful on appeal against the conviction.

2) Is it in the Public Interest to Prosecute?

Even where there is enough evidence for conviction, the CPS may not proceed with a prosecution if it considered that prosecuting the accused is not in the public interest. An example is where prosecuting a person(s) could lead to state secrets being revealed to the defence. If there is a chance of that happening, the CPS would not normally prosecute even though it was very clear that the accused committed a crime.

In recent times, however, the CPS has come under severe criticism and public scrutiny in the way that it has conducted itself over the years, and some are now calling for greater accountability on its part. This call for greater accountability is partly due to the fact that the CPS is not subject to judicial review.

Though the CPS is the main prosecuting body, other bodies such as local authorities and the Customs and Excise department can also prosecute offenders in their own right.

5. Private Prosecution

We have seen how the CPS will not prosecute if there is insufficient evidence that is unlikely to lead to conviction. Thus, a victim whose case the CPS refuses to proceed with for lack of evidence may, in rare circumstances, bring a private prosecution against the accused. It is important to note that a private prosecution route is only resorted to where the CPS fails to prosecute. A private prosecution, however, is not without problems. Some of these problems are:

a) The Private Prosecutor bears the bill

The taxpayer bears the cost on both the prosecution and the accused side in cases prosecuted by the CPS and other government agencies. However, the cost is borne by the private prosecutor in the case of a private prosecution.

This can be a very expensive process indeed, so only people with sufficient assets are likely to be able to initiate a private prosecution.

b) Malicious Prosecution

Another danger of a private prosecution is that where the prosecution fails, the accused could initiate a civil action against the individual for malicious prosecution. This action is intended to compensate the accused for the trouble he/she has been put through by the private prosecutor.

A successful malicious prosecution action could cause the private prosecution lasting financial damage.

Again a private prosecution can be a risky and expensive business especially for people with little or no assets.

6. Legal Aid

It is not the intention of this chapter to discuss the entire area of legal aid. Rather it is to inform readers that people who have little or no income may be entitled to legal aid from the Legal Aid Board.

It is therefore important to contact a solicitor, reputable legal advice or Citizen's Advice Bureau to ascertain whether you are entitled to legal aid.

Furthermore, it is important to note that not every area of legal advice is subject to legal aid. An example is defamation cases (libel and slander) where legal aid is not available.

B – Criminal Law Implications of HIV infection

1. Offences

Anyone who deliberately or intentionally transmits HIV or any other sexually transmitted disease (STD) to another, commits a criminal offence.

Section 20 Offences Against the Person Act 1861 states that:

> *"Whosoever shall unlawfully and maliciously would or inflict any grievous bodily harm upon any other person, either with or without any weapon or instrument, shall be guilty of an offence."*

If convicted on indictment, it carries a maximum sentence of 5 years imprisonment. On the other hand, it carries a maximum prison sentence of 6 months and/or a fine, on summary conviction.

A similar offence is also created under **section 18** of the legislation. According to **section 18** Offences Against the Person Act 1861:

> *"Whosoever shall unlawfully and maliciously by any means whatsoever wound or cause any grievous bodily harm to any person with intent to do some grievous bodily harm to any person, or with intent to resist or prevent the lawful apprehension or detainer or any person, shall be guilty of an offence."*

On conviction on indictment, the offence carries a maximum sentence of Life Imprisonment.

Though they are similar, this offence is different from that contained under Section 20 above, in that the intention to commit the crime under this section is much more specific than that contained under section 20. Also, the use of the phrase 'by any means whastsoever' means that the offence has a broader meaning.

Another appropriate offence is contained under **Section 23** Offences Against the Person Act 1861, which states that:

> *"Whosoever shall unlawfully and maliciously administer to or cause to be administered to or taken by any other person any poison or other destructive or noxious thing, so as thereby to endanger the life of such person, or so as thereby to inflict upon such a person any grievous bodily harm, shall be guilty of an offence."*

This offence carries a maximum sentence of 10 years imprisonment if convicted on indictment.

A further offence is contained under **section 24** Offences Against the Person Act 1861, which states that:

> *"Whosoever shall unlawfully and maliciously administer to or cause to be administered to or taken by any other person any poison or other destructive or noxious thing, with intent to injure, aggrieve, or annoy any such person, shall be guilty of an offence."*

It carries a maximum sentence of 5 years imprisonment, if convicted on indictment.

The difference between this and the section 23 offence is that, under this offence, there is no need to prove the consequences of the defendant's actions.

Under the offences, considered so far, it is clear that the deliberate transmission of HIV or any other STD to another is regarded as a criminal offence. The first ever person to be convicted in England and Wales was **Mr Mohammed Dica** on 14th October 2003.

In **R v Mohammed Dica (2003),** the defendant (Mr Dica) was convicted of **'biological' Grievous Bodily Harm** (GBH) by deliberately infecting two women with HIV. Though he was diagnosed as HIV positive in 1995, he had unprotected sex with them without revealing his HIV positive status.

Mr Dica convinced his first victim to have unprotected sex with him, saying that she could not be pregnant as he had had a vasectomy.

When confronted with his HIV positive status in court, Mr Dica responded that he could not possibly be responsible for her plight, as HIV was a "homosexual disease" and that the disease affects only people that are "cursed by God".

After the jury declared a guilty verdict, the trial Judge Nicolas Philpot said:

> "If I had to sentence him today there is no doubt he would be going to prison and for a long time."

One of the police officers who investigated the case, Detective Sergeant Jo Goodall, of Lambeth Community Safety Unit in South London, said after the trial:

> "This is a landmark case, being the first successful prosecution in England and Wales for the inflicting of a serious sexually transmitted disease, namely HIV." He continued:

> "I admire the courage of the two females in coming forward and respect the verdict of the jury in bringing to justice this man. Today's verdict means that those who are not prepared to take responsibility for themselves and who continue to recklessly infect sexual partners with this fatal and life-threatening disease will in future face prosecution in the criminal courts."

Mr Dica was sentenced to 8 years imprisonment on 3rd November 2003.

There was an earlier case in Scotland in February 2001; the case of **R v Stephen Kelly (2001).** In this case, Mr Kelly deliberately infected his girlfriend Anne Craig with the virus and was sentenced to 5 years imprisonment.

In 1997, a Cypriot court sentenced a fisherman from Cyprus **(Mr Paul Georgiou)** to 15 months imprisonment for deliberately infecting and English woman (Ms Janette Pink) when she was on holiday in Cyprus.

It is also an offence under section 3 Sexual Offences Act 1956 for a person to procure a woman, by false pretences or false representations, to have sexual intercourse in any part of the world.

Furthermore, a person may also commit the tort of battery (i.e. trespass to the person) where another person was deliberately infected with HIV or other STDs. The **tort of battery** - as defined by Trindale **(1982)** - is as follows:

> "A battery is a direct act of the defendant which has the effect of causing contact with the body of the plaintiff without the latter's consent."

However the tort of battery requires the existence of the following elements:

a)   a direct act

b)   an intentional act

c)   contact with the plaintiff

d)   contact without plaintiff's consent

Even where the victim consented to sex, it could be argued that he/she did not consent to sex with an infected person.

Some now argue that a charge of attempted murder (though never been applied) may also be brought against an infected person who deliberately or negligently infects others with HIV.

It is worth noting that deliberately infecting others with HIV may also be a breach of articles 2 and 3 of the European Convention on Human Rights, namely:

Article 2

Everyone's right to life shall be protected by law. No one shall be deprived of his life intentionally save in the execution of a sentence of a court following his conviction of a crime for which this penalty is provided by law …..

Article 3

No one shall be subjected to torture or to inhuman or degrading treatment or punishment.

2. Detention of Infected Persons

Section 38 Public Health (Control of Disease) Act 1984 [as amended by section 5 Public Health (Infectious Diseases) Regulation 1988] states that in its application to AIDS, Section 38(1) of the Act shall apply so that a justice of the peace (acting if he deems it necessary ex parte) may on the application of any local authority make an order for the detention in hospital of an inmate of that hospital suffering from HIV/AIDS, in addition to the circumstances specified in that section, if the justice is satisfied that on his leaving the hospital, proper precautions to prevent the spread of that disease would not be taken by him:-

a)   in his lodging or accommodation, or

b)   in other places to which he may be expected to go if not detained in the hospital.

Furthermore, **Article 5 (1) (e) of the European Convention on Human Rights** allows for the lawful detention of persons for the prevention of the spread of infectious diseases, of persons of unsound mind, alcoholics or drug addicts, or vagrants.

3. Controlling HIV/AIDS

In relation to controlling the spread of **HIV/AIDS, Section 1 AIDS (Control) Act 1987** requires district and regional health authorities to publish periodic reports to the secretary of state as outlined under the Schedule to the legislation.

According to the Schedule of the **AIDS (Control) Act 1987**, the content of the report should include:

1. The number of persons known to the Authority of Board to be persons with AIDS at the end of the period to which the report relates ("the reporting period") having been diagnosed as such-

    a)   in that period; and
    b)   up to the end of that period,

    by facilities or services provided by the Authority or Board.

2. The number of persons known to the Authority or Board to have been diagnosed as persons with AIDS by such facilities or services in the reporting period or a previous reporting period and to have died-

    a)   in the reporting period; and
    b)   up to the end of the reporting period.

3. Where the number to be reported under any of the foregoing provisions is between one and nine (inclusive) the report shall state only that the number is less than ten.

4. Particulars of the facilities and services provided by the Authority or Board, or known to it to been provided in its district or area by others, in the reporting period for testing for, and preventing the spread of, AIDS and HIV.

5. The number of persons employed by the Authority or Board wholly or mainly in providing in the reporting period such facilities and services as are mentioned in paragraph 4 above.

6. An estimate of the facilities and services which the Authority or Board will provide in the twelve months following the reporting period for the purposes mentioned in paragraph 4 above.

7. Particulars of the action taken by the Authority or Board, or known to it to have been taken in its district or area by others, in the reporting period to educate the public in relation to AIDS and HIV and to provide training for testing for AIDS and HIV and for the treatment, counselling and care of persons with AIDS or infected with HIV.

8. The number of positive results in the reporting period from blood samples taken for the purposes of HIV antibody tests by facilities or services provided by the Authority or Board [This last point (number 8) was added by The AIDS (Control) (Contents of Reports) order 1988].

Conclusion

A person found guilty of a criminal offence will normally be punished by the state. Thus, a person who deliberately transmits HIV or other STDs deserves to be punished and will be punished.

Self-Assessment Questions

1) *List as many differences as possible between civil liabilities and criminal offences.*

2) *Explain, referring to the example of O.J. Simpson, why some accused are prosecuted and sued in both criminal and civil courts.*

3) *Who else apart from the CPS may be able to prosecute?*

4) *Explain the nature of criminal liability.*

5) *It is possible for a person to bring a private prosecution? In what circumstances is that possible and what are some of the possible consequences of a private prosecution?*

6) *Why is the deliberate transmission of HIV or other STDs to another a criminal offence?*

Chapter 17

The Right to Self-Determination and Consent to Treatment

Contents of this Chapter

1.   **Right to Self-Determination**
2.   **Consent to Treatment**
3.   **Where consent may not be necessary**
4.   **Conclusion**
5.   **Self-Assessment Questions**

1. Right To Self-Determination

It is a moral requirement that the AUTONOMY of the individual be respected, as every adult and sane individual has a right to self-determination. As a result, nobody has a right to violate another person's body without his consent. Any such violation may constitute the criminal offence of assault and battery. In his famous speech, Justice Cardozo notes in Schloendorff v Society of New York Hospital (1914):

> "Every human being of adult years and sound mind has a right to determine what shall be done with his own body; and a surgeon who performs an operation without the patient's consent commits an assault, for which he is liable in damages."

Thus, he the individual alone can decide what he wants or does not want to do with his own body and no other person has a right to impose his views on him. Concerning this, the Declaration of Lisbon (1981) by the World Medical Association states that:

> "...the patient has the rights to choose his or her physician freely; to be cared for by a doctor whose clinical and ethical judgements are free from outside interference; to accept or refuse treatment after receiving adequate information; to have his or her confidences respected; to die in dignity; and to receive or decline spiritual and moral comfort including the help of a minister of an appropriate religion..."

Basically, the patient has a right to self-determination.

However, in discussing a person's right to self-determination, one issue that continues to split public opinion is the issue of 'CONFLICT OF RIGHT'. Consider the conflict between a woman's right to have an abortion and the foetus' right to life. It has become an unending argument and counter-argument in religious, political and social circles as to which of these two rights is superior.

Indeed, in the United States, this has become an election issue where a politician is expected to choose whether he/she is a pro-abortionist or an anti-abortionist (pro-life).

2. *Consent To Treatment*

The fact that a sane adult has a right to self-determination means he can decide to accept or refuse any medical treatment or advice. A doctor who ignores the wishes of the patient and proceeds with treatment commits the criminal offence of battery and possible assault. Only in a few circumstances can a doctor or physician administer such treatment without the patient's consent and not commit an offence. Thus, doctors or health officials should always seek consent from patients on the type of treatment that is proposed, before proceeding with it.

Even where consent was given, a doctor nevertheless commits an offence if he exceeds the limits of the consent. The following cases illustrate this principle:

a) In Hamilton v Birmingham RHB (1962), where a doctor, while performing a caesarean section, also went on to perform a sterilisation without the patient's consent.

b) In Michael v Molesworth (1950), where a medical operation was performed by a different surgeon from the one agreed.

c) In Cull v Royal Surrey Country Hospital (1932), where the patient consented to an abortion and the doctor carried out a hysterectomy instead.

d) In Devi v West Midlands RHA (1981) where the patient consented to an operation of the uterus, but the surgeon carried out a sterilisation as well.

e) In Mohr v Williams (1905), where the patient consented to an operation on her right ear. However, while she was unconscious under anaesthetic, the surgeon found that there was a more serious condition on the left ear, so he operated on it instead.

Thus, in the Ontario (Canada) Court of appeal case of Malette v Shulman (a case of blood transfusion given to an unconscious card-carrying Jehovah's Witness), the trial judge Robins JA notes:

> *"The right of a person to control his or her own body is a concept that has long been recognised at common law. The tort of battery has traditionally protected the interest in bodily security from unwanted physical interference. Basically, any intentional non consensual touching which is harmful or offensive to a person's reasonable sense of dignity is actionable. Of course, a person may choose to waive this protection and consent to the intentional invasion of this interest, in which case an action for battery will not be maintainable. No special exceptions are made for medical care, other than in emergency situations, and the general rules governing actions for battery are applicable to the doctor-patient relationship. Thus, as a matter of common law, a medical intervention in which a doctor touches the body of a patient would constitute battery if the patient did not consent to the intervention. Patients have the decisive role in the medical decision-making process. Their right of self-determination is recognized and protected by law..."*

Justice Robins adds:

> "At issue here is the freedom of the patient as an individual to exercise her right to refuse treatment and accept the consequences of her own decision. Competent adults, as I have sought to demonstrate, are generally at liberty to refuse medical treatment even at the risk of death. The right to determine what shall be done with one's own body is a fundamental right in our society. The concepts inherent in this right are the bedrock upon which the principles of self-determination and individual autonomy are body. Free, individual choice in matters affecting this right should, in my opinion, be accorded very high priority…"

Regarding consent to treatment, the US President's Commission, established by Congress in 1978 states:

> "The voluntary choice of a competent and informed patient should determine whether or not life-sustaining therapy will be undertaken, just as such choices provide the basis for other decisions about medical treatment. Health care institutions and professionals should try to enhance patient's abilities to make decisions on their own behalf and to promote understanding of the available treatment options……Health care professionals serve patients best by maintaining a presumption in favor of sustaining life, while recognizing that competent patients are entitled to choose to forego any treatments, including those that sustain life"

In the United States, there is also the concept of "Informed Consent" where not only should the patient be informed of the type of treatment that is proposed but also all the known possible consequences of such treatment, so that the patient can make an informed decision.

However, the strict rule of 'Informed Consent' does not apply in English Law. Thus, in Sidaway v Board of Governors of the Bethlem Royal Hospital (1985), it was held that no offence is committed by a doctor (as long as consent was not obtained by fraud) who fails to reveal to a patient all the possible consequences of a particular surgical procedure. In this case, Mrs Sidaway consented to an operation on her neck and shoulders, in order to relieve pain. Though the doctor informed her of the possibility of the procedure disturbing a nerve root and the implications of it, he failed to tell her the possibility of damage to the spinal cord and its consequences. She sued for compensation when the spinal cord was damaged during surgery and she became severely disabled.

Concerning Sidaway, the judge Sir John Donaldson said:

> "I am wholly satisfied that as a matter of English law a consent is not vitiated by a failure on the part of the doctor to give the patient sufficient information before the consent is given. It is only if the consent is obtained by fraud or by misrepresentation of the nature of what is to be done that it can be said that an apparent consent is not a true consent. This is the position in the criminal law and the cause of action based upon trespass to the person is closely analogous. I should add that the contrary was not argued upon this appeal."

Another judge, Dunn LJ adds:

> "The first argument was that unless the patient's consent to the operation was a fully informed consent the performance of the operation would constitute a battery on the patient by the surgeon. This is not the law of England. If there is consent to the nature of the act, then there is no trespass to the person."

It is now a normal practice for doctors, surgeons and health practitioners to require patients to sign a consent form before any major treatment or surgery.

3. *Where consent may not be necessary*

There are circumstances where the patient's consent may not be required before treatment is administered or surgery performed. These are briefly discussed below:

(i)   where the patient is unconscious

A medical practitioner is entitled to presume consent where an unconscious patient is admitted to a hospital for treatment.

However, a medical practitioner should not take advantage of the patient's unconsciousness by performing procedures that are not essential for the survival of the patient (Re: MARSHALL V CURRY, 1933). Any such unnecessary procedures would amount to trespass on the person.

Furthermore, a doctor commits battery by performing procedures on an unconscious patient where, before the procedures were performed, documentary evidence (e.g. non-consent card) signed by the patient clearly forbids any such procedure to be performed on him at any time.

(ii)   Proxy Consent

There are instances where close family members of an unconscious patient are known to have consented or refused treatment (proxy consent) of the patient. It is worth noting however, that the next of kin has no legal right to consent to or refuse treatment of an adult patient, so that doctors may proceed with treatment even where a family member refuses. The only exception would be where the patient had previously made his wishes known then he would accept a proxy consent in any such circumstances.

On the whole however, proxy consent is mostly applicable where the patient is a child.

(iii)   Children and Proxy Consent

In English Law, a child below the age of 18 is known as a minor. A parent therefore, can consent to or refuse treatment of such a minor.

However, under the Children Act 1989, medical practitioners may ignore a parent's refusal (which could be challenged in court) if it is in the best interest of the child to proceed with the treatment.

Furthermore, section 8(1) Family Reform Act 1969 states that:

> *"The consent of a minor who has attained the age of sixteen years to any ... medical ... treatment which, in the absence of consent, would constitute a trespass to the person, shall be as effective as it would be if he were of full age; and where a minor has by virtue of this section given effective consent to any treatment it shall not be necessary to obtain any consent for it from his parent or guardian."*

However, the case in Gillick V West Norfolk & Wisbech Health Authority (1986) now known as "Gillick Competence" establishes that in certain circumstances children under 16 years could accept or refuse treatment (i.e. ignoring their parent's wishes) in their own right, if it was found that the child achieved a significant understanding and has the intelligence to enable him or her to understand fully what is proposed. Without such clear demonstration of understanding and intelligence by the child, the parents continue to have the right to proxy consent unless the law thought otherwise.

In this case, Mrs Gillick sought a declaration from the court that a circular by the UK government which contemplated that contraceptive advice and treatment might, in exceptional circumstances, be given to girls under the age of 16 without parental consent was illegal, as children under 16 were unable to give effective consent and that any such advice by a doctor without parental consent would be considered as the criminal offence of battery. Besides, the circular was encouraging what was illegal anyway.

The Court of Appeal reversed an earlier decision by a lower court and rejected Mrs Gillick's assertions.

According to Lord Templeman:

"I accept also that a doctor may lawfully carry out some forms of treatment with the consent of an infant patient and against the opposition of a parent based on religious or any other grounds. The effect of the consent of the infant depends on the nature of the treatment and the age and understanding of the infant. For example, a doctor with the consent of an intelligent boy or girl of 15 could in my opinion safely remove tonsils or a troublesome appendix."

Lord Fraser agreed and adds:

"provided the patient, whether a boy or a girl, is capable of understanding what is proposed, and of expressing his or her own wishes, I see no good reason for holding that he or she lacks the capacity to express them validly and effectively and to authorise the medical man to make the examination or give the treatment which he advises."

(iv)   <u>Consent and Those that are Mentally Incompetent</u>

According to Section 63 Mental Health Act 1983, the consent of a patient shall not be required for any medical treatment given to him for the mental disorder from which he is suffering, if the treatment is given by or under the direction of the responsible medical officer.

This was confirmed in the case of RE: F (1990) where it was decided that treatment is possible without the patient's consent, as long as it was in his best interest to do so.

However, Section 57 Mental Health Act 1983 states that some forms of treatment for mental disorder requires the consent of the patient, namely:

a)   any surgical operation for destroying brain tissue or for destroying the functioning of brain tissue; or

b)   such other forms of treatment as may be specified for the purposes of this section by regulations made by the Secretary of State.

However, even where the patient had previously consented to such treatment, he may, according to Section 60, withdraw his consent at any time for the continuation of further treatment.

4. Consent and Negligence

Even where a patient had given consent to a particular mode of treatment, a doctor may still be liable, if he was negligent in administering the treatment.

Proof of negligence in relation to doctor-patient relationship requires the following:

a)   that the doctor owes his patient a duty of care;

b)   that this duty was broken by the doctor; and

c)   as a result of this duty being broken, the patient suffered loss or injury.

If all these three points are proven, the doctor may be liable in negligence. However, in the case of Bolam v Friern Barnet Hospital Management Committee (1957), now known as the 'Bolam Test', it was decided that a surgeon is not liable in negligence where the standard that he applied or the procedure that he used, is of a standard that is acceptable or practiced by a substantial body of medical opinion, and this body of medical opinion is both respectable and responsible, and experienced in this particular field of medicine.

Basically, a doctor cannot be penalised by adopting a procedure that is the norm in that field of medicine, even if it later transpires to be not so good.

Conclusion

Every human has certain rights and the right to determine what shall happen to his or her own body is a fundamental one. Closely linked to this is the right to have consent to treatment. Thus, if these rights are violated, then the person may have a right to legal redress. This is a vital area to understand for anyone involved in the treatment and advice of patients, in order to ensure that the rights of the individual are always respected.·

Self-Assessment Questions

1. Define the 'right to self-determination'

2. Explain 'consent to treatment'

3. Which categories are included within those who have the right to self-determination?

4. What offence might be committed if a doctor administers treatment without a patient's consent?

5. In what circumstances can a doctor or surgeon legally operate or administer treatment without a patient's consent?

6. What is the significance of the Sidaway case and that of Bolam?

Chapter 18

Assisted Suicide and Mercy Killing

Contents of this Chapter

1. Introduction

Assisted suicide and mercy killing come under the study of **EUTHANASIA.** The Webster's New World Dictionary defines Euthanasia as:

"the act of causing death painlessly, so as to end suffering"

Such causing of death is normally due to terminal illness.

Euthanasia my be broadly classified as:

a)   voluntary and involuntary euthanasia, or

b)   active and passive euthanasia

Voluntary euthanasia implies that the patient volunteered to end his or her life as a result of suffering.

Involuntary euthanasia implies the ending of the patient's life by doctors, carers, or family members, without the patient's or proxy consent. This may occur where the patient is unconscious so cannot give consent.

Active euthanasia implies that a physician, carer, family member, or friend actively ended the patient's life, for example by the administration of a lethal injection, by strangulation or withdrawing a life support system. Active euthanasia is normally regarded as murder in English Law.

Passive Euthanasia on the other hand, implies that there was no active ending of the patient's life but death was for example as a result of assisted suicide.

2. Assisted Suicide

Prior to 1961, it was an offence in the United Kingdom to attempt or to commit suicide. However, committing or attempting suicide is no longer an offence by virtue of the **Suicide Act 1961**. The question is, what about assisted suicide? That is enabling or assisting another person to commit suicide. While pamphlets and books with instructions on "self-deliverance" (suicide) are readily available in the UK, assisting another person to commit suicide continues to remain a criminal offence under the legislation.

Section 2(1) Suicide Act 1961 provides that:

> "A person who aids, abets, counsels or procures the suicide of another, or an attempt by another to commit suicide, shall be liable on conviction on indictment to imprisonment for a term not exceeding fourteen years."

Cases of assisted suicide may arise out of a desire to end prolonged pain and suffering as a result of terminal illness.

The Canadian case of **Rodriguez v A-G of British Columbia (1993)** seems to suggest that though actively assisting a person to commit suicide is an offence, the setting up of a mechanism that she (Ms Rodriguez) could use to end her life should she become paralysed from the motor neurone disease from which she was suffering, was on the whole, in line with Canadian Constitution. CORY J. declares:

> "Dying is an integral part of living...it follows that the right to die with dignity should be as well protected as is any other aspect of the right to life. State prohibitions that would force a dreadful, painful death on a rational but incapacitated terminally ill patient are an affront to human dignity."

However, an equally powerful counter argument is the possibility of abuse once assisted suicide is allowed in any form as was noted in the Rodriguez's case cited above:

> "There is no certainty that abuses can be prevented by anything less than a complete prohibition [of assisted suicide]. Creating an exception for the terminally ill might therefore frustrate the purpose of the legislation of protecting the vulnerable because adequate guidelines to control abuse are difficult or impossible to develop."

Both these arguments equally attract a great deal of support and the conclusion drawn by the Supreme Court was that it was up to the Canadian Parliament to decide.

A recent case (by judicial review) in the UK similar to the Canadian case was **R v DPP ex parte Diane Pretty (2001).**

Mrs Diane Pretty, a 42 year old mother from Bedfordshire, was diagnosed with the debilitating Motor Neurone Disease in 1999. Her condition deteriorated rapidly and she was now able to do virtually nothing for herself. She wished to die at home, with her family around her at the time of her choosing, rather than be condemned to suffer both physically and emotionally.

Mrs Pretty was entirely clear about her decision; but she was physically unable to take her own life without assistance. Under **Section 2 of the Suicide Act 1961**, if her husband (Mr Pretty) of 25 years were to help her, he could be prosecuted for aiding and abetting a suicide.

Thus, on 27th July 2001, Liberty, a civil rights organisation, wrote to the Director of Public Prosecution (DPP), asking for his assurance that Mr Pretty would not be prosecuted under the Suicide Act if he were to help his wife to take her own life. On 8th August the DPP wrote back saying that he could not guarantee that, despite conceding that Mrs Pretty and her family are having to endure "terrible suffering".

Although the Legal Services Commission admitted that the case is one of great public interest, they refused Mrs Pretty Legal Aid.

Liberty applied to the High Court, challenging the decision of the DPP under articles 3 and 8 of the European Convention on Human Rights.

Article 3

No one shall be subjected to torture or to inhuman or degrading treatment or punishment.

Article 8

1. Everyone has the right to respect for his private and family life, his home and his correspondence.

2. There shall be no interference by a public authority with the exercise of this right except such as is in accordance with the law and is necessary in a democratic society in the interests of national security, public safety or the economic well-being of the country, for the prevention of disorder or crime, for the protection of health or morals, or for the protection of the rights and freedoms of others.

Mrs Pretty said:

> *"I want the court to know that I want the right to die at the time of my choosing, with dignity, now that I have lost all functions apart from my mind. I hope the courts will give me the opportunity to fulfil this last request".*

On 31st August, the High Court agreed to judicially review the decision of the DPP. The lawyer for Liberty (representing Mrs Pretty), Mona Arshi said:

> *"Today, we obtained permission to apply for judicial review against the decision of the Director of Public Prosecutions. This is the first time in this country that the Suicide Act has been challenged in this way. It's the first stage of the legal process and we look forward to presenting the case at the full judicial review hearing.*
>
> *We believe this case has a tremendous importance not just for the Prettys themselves but for a small but significant number of people who, though in dire circumstances and fully able to take a rational decision to end their lives are prevented from doing so legally by their physical disability.*

We believe that effectively Mrs Pretty is being discriminated against by the State because she is physically unable to take her own life, as a result of the extreme state of her terminal illness. We hope that, given today's decision in the High Court, the DPP will reconsider his position.

The case does raise broad and emotive issues that need open debate. But we would ask people to remember that it is principally about one person, Mrs Pretty, and how she believes she can best meet the end of her life with dignity.

Given the severity of Mrs Pretty's condition, we will be requesting a hearing at the earliest possible date."

On 18th October 2001, the High Court, though sympathising with the suffering of Diane Pretty, upheld the decision of the Director of Public Prosecution and added that this is a situation that only Parliament at Westminster can resolve by legislation.

Disappointed and, reacting to the decision by the High Court, Deborah Annetts, Director of the Voluntary Euthanasia Society, UK says:

"The case has highlighted the current law on assisted suicide and shown that it needs to be radically overhauled. With over 90% public support for a change in the law, there is widespread recognition that the current law is inhumane because it denies the terminally ill the choice to end their lives how and when they want. The public recognises the importance of human rights even if the courts do not."

Diane Pretty appealed to the House of Lords, the Supreme Court of Britain. While it expressed great sympathy for the pain and suffering that she was experiencing, the House rejected her appeal on 29th November 2001, and upheld the provisions of the Suicide Act. Not willing to give up her fight till her death, Diane appealed to the European Court of Human Rights (ECHR) in Strasburg, France to let her die in dignity. On 29th March 2002, the ECHR, though sympathetic with her plight, upheld the decision of the House of Lords, stating that the House's decision did not breach articles 3 or 8 of the European Convention of Human Rights.

Having lost the legal battle, Diane Pretty died on 11th May 2002. However, the legacy created by her case continues to fan great passions amongst the people of the United Kingdom.

However, in the case of **Miss B** (2002), the High Court allowed her to refuse consent to medical treatment which eventually led to her death.

Concerning this case, the BBC notes:

"A woman known as 'Miss B', who was paralysed from neck down, died peacefully in her sleep on 29th April 2002 after winning the legal right to have medical treatment withdrawn.

Dame Elizabeth Butler-Sloss, President of the High Court family division, ruled last month that Miss B had the 'necessary mental capacity to give consent or refuse consent to life-sustaining medical treatment.'

It was the 43 year old former social care professional's case that it was her decision, not her doctor's whether the ventilator which kept her alive should be switched off.

In a landmark ruling, Dame Elizabeth gave Miss B the right to be transferred to another hospital and be treated in accordance with her wishes, including drug treatment and care to 'ease her suffering and permit her life to end peacefully and with dignity.'"

3. Mercy Killing

An act of mercy-killing occurs where doctors, carers, relatives or friends kill, or allow the patient to die out of mercy and love. It could be that those caring for the patient, who may have devoted a great deal of effort towards the patient, have finally decided to free themselves of the misery.

Mercy killing involves both actively killing the patient or allowing the person to die, for instance, by withdrawing life support system. Mercy killing - which is active euthanasia - is generally regarded as murder under UK law.

In the words of Devlin J (1957):

> "If the acts are intended to kill and do, in fact kill, it does not matter if a life is cut short by weeks or months, it is just as much murder as if it were cut short by years."

This view was confirmed in the case of **R v Cox (1992).** Dr Nigel Cox was charged and convicted of attempted murder of Ms Boyes. Ms Lillian Boyes was a 70 year old terminally ill patient, who was in excruciating pain as a result of her illness. She had on many occasions asked Dr Cox and others to kill her in order to relieve her of the endless pain. In the end, Dr Cox administered a lethal dose of potassium chloride which killed her almost immediately.

In summing up to the jury for a verdict, the trial judge, OGNALL J. Stated:

> "The prosecution allege that Dr Cox attempted to murder Lillian Boyes. They say that he deliberately injected her with potassium chloride in a quantity and in a manner which had no therapeutic purpose and no capacity to afford her any relief from pain and suffering whilst alive. They submit that Dr Cox must have known that and that in truth his conduct in giving that injection was prompted solely and certainly primarily by the purpose of bringing her life to an immediate end.
>
> Proof of murder, members of the jury, would require proof that the doctor's conduct actually caused her death. The prosecution have told you that having regard to Ms Boyes' condition on that morning, they cannot exclude the possibility though they, no doubt, would say it was remote, that in fact, she died of natural causes between the actual injection of potassium chloride and her death. That is before the potassium chloride took its effect. It is for that reason, because they cannot exclude that possibility, however remote, that as you know, the charge you gave to make up your minds about is not one of murder but of attempted murder, and I am sure you understand.
>
> If it is proved that Dr Cox injected Lillian Boyes with potassium chloride in circumstances which make you sure that by that act he intended to kill her, then he is guilty of the offence of attempted murder, You know, in this case, from the earliest stage that it has been admitted that he did indeed inject her intravenously with two ampoules of undiluted potassium chloride. Which no doubt you remember without looking at it ever again. His note at page 70 of the medical records clearly indicates.
>
> According to her younger son Patrick, after that injection she just, and I quote, 'faded away' within minutes. According to Staff Nurse Creasey she died, so she said, in a few minutes. Later, she said about one minute after the injection.
>
> Thus, the giving of the potassium chloride in that form, intravenously, is admitted, as I have said. The only question, therefore, for your consideration, ladies and gentlemen, in arriving

at your verdict, is this. Is it proved that in giving that injection Dr Cox intended thereby to kill his patient? In the context of this particular case, what is meant, what do I mean, as a matter of law by proof of an intention to kill?...

We all appreciate do we not, and certainly the evidence you have heard in this case demonstrates it, that some medical treatment, whether of a positive, therapeutic character or solely of an analgesic kind, by which I mean designed solely to alleviate pain and suffering, carries with it a serious risk to the health or even the life of the patient. Doctors, as you know, are frequently confronted with, no doubt, distressing dilemmas. They have to make up their minds as to whether the risk, even to the life of their patient, attendant upon their contemplated form of treatment, is such that the risks or is not medically justified. Of course, if a doctor genuinely believes that a certain course is beneficial to his patient, either therapeutically or analgesically, even though he recognises that the course carries with it a risk to life, he is fully entitled, nonetheless to pursue it. If sadly, and in those circumstances the patient dies, nobody could possibly suggest that in that situation the doctor was guilty of murder or attempted murder.

And the problem, you know, is obviously particularly acute in the case of those who are terminally ill and in considerable pain, if not agony. Such was the case of Lillian Boyes. It was plainly Dr Cox's duty to do all that was medically possible to alleviate her pain and suffering even if the course adopted carried with it an obvious risk that as a side effect - note my emphasis, and I will repeat it - even if the course adopted carried with it an obvious risk that as a side effect if that treatment, her death would be rendered likely or even certain.

There can be no doubt that the use of drugs to reduce pain and suffering will often by fully justified notwithstanding that it will, in fact, hasten the moment of death, but please understand this, ladies and gentlemen, what can never be lawful is the use of drugs with the primary purpose of hastening the moment of death.

And so, in deciding Dr Cox's intention, the distinction the law requires you to draw is this. Is it proved that in giving that injection in that form and in those amounts Dr Cox's primary purpose was to bring the life of Lillian Boyes to an end?

If it was, then he is guilty. If, on the other hand, it was or may have been his primary purpose in acting as he did to alleviate her pain and suffering then he is not guilty, and that is so he recognised that in fulfilling that primary purpose he might or even would hasten the moment of her death.

That is the crucial distinction in this case. In shorthand form, the question of primary purpose. It is relatively easy for me to define for you. It is, however, submitted to you that for any doctor it can be, and was in this case, extraordinarily difficult to apply. Certain it is, it must confront you, members of the jury, with a most exacting task in striving to reach, as I know you will, a true verdict according to the evidence.

I have told you that if Dr Cox's primary purpose was to hasten her death, then he is guilty. In using the words 'hasten her death' I do so quite deliberately, members of the jury. It matters not by how much or by how little her death was hastened or intended to be hastened. I am sure you understand. You may recall Staff Nurse Creasey agreeing with [counsel for Dr Cox] that at the time Lillian Boyes received the first injection, not the potassium chloride, but you remember the earlier one of diamorphine and diazepam, that at the time she received that first injection from Dr Cox that morning, she, Staff nurse Creasey, considered that Lillian Boyes was only hours from death at best and possibly only minutes away.

Of course, there can be no certainty in that regard, but even if that be the case, no doctor can lawfully take any step deliberately designed to hasten that death by however short a period of time.

Of course, members of the jury, to hasten the death, not merely alleviate suffering, it brings it to an end, does it not? A dead person suffers no more. But that is not what I mean by alleviation of suffering, nor, I am confident, what you understand me to mean by it. Alleviation of suffering means the easing of it for so long as the patient survives, not the easing of it in the throes of and because of deliberate purposed killing.

You will remember Professor Blake's evidence. A doctor's duty is to alleviate suffering for so long as the patient survives but, he said, he must never kill in order to achieve relief from suffering. To shorten life intentionally as one's prime purpose. He agreed, is unlawful, even though it may be the only means of alleviating the patient's suffering or pain...

You must understand, members of the jury, that in this highly emotional situation, neither the express wishes of the patient nor of her loving and devoted family can affect the position. You will understand, and I tell you, that Lillian Boyes was fully entitled to decline any further active medical treatment and to specify that thereafter she should only receive painkillers. You remember she did that on 11th August. It is recorded in the notes and there is no doubt that that was universally respected by the doctors and nursing staff thereafter. That was her, Lillian Boyes, absolute right and doctors and nursing staff were obliged to respect her wishes... [Dr Burne, a senior house officer] told you that he had told Lillian Boyes on that day when she had said 'no more active intervention, please, only painkillers from now on' he had said to her, in effect, these are my words but I hope they reflect what he told you he said to her: 'thus far and no further. We will stop your positive medical treatment. We will confine ourselves to giving you only analgesics, only painkillers, but we cannot accede to your request that we give you something to kill you.'

How then, members of the jury, do you test what the Crown say were Doctor Cox's intentions so as to answer that central question, namely was his primary purpose to bring her life to an end or was it, or may it have been, on the other hand, directed primarily to alleviating her pain and her suffering?

The answer is that you do so by looking at all the circumstances of this case as you find them proved. You will look at Lillian Boyes' medical history, especially in those last days up to the day she died, 16th August and, of course, especially including that day. You will look at the expert evidence from the doctors and others experienced in drugs and toxicology. And you may think it of fundamental importance, it is a matter for you, like all questions of fact, but you may think of fundamental importance to consider the nature of the substance finally injected by Dr Cox in those quantities into Lillian Boyes' body.

If you reach the certain conclusion that potassium chloride injected undiluted and intravenously as it was can only in Dr Cox's mind have been with the purpose of bringing her life to an end, then the charge is made out. Dr Cox, as you know, is a highly-qualified, experienced and respected consultant physician. What did he know of the properties and potential of potassium chloride used in this way?...".

On appeal, the House of Lords upheld Dr Cox's conviction.

Concerning mercy killing, Lord Goff comments in the case of **Airedale NHS Trust v Bland (1993)**:

"It is not lawful for a doctor to administer a drug to his patient to bring about his death, even though that course is prompted by a humanitarian desire to end his suffering, however great that suffering may be. So to act is to cross the Rubicon which runs between

on the one hand the care of the living patient and on the other hand euthanasia – actively causing his death to avoid or to end his suffering. Euthanasia is not lawful at common law."

There are, however, exceptional circumstances where this may be allowed. The Bland case mentioned above was a case of active euthanasia. **Anthony Bland**, a seventeen year old Liverpool Football Club supporter was one of the Victims of the **Hilsborough disaster in 1989**. This was when 96 fans of Liverpool football club died at the Hillsborough stadium in Sheffield, England when a wall of people fell on other fans by accident. As a result, Anthony Bland's lungs were crushed and punctured which stopped oxygen supply to his brain, thus causing an irreversible coma; a Persistent Vegetative State (PVS). As a result, he was on a life support machine for four years. All this while, his family was at his bedside. They have lost their home, jobs and both the parents and the taxpayer has spent much money to keep Anthony on the life support system for all these years with no single sign of improvement.

The family and the hospital therefore agreed to discontinue the life support system to let Tony die peacefully. This decision was challenged in court and later came all the way to the House of Lords, after the court of Appeals dismissed the appeal and upheld the parents and hospitals decision to end his life.

Lord Mustill comments on the Bland case:

"The conclusion that the declarations can be upheld depends crucially on a distinction drawn by the criminal law between acts and emissions, and carries with it inescapably a distinction between, on the one hand what is often called 'mercy killing' where active steps are taken in a medical context to terminate the life of a suffering patient, and a situation such as the present, where the proposed conduct has the aim for equally humane reasons of terminating the life of Anthony Bland by withholding from him the basic necessities of life. The acute unease which I feel about adopting this way through the legal and ethical maze is I believe due in an important part to the sensation that however much the terminologies may differ the ethical status of the two courses of action is for all relevant purposes indistinguishable. By dismissing this appeal I fear that your Lordship's House may only emphasise the distortions of a legal structure which is already both morally and intellectually misshapen. Still, the law is there and we must take it as it stands".

Lord Browne-Wilkinson adds:

"The conclusion I have reached will appear to some to be almost irrational. How can it be lawful to allow a patient to die slowly, though painlessly over a period of weeks from lack of food but unlawful to produce his immediate death by a lethal injection, thereby saving his family from yet another ordeal to add to the tragedy that has already struck them. I find it difficult to find a moral answer to that question. But it is undoubtedly the law and nothing I have said cast doubt on the proposition that the doing of a positive act with the intention of ending life is and remains murder".

In the end, the House of Lords reluctantly accepted the desire of the patients and Airedale hospital and allowed the discontinuation of the intravenous feeding and life-support system. However, the Law Lords made very clear that the rules in judicial precedent will not apply to this case; and that similar cases in the future will be individually decided on their own merits.

Expressing an overall view of euthanasia and the likely reform of the law, Lord Goff stated:

"It is of course, well known that there are many responsible members of our society who believe that euthanasia should be made lawful; but that result could, I believe, only be

achieved by legislation which expresses the democratic will so that fundamental change should be made in our law, and can, if enacted, ensure that such legalised killing can only be carried out subject to appropriate supervision and control".

Basically, like the Canadian case, Lord Goff said that parliament alone could resolve the problem by legislation.

An American case that has caused a big debate is that of **Mrs Terri Schiavo**. Mrs Schiavo, a 39 year old woman from Florida, was brain damaged as a result of a heart attack and has been in a Persistent Vegetative State (PVS) since 1990, with no clear hope of recovery. Her husband, Mr Michael Schiavo, wants the life support system to be switched off, so that his wife can die in dignity.

However, Mrs Terry Schiavo's parents disagree, hoping that their daughter will one day recover from her coma. This has caused sharp divisions in the United States. In an article titled: The Right to Die – But Who Says? (an agonising quarrel between parents and husband) – 18th October 2003, The Economist Magazine notes:

> *"For those unfamiliar with right-to-die decisions, the web videos of 39-year-old Terri Schiavo are painful to watch. Here is a woman whose expression appears to go from stupor to joy at the sound of her mother's voice. She opens her eyes wide on command and moves her head to track a floating balloon. Although clearly mentally impaired, she does not look like the vegetable one normally associates with debates over withdrawing life-support.*
>
> *But on Wednesday, to the horror of thousands of web surfers worldwide, doctors removed the feeding tube that has been keeping her alive. The formerly healthy Mrs Schiavo was left brain-damaged and dependent on the tube by a heart attack in 1990. Without it, she is expected to die within two weeks.*
>
> *The decision, by Judge George Greer in Clearwater, Florida, ended a long legal battle between parents who wanted to take care of Mrs Schiavo and a husband who pleaded for her death. Bob and Mary Schindler believed that, with therapy, their daughter could eat and speak. Michael Schiavo said his wife had permanently lost all awareness and should be allowed to die. In November 2002 Judge Greer cleared the way for her death by siding with three of five doctors who testified that her movements were the normal reflexes of someone in a persistent vegetative state, not conscious responses.*
>
> *Until recently, it seemed a tragic family feud. News reports described her as vegetative, leaving many casual observers to wonder whether grief had overridden logic in the parents' decision to fight for life-support. But the videos, taken a year ago and posted on the web in July, have rattled this ideas. Although other patients in Mrs Schiavo's condition have been taken off life-support, outsiders rarely saw them. Mrs Schiavo smiles and laughs on home computers around the world.*
>
> *Visitors to the website have sent some 57,000 e-mails to the office of Florida's Catholic governor, Jeb Bush, asking him to keep Mrs Schiavo alive. Some viewers expressed shock at finding her moving and making sounds, not just lying there completely comatose. The governor did ask both federal and state courts to review her case before the feeding tube was removed, but his arguments were rejected.*
>
> *For her husband's supporters, the video clips were patently misleading: a few seconds of coincidental movement and sound in more than a decade of unresponsiveness. "The video clips don't show the 99 other times out of 100 when the mother came in and said 'Hi Terri, hi Terri' and nothing happened," says George Felos, Mr Schiavo's lawyer. "Any person who has spent any time with Terri knows she has no consciousness."*

Having lost the court battle last year, the Schindlers have fallen back on legal technicalities. In a hearing on October 10th their lawyer, Patricia Anderson, asked a federal judge for therapy that might teach Mrs Schiavo to eat by mouth before her feeding tube was removed. Mr Schiavo refuses to allow such therapy, citing doctors who say she cannot do it, and could choke if she tried. This puzzles those who want to keep Mrs Schiavo alive. "It's like saying, there's a woman drowning, but don't rescue her... you might hurt her neck," a frustrated Ms Anderson argued in court. The judge sympathised, but ruled he had no power to stop the tube removal.

Some doctors say that whether or not Mrs Schiavo can use a spoon was not the real issue. "The question is, what did she really want?" says Dr Linda Emanuel, a specialist in end-of-life issues at North-Western University in Chicago. "Anyone has the right to avoid unwanted life-sustaining treatments. That goes for people in persistent vegetative states as well as patients with full consciousness."

Mr Schiavo insists that his wife made it clear before the heart attack that she would not want to live hooked up to a tube. His still numerous supporters say the parents showed no mercy by taking 13 years to carry out her wish. But the Schindlers argued that she would have wanted help, at least the chance at getting better with therapy: to deny her that constitutes cruelty to a disabled person.

Some of those who wanted Mrs Schiavo to live gathered this week for a vigil outside her hospice. On the internet, the videos continue to play, illustrations of the fine line between mercy and cruelty."

On 21st October 2003, the Florida Legislature and House passed a bill 35E (known as Terri's Bill) into law. This law allows Florida State governor, Jeb Bush (younger brother of President George Bush Jnr), to issue an Executive Order allowing nutrition and hydration to be returned to Terri Schiavo, after she had been left without it for more than 6 days.

The Netherlands (Holland) is one country where euthanasia has been tolerated and openly practiced. Thus, on 28th November 2000, the Dutch Parliament voted in favour of legalising euthanasia in certain circumstances.

In an article entitled: " Dutch MPs vote to legalise mercy killing", the GUARDIAN (29 November 2000) note:

"The Netherlands, where the authorities have for decades turned a blind eye to euthanasia, yesterday became the first country to legalise it.

In a historic vote, the lower house of parliament in the Hague approved by 104 to 40 a bill backed by most Dutch doctors that will, its supporters say, put the country at the forefront of patient's rights.

"Doctors should not be treated as criminals. This will create security for doctors and patients alike". Said the health minister, Els Borst who drafted the bill. "Something as serious as ending one's life deserves openness".

But religious and pro-life groups were hostile, saying the law was open to abuse. Some even drew parallels with Nazi Germany in 1935...Your life is no longer safe," said Burt Dorenbos of Scream for Life. "If doctors are not hesitating to kill people, they will not hesitate to withdraw treatment from people they do not like."

Rita Marker, the head of another anti-euthanasia group, said the law would "tell people that if it's legal, it's right - what is a crime now will be transformed into a medical treatment."

The Catholic church, too, was quick to criticise the move "it is a sad record for the Netherlands to become the first to want to approve a law that goes against human dignity," said the Vatican's spokesman, Joaquin Navarro-Valls. "We are faced with a law of the state which opposes the natural law of human conscience."

Following a series of court rulings and government directives since the 1970s including a carefully worded "codification" of mercy killing adopted in 1993, Dutch doctors already had virtual immunity from prosecution in euthanasia cases, provided they followed strict guidelines.

But the criminal code had never been amended, theoretically allowing them to be charged with murder. Under the new bill, the public prosecutor's office will not review euthanasia cases unless misconduct is suspected.

"This vote simply takes euthanasia out of the criminal arena," said a justice ministry spokesman. "Providing the regulations have all been met, there can be no threat of criminal charges."

While euthanasia is tolerated on certain conditions in several countries including Switzerland, Colombia and Belgium, none has yet sought to legalise it.

The US state of Oregon legalised medically assisted suicide - in which the doctor gives the patient the lethal drugs, but does not administer them - in 1994, and the Northern Territory in Australia followed in 1996, only to repeal the law a year later.

The Dutch bill, backed by all three ruling coalition parties, is set to become law next year. It sets much the same conditions as those laid down in 1993: patients must be in continuous, unbearable and incurable suffering, be aware of medical options and have sought a second professional opinion.

The request to die must be made voluntarily, independently, persistently and only after careful consideration by a patient judged to be of sound mind. The doctor is not supposed to suggest euthanasia, and the patient's life must be ended in a medically appropriate manner.

The law also allows a patient to make a prior written request for euthanasia, giving doctors the right to use their own discretion when patients become too ill physically or mentally to decide for themselves.

But a highly controversial clause that would have allowed children as young as 12 to demand a mercy killing even if their parents disagreed was dropped earlier this year. Children between the ages of 12 and 16 will be able to ask for help to die, but only with parental consent.

According to new data from the health and justice ministries, Dutch doctors helped 2,216 patients, mostly with cancer, to die last year through active euthanasia or assisted suicide. The actual numbers are thought to be higher as some experts claim that 60% of cases go unreported.

Some in the UK are now calling on the UK government to follow the Dutch example. There is however, very strong opposition against any such move in the UK.

Those against euthanasia fear that any such legalisation will create an environment of lack of trust, as doctors could be viewed as potential killers. This view was previously expressed by CAPRON (1986):

> "I never want to have to wonder whether the physician coming into my hospital room is wearing the white coat (or the green scrubs) of a healer, concerned only to relieve my pain and restore me to health, or the black hood of the executioner. Trust between patient and physician is simply too important and too fragile to be subjected to this unnecessary strain".

Others worry that if not checked properly, some unscrupulous doctors and nurses might decide to kill a patient that is seen to be 'trouble-making'. Or family members tempted to kill to quickly inherit property or money.

Nevertheless, a recent survey show that about 90% of the UK population are in favour of some form of well controlled euthanasia. The problem however, is controlling has never been easy.

In April 2001, the Dutch parliament finally passed legislation making euthanasia legal within the control guidelines that are discussed above, namely that:

a)   Patients are undergoing irremediable and unbearable suffering.

b)   Patients are aware of all other medical options and have sought a second professional opinion.

c)   A request for euthanasia has been made voluntarily, persistently and independently while the patient is of sound mind.

d)   Parental consent is given for children between 12 and 16 seeking euthanasia.

e)   Doctors do not suggest euthanasia as an option.

f)   The patient's life is ended in a medically appropriate manner.

Furthermore, it is also possible for patients to leave a living will requesting for euthanasia. This gives doctors the option to use their discretion on whether or not euthanasia may be used when patients become too ill.

Conclusion

Although assisting someone to end their own life is highly controversial, even where it can clearly put an end to someone's suffering, it looks likely that many countries will increasingly seek to legalise it in some form as society seeks to uphold the patient's right to self-determination. This will most probably be in a highly regulated way. However, it is certain that there will still be fierce opposition from those who oppose euthanasia, regarding it as murder.

Nevertheless, though illegal, some commentators believe that thousands of secret cases of euthanasia take place each year in the United Kingdom.

Self-Assessment Questions

1. What is the difference between voluntary and involuntary euthanasia?

2. What is the difference between active and passive euthanasia?

3. What important UK Act means that it is no longer an offence to commit suicide, but an offence to assist a person to assist suicide?

4. Why do you think it is so difficult for judges to rule on cases concerning Assisted Suicide and Mercy Killing and what do you think could be done to make such complicated rulings easier?

5. Why do you think that the opponents of mercy killing are so worried about the possible legalisation of it, especially when there are so many people who are in terrible pain and suffering from terminal illness?

6. What are the legal requirements imposed by the Dutch on doctors who assist people to die?

7. Do you think euthanasia should ever be legalised? Justify your answer.

Chapter 19

Terminal Illness and Bereavement

Contents of this Chapter

A. Terminal Illness

To fully understand terminal illness, it would be wise to first understand the meaning of the words 'terminal' and 'illness'.

The concise Oxford Dictionary defines 'terminal' as:

> "(of a disease) ending in death, fatal; or (of a patient) in the last stage of a fatal disease; or (of a morbid condition) forming the last stage of a fatal disease".

The same dictionary defines 'illness' as:

> "a disease, ailment or malady."

Thus, terminal illness can be described as an incurable and irreversible disease as a result of illness or injury that a recognised and qualified medical practitioner would agree will probably result in the death of the person. This means that society expects the terminally ill patient to die of the disease, ailment or malady. It is important to note that this is only an expectation. In reality, however, a person with a terminal illness may never die of it at all and may live long enough to die of natural causes.

Amongst others, terminal illness would therefore include cancer and HIV.

Being diagnosed as terminally ill can be extremely distressing for the patient, family members and friends. Sadly, on top of the distressing times the patient, as well as family members, may be despised and discriminated against and stigmatised by society, because of the disease itself.

While some terminally ill people may continue to live within wider society, others would end up in hospice care, probably with no friends or relatives visiting to give encouragement and hope.

In some cases, it may be necessary for both patient and family members to undergo counselling on how to live and cope with terminal illness in the family.

B. Bereavement

The International Work Group (IWG) on Deaths, Dying, and Bereavement of King's College, University of Western Ontario, Canada defines bereavement as:

> *"the state of deprivation following the loss of something held to be significant, whether positive or negative."*

Thus, bereavement could occur at the death of a loved one. In this chapter, the examination of bereavement will be limited to the loss of a person through death.

The Oxford Concise dictionary defines death as:

> *"the final cessation of vital functions in an organism; the ending of life".*

1. Some Determinants of Degree of Grief

The degree to which a person grieves for the death of another may depend on several factors like:

a) Closeness/relationship

It is accepted that it would be more painful to lose a close relative like husband, wife, brother, sister, mother, father, cousin, niece, uncle, aunt, or close friend, than it would a distant relative.

Furthermore, the degree of pain experienced would also depend on the level of familiarity a person had with the dead one. Thus, the closer you were to the deceased (whether relative or non-relative), the more painful it is likely to be.

b) Age of the dead one

The age at which a person dies could also determine the extent to which surviving relatives and friends may grieve and mourn.

Thus, the death of a young person is likely to be more painful than the death of an elderly person. The death of children can be particularly painful for parents for the waste of life at that young age. Parents may also experience feeling of guilt, anger, confusion and frustration finding it difficult to understand the death of a child.

c) Cause of death

Another possible determinant of the level of grieving is the cause of death. The more traumatic the death, the more painful it is likely to be for others.

People are less likely to come to terms with death by suicide than death as a result of an illness. Suicide could result in feelings of shame, guilt, anger and disbelief.

Other causes of death that can be seen in some societies and communities as bringing shame to surviving relatives would include death from AIDS, alcoholism and drug addiction.

d) Level of dependency

In some circumstances, the degree to which survivors were dependent (e.g. financially) on the deceased would determine the level of grief.

Thus, the greater the level of dependency, the more likely that survivors will feel the loss.

e) Status in life

A person's status in life before death can play a major role in the way that people mourn for that person's death.

People, and indeed society as a whole is much more affected by the death of a caring person, well liked celebrity or a wealthy person than the death of a poor or an unpopular person. The pain would also be longer lasting if the deceased was expected to be prosperous in life.

f) Absence of the Corpse

Another cause for grief and anxiety is where a loved one dies and the body is not found for proper burial. This may be the case when a person dies in a war, plane crash, ship wreck, or is murdered.

In either case, it could prolong the agony and grief of the survivors.

g) Culture and Religion

Culture and religion can play an important role in the extent to which people mourn for the dead. In some cultures, while people may mourn for the dead, it is also a time for celebration of a life well spent.

In other cultures, however, the period for mourning the dead can last for weeks or months.

Religious beliefs about the dead could be a source of strength and hope for the survivors, for instance the belief by Christians of Jesus' promise of a resurrection of the dead can give people hope and the possibility of seeing their loved ones again. It is also believed by some that their loved ones are in heaven as they were good people before their death.

On the other hand, it could be a disturbing time for others, because of the belief in some religions that the 'not-so-good' would go to a place of eternal torment at death.

h) Age of the Survivors

Children's reaction to death is unlikely to be as dramatic as adults. However, research (see below) shows that children, though hurt by the death of someone close, may hide their feelings.

On the other hand, it could be very painful to lose a partner in old age, as the surviving partner may not have anyone else to share life-long experiences with.

g) Suddenness of Death

Sudden death can cause great deal of shock, disbelief, anger and pain.

The more unexpected the death was, the more agonising it is likely to be for survivors.

2. *Reaction to Death*

People react in different ways to the death of a loved one. The manner of reaction could be influenced by the points discussed above and the manner in which the news about the death was communicated to the survivor(s). Thus, it would be shocking to hear about the death of a loved one on television rather than being told personally by a caring and loving person. Effective communication will therefore be important here.

The National Mental Health Association, USA in one of its fact sheets "Coping with Loss - Bereavement and Grief" - 1997 states that the following are some emotions that people may experience at the death of a loved one:

a)   Denial

b)   Yearning

c)   Disbelief

d)   Anger

e)   Confusion

f)   Humiliation

g)   Shock

h)   Despair

i)   Sadness

j)   Guilt

In its magazine, "Redcross Crescent", Amanda Williams, a press officer of the International Committee of the Red Cross (ICRC) in an article "Bearing Bad News" (issue 1 1997) describes the difficulty in explaining to people that their loved ones are dead. She wrote in relation to the Bosnian war:

> *"In Bosnia and Herzegovina, the Red Cross emblem is taking on a new connotation. For the families of the missing, the sight of it on their doorstep can mean news, the thing they want and dread most in life.*

Slowly, the tracing process is finding answers for the families of more than 18,000 people reported missing on all sides of the Bosnian conflict. And, as it yields results, ICRC delegates are dealing with one of the most difficult tasks they can face - telling a mother, wife, or daughter that a man she loves is dead. It is a moment charged with emotions as families confront the horror or the reality of death, and the destruction of the hope which has sustained them for months.

ICRC stress management consultant, Barthold Bierens de Haan, describes a scene he says is typical of those now confronting delegates daily. The location is Tuzla, where many families of the missing are living, many of them from Srebrenica. A young woman who is searching for her husband is visited, and, as a delegate prepares her, explaining the tracing mechanisms, her face gradually falls. She balls up her fist and her breathing becomes more rapid.

The ICRC is now sure, she is told, and she suddenly turns pale. The tragic news of her husband's death is then given, and the circumstances in which it occurred. She bursts into tears and buries her face in her skirt. Her mother-in-law, sitting on the ground at the delegate's feet, so dignified before, rocks back and forth moaning. Soon all the women in the room are weeping.

"The shock and grief may come out in more violent and demonstrative ways", says Bierens de Haan. "Some people scream or moan, other choke or faint, others still run from the room."

The psychiatrist is now convinced that the work, although extremely difficult, is an important step in helping families begin the mourning process. The release of emotions can last many months before a kind of acceptance is reached.

Nothing more humanitarian

In Tuzla, the enormity of the responsibility so concerned sub-delegation head Florent Cornaz that he called in Geneva experts to help him find ways to ensure the work was approached as professionally as possible, and that his staff were protected from potential psychological consequences. "There is nothing more humanitarian," he says, "than having to sit face to face with another human being, and deliver news of this enormity. It demands that we are at our most professional."

Since the Dayton Agreement, which entrusted the ICRC with the issue, just over 18,000 have been registered by their families as missing in Bosnia and Herzegovina. Finding out what happened to them is principally down to a working group, set up and chaired by the ICRC, in which all three parties from the Bosnian conflict are supposedly compelled by Dayton - and international humanitarian law - to disclose any information they have about people killed by their side. So far, answers have been slow in coming. There are other sources. Individuals have responded to a worldwide ICRC campaign urging those who have information to come forward. At the time of writing, the fate of 1,000 men had been discovered. Only a handful were confirmed as still alive.

Any answers are double-checked against information given by the families themselves before a formal letter is drafted and delivered by delegates. The letter is essential: it may become an important document for social and legal benefits. It does not, of course, address the problem which the revelation brings - the right of the families to have the body returned, a question currently being tackled by the international community.

Psychological burden

The process exposes delegates to the full impact of human suffering, stripping away the protective shield that comes of avoiding emotional involvement. Here, the very essence of the work is compassion - delegates must forge a human connection, spend time, listen, even hug or hold hands. It exposes them to the necessary emotional and psychological burden which the sub-delegation in Tuzla has been at pains to tackle.

At the outset, a seminar was organised with leading psychiatrists, where expatriates were taught about mourning customs, and encouraged to explore their own feelings. In the wake of the first, sometimes shocking, experiences, the help of qualified local nurses was enlisted to deal with extreme reactions.

Teams now work in rotation, to avoid emotional burn-out, local staff are compelled to take time off in between, and expatriates are recruited from other offices. To limit possible damage, regular debriefings are held in which delegates share experiences. It means that new, effective ways can be found to deal with the unpredictable. As Florent Cornaz says, "You learn as you go along. You cannot write a guide book for something like this."

Crippling reality

Despite the preparation, despite ending an agonising limbo, the news that a loved one is dead presents families with a crippling reality in which the ICRC and the international community can offer little comfort. Some women refuse to believe the news - their hope extinguishes rationale - and they find comfort in powerful rumours that their men are hidden in secret prisons. For all the ICRC's constant work in following up these allegations, and finding nothing, the rumours keep hope alive, for the alternative is almost unbearable.

"Think of the women of Srebrenica," says Cornaz. "They lost all touch with time, obsessed as they became with what happened in July 1995. The news forces the clock to start again. They have to confront a future without their menfolk, to accept an unwanted emancipation. They have to think about their lives as displaced people relying completely on outside help for survival, and of confronting their children who ask: 'When is daddy coming home?'"

"For others it isn't only the circumstances of losing a relative that they have to deal with, but the whole horror of what happened to them during the war. Some lost their homes four or five times, lived under siege in terrible conditions, and went through many traumatising events. They are so vulnerable, which makes it absolutely essential for the ICRC to deal with what we do as sensitively as possible."

It is pioneering work and the effects will not be known for a long time. As for the impact on delegates, Bierens de Haan says, "They will probably never be the same people again. It is normal in some ways to be hurt by an experience like this, but it is also a very important human lesson."

History seemed to have repeated itself in another Yugoslavian State (Kosovo) where some of the most horrendous crimes, similar to those committed in Bosnia-Herzegovina were reported in the Balkan War, namely, extreme degrees of man's inhumanity against man.

Even worse atrocities were committed against humanity in 1994 in Rwanda when 1 million people were massacred in just 100 days during the Rwandan ethnic conflict.

Atrocities of similar nature are committed almost each year in different parts of the world.

3. *Children and Death in the Family*

Though they may not show it as blatantly as adults, children can be severely affected by death in the family. It is therefore, essential for adults to recognise the signs of distress, anger and pain in children as a result of death in the family.

The Royal College of Psychiatrists, London in (fact sheet 11, for Parents and Teachers) "Death in the family - helping children to cope" states:

"When a family member dies, everyone in the family is affected. Children react very differently from adults. Their response will depend upon a number of factors.

Relationship: What type of relationship the person who has died had with the child and the family will affect the response. Loss of a parent, brother or sister will have a very different impact from the loss of a more distant relative. The impact on the child will depend a lot on how closely involved the dead person was in the daily life of the child and family.

Age and level of understanding: The child's level of understanding and how the death affects life in practical terms are major factors. Infants may feel the impact of loss mainly in the way it affects the way in which they are handled, and their daily routine. They are very sensitive to the unhappy feelings of those around them, and may become anxious, difficult to settle and needy of attention. Pre-school children usually see death as temporary and reversible - a belief reinforced by cartoon characters who 'die' and 'come to life' again.

Children between the ages of five and nine begin to think more like adults about death. They are able to understand basic facts, for example that death happens to all living things, has a cause, and involves permanent separation. They can also understand that dead people do not need to eat, drink, do not see, hear, speak or feel. Teenagers are able to understand death in much more adult terms, and to be aware of the feelings of others.

Young children often do not appear sad. They may show their sadness briefly, and at unexpected moments. This may mislead adults into thinking that they have not been affected by the death. Children tend to express their feelings through behaviour rather than words. Most children show anger and anxiety as well as sadness about death. Anger is a natural reaction to the loss of someone who was essential to the child's sense of stability and safety. Anger may be shown in boisterous play, nightmares, or irritability. Often, the child will show anger to surviving family members. Anxiety is shown in 'babyish' talk and behaviour, and demanding food, comfort and cuddles. Younger children believe that they cause what happens around them. They may fear that they caused the death by being naughty. Teenagers may find it difficult to put their feelings into words, and may not show their feelings openly, for fear of upsetting others."

Death in the family - helping children cope

Circumstances of the death: The circumstances of the death affects the impact on the child. Each family responds in its own way to death. Religion and culture will have an important influence on what happens. Other factors that can make a big difference from the child's point of view are:

- *How traumatic the death was. A traumatic death is harder to cope with.*

- *Whether the death was sudden or expected, a relief from suffering or a crushing blow.*

- *The effect of grief on other family members may mean that they are not able to cope with giving the child the care that is needed.*

- *How much practical support is available to help the family cope".*

4. What can be done to Help?

There is a lot that can be done to cope with bereavement. It is important that effort is made to deal with it. The US National Mental Health Association (1997) comments:

"Coping with death is vital to your mental health. It is only natural to experience grief when a loved one dies. The best thing you can do is allow yourself to grieve. There are many ways to cope effectively with your pain.

- ***Seek out caring people.*** *Find relatives and friends who can understand your feelings of loss. Join support groups with others who are experiencing similar losses.*

- ***Express your feelings.*** *Tell others how you are feeling; it will help you to work through the grieving process.*

- ***Take care of your health.*** *Maintain regular contact with your family physician and be sure to eat well and get plenty of rest. Be aware of the danger of developing a dependence on medication or alcohol to deal with your grief.*

- ***Accept that life is for the living.*** *It takes effort to begin to live again in the present and not dwell on the past.*

- ***Postpone major life changes.*** *Try to hold off on making any major changes, such as moving, remarrying, changing jobs or having another child. You should give yourself time to adjust to your loss.*

- ***Be patient.*** *It can take months or even years to absorb a major loss and accept your changed life.*

- ***Seek outside help when necessary.*** *If your grief feels like it is too much to bear, seek professional assistance to help come to terms with your loss and work through your grief. It's a sign of strength, not weakness, to seek help.*

Helping Others Grieve

If someone you care about has lost a loved one, you can help them through the grieving process.

- ***Share the sorrow.*** *Allow them, even encourage them to talk about their feelings of loss and share memories of the deceased.*

- **Don't offer false comfort.** It doesn't help the grieving person when you say "it was for the best" or "you'll get over it in time." Instead, offer a simple expression of sorrow and take time to listen.

- **Offer practical help**. Baby-sitting, cooking and running errands are all ways to help someone who is in the midst of grieving.

- **Be patient.** Remember that it can take a long time to recover from a major loss. Make yourself available to talk.

- **Encourage professional help when necessary.** Don't hesitate to recommend professional help when you feel someone is experiencing too much pain to cope alone.

<u>Helping Children Grieve</u>

Children who experience a major loss may grieve differently than adults. A parent's death can be particularly difficult for small children, affecting their sense of security or survival. Often, they are confused about the changes they see taking place around them, particularly if well-meaning adults try to protect them from the truth or from their surviving parent's display of grief.

Limited understanding and an inability to express feelings puts very young children at a special disadvantage. Young children may revert to earlier behaviours (such as bed-wetting), ask questions about the deceased that seem insensitive, invent games about dying or pretend that the death never happened. Coping with a child's grief puts added strain on a bereaved parent. However, angry outbursts or criticism only deepen a child's anxiety and delay recovery. Instead, talk honestly with children in terms thy can understand. Take extra time to talk with them about death and the person who has died. Help them work through their feelings and remember that they are looking to adults for suitable behaviour.

<u>Looking To The Future</u>

Remember, with support, patience and effort, you will survive grief. Some day the pain will lessen, leaving you with cherished memories of your loved one."

Furthermore, regarding helping children to cope with death, The Royal College of Psychiatrists adds:

"Being aware of how children normally respond to death makes it easier for an adult to help. It also makes it easier to identify danger signals.

Early stages: Adults sometimes try to shield children from what has happened by withholding information from them. However, experience shoes that children benefit from knowing what has happened as soon as possible, and may want to see the dead relative. The closer the relationship, the more important this is. Adults can also help children to cope by listening to the child's experience of the death, answering their questions, and reassuring them. Children often fear abandonment by loved ones, or fear that they are to blame for the death. Being able to talk about this, and express themselves through play, helps them to cope and also prevents emotional disturbances later in life.

Young children often find it difficult to recall memories of a dead person without being reminded of them. This lack of memory can be very distressing for them. A photograph can be a great source of comfort. Children usually find it helpful to be included in family activities such as attending the funeral. Thought may need to be given as to the support and preparation a child will need in order to be able to do this. A child who is frightened about attending a funeral should not be forced to go. However, (except for very young children) it is usually important to find a way to enable them to say goodbye. For example, lighting a candle, saying a prayer or visiting the grave.

Later on: Once children accept the death, they are likely to display their feelings of sadness, anger and anxiety on and off over a long period of time, and often at unexpected moments. The surviving relatives should spend as much time as possible with the child, making it clear that the child has permission to show his or her feelings openly or freely. Sometimes a child may 'forget' that the family member has died, or persist in the belief that he or she is still alive. This is normal in the first few weeks following a death, but may cause problems if it continues."

Conclusion

At some point in their lives, everyone will have to face the prospect of a loved one either being diagnosed as having a terminal illness, or dying. An understanding of the feelings and emotions which people experience in these most traumatic of circumstances can sometimes help to give them some comfort as they undergo the difficult grieving process.

Self-Assessment Questions

1. What is a 'terminal' illness?

2. What is 'bereavement'?

3. List the 9 main determinants of degree of grief.

4. Referring to the Red Cross Article "Bearing Bad News", and also drawing on any personal experience you may have, imagine you have to tell a family that one of their children, a young girl, has been killed in a road accident. There is a father, a mother and a brother aged 4.

  i)   How would you prepare yourself to tell them the news in the most sensitive way?
  ii) If the family refuses to believe you, how can you ensure that they finally accept the truth?
  iii) How can you ensure that the 4 year old boy understands what has happened to his sister?

Chapter 20

Access to and Disclosure of Medical Records

Contents of this Chapter

1. Introduction

This chapter is intended to be a brief examination of some of the rules regarding access to and the disclosure of medical records of patients and also the levels of confidentiality expected of those who have access to them.

2. General Concept

In the absence of a specific contractual agreement on confidentiality, there is a general common law duty imposed on doctors and other health professionals to respect the confidences of their patients at all times.

It was established in the Court of Appeal case in A-G v Guardian Newspapers Ltd (1988) *that not just medical records but all other confidences of the patient should be respected. This view had earlier being expressed by the court in the case of* Hunter v Mann (1974):

> "the doctor is under a duty not to (voluntarily) disclose, without the consent of the patient, information which he, the doctor, has gained in his professional capacity".

This inherent respect for the patient's confidences is reflected both in the International Code of Medical Ethics and the Declaration of Geneva produced by the World Medical Association as shown below.

a) International Code of Medical Ethics

Duties to the Patient

- A doctor must always bear in mind the obligation of preserving human life.

- A doctor owes to his patient complete loyalty and all the resources of his science.

- Whenever an examination or treatment is beyond his capacity he should summon another doctor who has the necessary ability.

- **A doctor shall preserve absolute secrecy on all he knows about his patients because of the confidence entrusted in him.**

- A doctor must give emergency care as a humanitarian duty unless he is assured that others are willing and able to give such care.

b) Declaration of Geneva (as amended at Sydney, 1968)

At the time of being admitted as a member of the medical profession:

- I will solemnly pledge myself to consecrate my life to the service of humanity;

- I will give to my teachers the respect and gratitude which is due;

- I will practice my profession with conscience and dignity;

- The health of my patient will be my first consideration;

- **I will respect the secrets which are confided in me, even after the patient has died;**

- I will maintain by all the means in my power the honour and the noble traditions of the medical profession;

- My colleagues will be my brothers;

- I will not permit considerations of religion, nationality, race, party politics or social standing to intervene between my duty and my patient;

- I will maintain the utmost respect for human life from the time of conception; and even under threat, I will not use my medical knowledge contrary to the laws of humanity;

- I make these promises solemnly, freely and upon my honour.

Furthermore, the Hippocratic Oath for doctors cited at graduation ceremonies at the University of Edinburgh, Scotland, also makes interesting reading:

"Whatever things seen or heard in the course of medical practice ought not be spoken of, I will not, save for weighty reasons, divulge".

The general concept of respect for confidentiality is also contained under the Data Protection Act 1998.

3. *When Disclosure may be possible*

Despite the rules mentioned above, there are circumstances where disclosure may be possible. The General Medical Council in Great Britain provides some possible exceptions to the confidentiality rules already discussed. These are highlighted below:

(a) Consent of the Patient

Disclosure may be possible where the patient or his lawyer consents to it.

However, it is advisable for such consent to be in writing.

Nevertheless, before such disclosure is affected, it is also advisable to confirm that the patient has the mental ability to consent.

(b) In the Patient's Interests

This may be necessary where it is seen to be in the best interest of the patient to disclose information, for instance to close relatives or other parties.

Such disclosure may be regarded as facilitating better understanding of the patient's illness and the care required of such relatives or appropriate parties.

It is however, advisable to persuade the patient to consent to the disclosure rather than imposing it on him.

(c) In the Public Interest

While cases under this heading should be rare, public interest is a possible ground for disclosure. In the words of AVORY J:

> *"There are cases where the desire to preserve [the confidential relation which exists between the medical man and his patient] must be subordinated to the duty which is cast on every good citizen to assist in the investigation of serious crime"*

This view was upheld in the case of **W v EGDELL (1990)** where the trial Judge, Scott J, comments:

> *"The question in the present case is not whether Dr Egdell was under a duty of confidence; he plainly was. The question is as to the breadth of that duty".*

Accordingly, paragraph 86 of the new **Blue Book** of the General Medical Council, states:

> *"Rarely, cases may arise in which disclosure in the public interest may be justified, for example, a situation in which the failure to disclose appropriate information would expose the patient, or someone else, to a risk of death or serious harm".*

(d)   Medical Research

Where a medical research project has been approved by a recognised ethical committee, disclosure may be possible for such research.

(e)   Statutory Provisions

Information can be disclosed where legislation provides for the disclosure of such records. An example of one such legislation is Section 172 Road Traffic Act 1988, where a doctor is under obligation to provide on request any evidence that may lead to identifying a driver involved in an accident.

(f)   Justification

Justification may be another ground for disclosure. Such cases may occur in a situation where for example a doctor employed by a football team discloses medical information about a player to the management of the football club. The reasoning here is that there is an express or implied understanding that such records would be disclosed.

(g)   Necessity

Quite similar to (f) above, this concept is that it was necessary to disclose such information. Such a situation as provided by the General Medical Council can be:

> *"Where a doctor believes that a patient may be the victim of physical or sexual abuse [and the patient cannot be judged capable of giving or withholding consent to disclosure], the parent's medical interests are paramount and may require the doctor to disclose information to an appropriate person or authority".*

Thus, examples of such victims would include children and those who have mental or severe physical disabilities.

4. HIV and Confidentiality

a)   General Rules

Confidentiality is increasingly tested to the limits with the prevalence of HIV/AIDS and other sexually transmitted diseases. To what extent should the principles of confidentiality and non-disclosure of medical records be maintained considering the possible devastating implications of HIV infection?

One big dilemma which is particular to HIV infection, is the potential consequences to the patient of disclosure, namely:

(a)   stigma, discrimination, ostracisation and possible hostilities from the public;

(b)   the patient may refuse to seek medical advice and care as a result of the disclosure or possible disclosure; and

(c)   the possible increase in the spread of the disease as a result of the patient's refusal to seek medical advice.

The argument for disclosure on the other hand is that this will prevent others from being infected as they can stay away from the infected person.

However, both government policy and public opinion favour the non-disclosure rules. This view was reinforced in the case of X v Y (1988) where Rose, J states:

"The public in general and patients in particular are entitled to expect hospital records to be confidential and it is not for any individual to take it upon himself or herself to breach that confidence whether induced by a journalist or otherwise".

Concerning confidentiality and disclosure, the General Medical Council (GMC) guidance states:

"Doctors are familiar with the need to make judgement about whether to disclose confidential information in particular circumstances, and the need to justify their action where such a disclosure is made. The Council believes that where HIV infection or AIDS has been diagnosed, any difficulties concerning confidentiality which arise will usually be overcome if doctors are prepared to discuss openly and honestly with patients the implications of their condition, the need to secure the safety of others, and the importance for continuing medical care of ensuring that those who will be involved in their care know the nature of their condition and the particular needs which they will have. The Council takes the view that any doctor who discovers that a patient is HIV positive or suffering from AIDS has a duty to discuss these matters fully with the patient."

In relation to confidentiality of an infected doctor, The General Medical Council (GMC) states that:

"Only in the most exceptional circumstances, where the release of a doctor's name is essential for the protection of patients, may a doctor's HIV status be disclosed without his or her consent".

However The GMC continues (June 1993):

"It is unethical for doctors who know or believe themselves to be infected with HIV to put patients at risk by failing to seek appropriate counselling or by failing to act upon it when given. Such behaviour may result in proceedings by the Council which could lead to the restriction or removal of a doctor's registration if this were necessary to protect patients or the doctor's own health. The Council has already given guidance...in the booklet "Professional Conduct and Discipline: Fitness to Practise" on doctors' duty to inform an appropriate person or authority about a colleague whose professional conduct or fitness to practise may be called into question. A doctor who knows that a health care worker is infected with HIV and is aware that the person has not sought or followed advice to modify his or her professional practice, has a duty to inform the appropriate regulatory body and an appropriate person in the health care worker's employing authority, who will usually be the most senior doctor."

b) Passing Information to other Healthcare Professionals

In relation to revealing confidential information about patients to other health care professionals, the GMC provides these guidelines:

"When a patient is seen by a specialist who diagnoses HIV infection or AIDS and a general practitioner is or may become involved in that patient's care, then the specialist should explain to the patient that the general practitioner cannot be expected to provide adequate clinical management and care without full knowledge of the patient's condition. The Council believes that the majority of such patients will readily be persuaded of the need for their general practitioners to be informed of the diagnosis.

If the patient refuses consent for the general practitioner to be told, then the doctor has two sets of obligations to consider: obligations to the patient to maintain confidence, and obligations to other carers whose own health may be put unnecessarily at risk. In such circumstances the patient should be counselled about the difficulties which his or her condition is likely to pose for the team responsible for providing continuing health care and about the likely consequences for the standard of care which can be provided in the future.

If, having considered the matter carefully in the light of such counselling, the patient still refuses to allow the general practitioner to be informed then the patient's request for privacy should be respected. The only exception to that general principle arises where the doctor judges that failure to disclose would put the health of any of the health care team at serious risk.

The Council believes that, in such a situation, it would not be improper to disclose such information as that person needs to know. The need for such a decision is, in present circumstances, likely to arise only rarely, but if it is made the doctor must be able to justify his or her action.

Similar principles apply to the sharing of confidential information between specialists or with other health care professionals such as nurses, laboratory technicians and dentists. All persons receiving such information must of course consider themselves under the same general obligation of confidentiality as the doctor principally responsible for the patient's care."

c) Informing Patient's Spouse and other Sexual Partners

There is another difficulty as to whether or not an HIV infected patient's spouse or sexual partner(s) is informed of the patient's HIV positive status. The GMC provides these guidelines in such circumstances:

"Questions of conflicting obligations also arise when a doctor is faced with the decision whether the fact that a patient is HIV positive or suffering from AIDS should be disclosed to a third party, other than another health care professional, without the consent of the patient. The Council has reached the view that there are grounds for such disclosure only where there is serious and identifiable risk to a specific individual who, if not so informed, would be exposed to infection. Therefore, when a person is found to be infected in this way, the doctor must discuss with the patient the question of informing a spouse or other sexual partner. The Council believes that most such patients will agree to disclosure in these circumstances, but where such consent is withheld the doctor may consider it a duty to seek to ensure that any sexual partner is informed, in order to safeguard such persons from a possible fatal infection."

Health care practitioners who are unsure of what to do in these circumstances should seek the opinion of their respective regulatory authority in their country.

5. Patient's Right of Access

A patient has the right of access to personal data held by health authorities under the following legislations:

(a)   Data Protection Act 1998;

(b)   Freedom of Information Act 2000;

(c)   Access to Health Records Act 1990, and

(d)   Access to Medical Reports Act, 1988

Under all these legislations a patient can not only have access but also have a right to seek correction or amendment of inaccurate information or report about him that is held by health authorities.

Conclusion

The respect for the confidences of the patient is fundamental and paramount at all times even after the death of the patient, as advocated at the Declaration of Geneva, as amended in Sydney.

Although there are circumstances where the patient's confidences may be compromised, as discussed earlier, public opinion is overwhelmingly against it. Even where there is disclosure at all, it should be an extremely minimal and rare occurrence.

Thus, even in cases where national legislation forces disclosure, it may turn out to be a contravention of Article 8 of the European Convention on Human Rights which advocates respect for the individual's privacy and family life, which is not only enforceable in all countries on the European Continent but is also superior to national laws.

HIV infection is such a sensitive issue that AIDS as the cause of death written on a person's death certificate could continue to cause social stigma. In such a situation, the recommendation is that death certificates are made available only to those who legitimately need them so that confidentiality continues to be respected even after the death of the patient.

Self-Assessment Questions

1. Why do doctors have a duty to protect the confidentiality of their patients?

2. What are the two main forms of guidance relating to this?

3. List the main situations in which a doctor may disclose information about a patient.

4. What are the implications of confidentiality relating to those infected with HIV/AIDS?

Chapter 21

Discrimination and Equal Opportunities

Contents of this Chapter

1. Introduction

The fair and equal treatment of all people is a fundamental requirement of a just society. This means that people should always be assessed based on fair and objective criteria. However, certain groups in society are considered more vulnerable to discrimination. This chapter will explore the different types of discrimination and the groups covered by equal opportunities rules.

A) DISCRIMINATION

2. Types of Discrimination

There are 3 main types of discrimination:

1) Harassment

Harassment can be defined as physical or verbal abuse against a person, their possessions or their property. It can also occur against someone who knows the victim – for example a family member, friend or acquaintance or their possessions or property. Examples of harassment could be: beating someone up, writing graffiti on someone's house, sending hate mail, making nuisance telephone calls or destroying property. Threats or actual acts of violence are covered by the Criminal Law and should be reported to the police.

2) Direct Discrimination

Direct discrimination occurs when people are treated differently. For example specifying in a job advert that only men can apply for the job or that no disabled people can apply for a job. Direct discrimination can also take the form of paying different people different wages for the same or similar work, or on the grounds of something which is inseparably linked to gender, for example refusing a woman a job, training or promotion solely because she is pregnant. It could also mean that someone is refused employment, housing or membership of a club. Or they may be offered these things but on different terms to other people, simply because they are from a different racial group are a different colour.

3) Indirect Discrimination

This is when discrimination occurs through some seemingly neutral provision to do with working conditions or allocation of services. This provision, if it practically disadvantages a particular group of people, can result in indirect discrimination. An example might be linking access to certain types of benefits to criteria such as 'only the head of the household' can apply. Another example could be that a company is advertising a job and the advert specifies that it is a requirement for all candidates to have a degree from a British University. This would then exclude all candidates who gained their degrees in other countries. If the company is then unable to justify the rule on grounds other than race, then this would be indirect discrimination.

Although it is not officially considered a type of discrimination, there is a fourth category which it is important to be aware of.

Victimisation

Victimisation is when a person is treated less favourably than others because he or she has brought about a complaint of discrimination or has supported such a complaint. In addition, it is unlawful for a person to use their authority to get someone else to discriminate against a person, or to put pressure on them to do so.

3. Main Areas covered by Discrimination and Equal Opportunities legislations

In the UK there are 3 main groups covered by Discrimination and Equal Opportunities Legislation. These are:

- Race
- Sex
- Disability

There are several different Acts of Parliament, which cover Equal Opportunities Legislation. These are:

i)   The Race Relations Act 1976 as amended by Race Relations (Amendment) Act 2000
ii)   The Sex Discrimination Act 1975
iii)   The Equal Pay Act 1970
iv)   The Disability Discrimination Act 1995

The main points covered by these Acts are discussed below, linked to the particular groups of people protected by the legislation.

4. Racial Discrimination

Probably the most painful and disturbing of all the types of discrimination is that which is based on race, colour, tribe or ethnicity. This is because of the terrible and appalling things that have been done in history because of racial differences, for example, the tens of millions of people tortured and massacred in the world wars, the evils and atrocities committed in Bosnia-Herzegovina, Kosovo and Rwanda.

In Rwanda, there was a race-hate massacre in 1994 where 1 million people were killed in just 100 days.

Right up until the present, such terrible acts or incitement to such acts and racism continue to be committed all over the world in both developing and developed countries.

Even in the UK, racial discrimination and harassment can be a significant problem for many people from ethnic minority groups or those who are visibly from African, Asian, Caribbean or oriental descent. For example, the Commission for Racial Equality (which was set up under the Race Relations Act 1976) quotes the following statistics:

- "The unemployment rate among people from ethnic minorities (19%) is more than twice the rate among white people (8%). 51% of ethnic minority 16-24 year-olds were unemployed in 1994 compared with only 18% of whites.

- On average, pay rates for people from ethnic minorities are 10% less than for white people.

- The proportion of ethnic minority families who are homeless is three times as high as the proportion of white families who are homeless.

- The Home Office has accepted that there may be as many as 130,000 racially motivated incidents in a year.

Race Relations Act 1976

Section 1 (1) states that a person discriminates against another in any circumstances relevant for the purposes of any provision of this Act if:

a)   on racial grounds he treats that other less favourably than he treats or would treat other person; or

b)   he applies to that other a requirement or condition which he applies or would apply equally to persons not of the same racial group as that other but:-

    (i)   which is such that the proportion of persons of the same racial group as that other who can comply with it is considerably smaller than the proportion of persons not of that racial group who can comply with it; and

    (ii)   which he cannot show, to be justifiable irrespective of the colour, race, nationality or ethnic or nationality or ethnic or national origins or the person to whom it is applied; and

    (iii)   which is to the detriment of that other because he cannot comply with it

It is hereby declared that, for the purposes of this Act, segregating a person from other persons on racial grounds is treating him less favourably than they are treated [section 1 (2)].

In this Act, "racial group" means a group of persons defined by reference to colour, race, nationality or ethnic or national origins, and references to a person's racial group refers to any racial group into which he falls [section 3 (1)].

Under section 2 (1) a person ("the discriminator") discriminates against another person ("the person victimised") in any circumstances relevant for the purposes of any provision of this Act if he treats the person victimised less favourably than in those circumstances he treats or would treat other persons, and does so by reason that the person victimised has:-

a)   brought proceedings against the discriminator or any other person under this Act; or

b)   given evidence or information in connection with proceedings brought by any person against the discriminator or any other person under this Act; or

c)   otherwise done anything under or by reference to this Act in relation to the discriminator or any other person; or

d)   alleged that the discriminator or any other person has committed an act, which (whether or not the allegation so states) would amount to a contravention of this Act,

    or by reason that the discriminator knows that the person victimised intends to do any of those things, or suspects that the person victimised has done, or intends to do, any of them.

However, section 2 (2) states that the provisions of subsection (1) does not apply to treatment of a person by reason of any allegation made by him if the allegation was false and not made in good faith.

Under section 4 (1), it is unlawful for a person, in relation to employment by him at an establishment in Great Britain, to discriminate against another:-

a)   in the arrangements he makes for the purpose of determining who should be offered that employment; or

b)   in the terms on which he offers him that employment; or

c)   by refusing or deliberately omitting to offer him that employment

Furthermore, it is also unlawful under section 4 (2), for a person, in the case of a person employed by him at an establishment in Great Britain, to discriminate against that employee:-

a)   in the terms of employment which he affords him; or

b)   in the way he affords him access to opportunities for promotion, transfer or training, or to any other benefits, facilities or services, or by refusing or deliberately omitting to afford him access to them; or

c)   by dismissing him, or subjecting him to any other detriment.

Exceptions for Genuine Occupational Qualifications

Section 5 (1) states that in relation to racial discrimination:-

a)   section 4 (1) (a) or (c) above does not apply to any employment where being of a particular racial group is a genuine occupational qualification for the job; and

b)   section 4 (2) (b) above does not apply to opportunities for promotion or transfer to, or training for, such employment

However, section 5 (2) states that being of a particular racial group is a genuine occupational qualification for a job only where:-

a)   the job involves participation in a dramatic performance or other entertainment in a capacity for which a person of that racial group is required for reasons of authenticity; or

b)   the job involves participation as an artist's or photographic model in the production of a work of art, visual image or sequence of visual images for which a person of that racial group is required for reasons of authenticity; or

c)   the job involves working in a place where food or drink is (for payment or not) provided to and consumed by members of the public or a section of the public in a particular setting for which, in that job, a person of that racial group is required for reasons of authenticity; or

d)   the holder of the job provides persons of that racial group with personal services promoting their welfare, and those services can most effectively be provided by a person of that racial group.

Institutional Racism

The concept of 'Institutional Racism' was first introduced in the "Stephen Lawrence Report" which is part of an inquiry by Sir William MacPherson into Police conduct and investigation at the unprovoked racial attack and murder of a black teenager Stephen Lawrence in 1993 by five white youths.

"Stephen Lawrence had been with his friend Duwayne Brooks during the afternoon of 22ⁿᵈ April. They were on their way home when they came at around 22.30 to a bus stop in Well Hall Road with which we are all now so familiar. Stephen went to see if a bus was coming, and reached a position almost in the centre of the mouth of Dickson Road. Mr Brooks was part of the way between Dickson Road and the roundabout when he saw the group of five or six white youths who were responsible for Stephen's death on the opposite side of the road....."

Stephen had been stabbed to a depth of about five inches on both sides of the front of his body to the chest and arm. Both stab wounds severed auxiliary arteries, and blood must literally have been pumping out of and into his body as he ran up the road to join his friend. In the words of Dr Shepherd, the pathologist, "it is surprising that he managed to get 130 yards with all the injuries he had, but also the fact that the deep penetrating wound of the right side caused the upper lobe to partially collapse his lung. It is therefore a testimony to Stephen's physical fitness that he was able to run the distance he did before collapsing"....

No body had been convicted of this awful crime...what followed had ultimately led to this public inquiry. Little did those around Stephen, or the police officers, or indeed the public expect that five years on this inquiry would deal with every detail of what occurred from the moment of Stephen's death until the hearings at Hannibal House, where this inquiry has taken place."

The police investigation into the murder was flawed and severely criticised by the report:

"The underlying causes of that failure are more troublesome and potentially more sinister. The impact of incompetence and racism, and the aura of corruption or collusion have been the subject of much evidence and debate." (Source: The Stephen Lawrence Report)

In one of her statements, Doreen Lawrence, Stephen's mother said:

"Basically we were seen as gullible simpletons. This is best shown by Detective Chief Superintendent Ilsley's comment that I had obviously been primed to ask questions. Presumably, there is no possibility of me being an intelligent, black woman with thoughts of her own who is able to ask questions for herself. We were patronised and were fobbed off..."

I thought that the purpose of the meetings was to give us progress reports, but what actually happened was that they would effectively say: "stop questioning us. We are doing everything"......

...we hoped to get some feedback from the Barker review....

...he promised that we would meet again so that he could tell us what he had found out. That was the first and last time we ever saw him."

The detailed inquiry into the murder and police conduct that followed led the creation of the concept of institutional racism.

The following definitions of institutional racism are 'lifted' directly from the report:

1. The Commission for Racial Equality (CRE) in their submission stated:-

"Institutional racism has been defined as those established laws, customs, and practices which systematically reflect and produce racial inequalities in society. If racist consequences accrue to institutional laws, customs or practices, the institution is racist whether or not the individuals maintaining those practices have racial intentions."

"...organisational structures, policies, processes and practices which result in ethnic minorities being treated unfairly and less equally, often without intention or knowledge".

2. The oral evidence of the three representatives of the Metropolitan Police Service (MPS) Black Police Association was illuminating. It should be read in full, but we highlight two passages from Inspector Paul Wilson's evidence:-

"The term institutional racism should be understood to refer to the way the institution or the organisation may systematically or repeatedly treat, or tend to treat, people differentially because of their race. So, in effect, we are not talking about the individuals within the service who may be unconscious as to the nature of what they are doing, but is the net effect of what they do".

"A second source of institutional racism is our culture, our culture within the police service. Much has been said about our culture, the canteen culture, the occupational culture. How and why does that impact on individuals, black individuals on the street? Well, we would say the occupational culture within the police service, given the fact that the majority of police officers are white, tends to be the white experience, the white beliefs, the white values.

Given the fact that these predominantly white officers only meet members of the black community in confrontational situations, they tend to stereotype black people in general. This can lead to all sorts of negative views and assumptions about black people, so we should not underestimate the occupational culture within the police service as being a primary source of institutional racism in the way that we differentially treat black people.

Interestingly, I say we because there is no marked difference between black and white in the force essentially. We are all consumed by this occupational culture. Some of us may think we rise above it on some occasions, but, generally speaking, we tend to conform to the norms of this occupational culture, which we all say is all powerful in shaping our views and perceptions of a particular community".

3. We are also grateful for the contribution to our Inquiry made by Dr Benjamin Bowling. Again it must be said that the summaries of such work can be unhelpful. But we hope that he will forgive us for quoting here simply one important passage:-

*"Institutional racism is the **process** by which people from ethnic minorities are systematically discriminated against by a range of public and private bodies. If the result or **outcome** of established laws, customs or practices is racially discriminatory, then institutional racism can be said to have occurred. Although racism is rooted in widely shared attitudes, values and beliefs, discrimination can occur irrespective of the intent of the individuals who carry out the activities of the institution. Thus policing can be*

*discriminatory without this being acknowledged or recognised, and in the face of official policies geared to removal of discrimination. However, some discrimination practices are the product of **uncritical** rather than unconscious racism. That is, practices with a racist outcome are not engaged in without the actor's knowledge; rather, the actor has failed to consider the consequences of his or her actions for people from ethnic minorities. Institutional racism affects the routine ways in which ethnic minorities are treated in their capacity as employees, witnesses, victims, suspects and members of the general public." Violent Racism: Victimisation. Policing and Social Context. July 1998.*

4. We are also encouraged by the letters from the new President of ACPO. Chief Constable John Newing. In his first letter (16 October 1998) he said:-

"... I define institutional racism as the racism which is inherent in wider society which shapes our attitudes and behaviour. Those attitudes and behaviour are then reinforced or reshaped by the culture of the organisation a person works for. In the police service there is a distinct tendency for officers to stereotype people. That creates problems in a number of areas, but particularly in the way officers deal with black people. Discrimination and unfairness are the result. I know because as a young police officer I was guilty·of such behaviour.

My definition is very similar to the way David Wilmot defined institutional racism in response to you and the press...

... We take the view that the important issue now is to stop arguing about definitions and do something about the racism within the service. Having said that it would be entirely unrealistic to think that the phrase 'institutional racism' will not continue to be used to describe a certain type of racist behaviour. Our hope is therefore is that your report will bring greater clarity to its meaning and use."

5. The 1990 Trust in their submission wrote:-

"...racism can be systemic and therefore institutional without being apparent in broad policy terms. Racism within the police can be both covert and overt, racism can be detected in how operational policing decisions are carried out and consequently implemented, and indeed how existing policy is ignored or individual officers' discretion results in racist outcomes".

6. Dr Robin Oakley has submitted two helpful Notes to our Inquiry. It is perhaps impudent to cite short extracts from his work, but these passages have particularly assisted us:-

"For the police service, however, there is an additional dimension which arises from the nature of the policing role. Police work, unlike most other professional activities, has the capacity to bring officers into contact with a skewed cross-section of society, with the well-recognised potential for producing negative stereotypes of particular groups. Such stereotypes become the common currency of the police occupational culture. If the predominantly white staff of the police organisation have their experience of visible minorities largely restricted to interactions with such groups, then negative racial stereotypes will tend to develop accordingly."

In Dr Oakley's view, if the challenges of 'institutional racism' which potentially affect police officers are not addressed, this will:-

"result in a generalised tendency, particularly where any element of discretion is involved, whereby minorities may receive different and less favourable treatment than the minority. Such differential treatment need be neither conscious nor intentional, and it may be practised routinely by officers whose professionalism is exemplary in all other respects. There is great danger that focussing on overt acts of personal racism by individual officers may deflect attention from the much greater institutional challenge... of addressing the more subtle and concealed form that organisational-level racism may take. Its most important challenging feature is its predominantly hidden character and its inbuilt pervasiveness within the occupational culture."

He goes on:-

"It could be said that institutional racism in this sense is in fact pervasive throughout the culture and institutions of the whole of British society, and is in no way specific to the police service. However, because of the nature of the police role, its impact on society if not addressed in the police organisation may be particularly severe. In the police service, despite the extensive activity designed to address racial and ethnic issues in recent years, the concept of 'institutional racism' has not received the attention it deserves." (Institutional Racism and Police Service Delivery, Dr Robin Oakley's submission to this Inquiry).

Dr Oakley in his second Note (17 December 1998) echoes the view of Professor Holdaway who has argued rightly that emotively powerful words such as "racism" must not be used simply as rhetorical weapons:-

"Such terms need to be given a clear analytic meaning which can demonstrably help illuminate the problem at hand".

"The term institutional racism should be understood to refer to the way institutions may systematically treat or tend to treat people differently in respect of race. The addition of the word 'institutional' therefore identifies the source of the differential treatment; this lies in some sense within the organisation rather than simply with the individuals who represent it. The production of differential treatment is 'institutionalised' in the way the organisation operates."

Towards the end of his Note Dr Oakley says this:-

"What is required in the police service therefore is an occupational culture that is sensitive not just to the experience of the majority but to minority experience also. In short, an enhanced standard of police professionalism to meet the requirements of a multi-ethnic society."

7. Sir Paul Condon (Commissioner of the Metropolitan Police Service) himself said this in his letter to the Inquiry dated 2 October 1998:-

"I recognise that individual officers can be, and are, overtly racist. I acknowledge that officers stereotype, and differential outcomes occur for Londoners. Racism in the police is much more than 'bad apples'. Racism, as you have pointed out, can occur through a lack of care and understanding. The debate about defining this evil, promoted by the Inquiry, is cathartic in leading us to recognise that it can occur almost unknowingly, as a matter of neglect, in an institution. I acknowledge the danger of institutionalisation of racism. However, labels can cause more problems than they solve."

8. Institutional racism is in our view primarily apparent in what we have seen and heard in the following areas:-

a)   in the actual investigation including the family's treatment at the hospital, the initial reaction to the victim and witness Duwayne Brooks, the family liaison, the failure of many officers to recognise Stephen's murder as a purely "racially motivated" crime, the lack of urgency and commitment in some areas of the investigation.

b)   countrywide in the disparity in "stop and search figures". Whilst we acknowledge and recognise the complexity of this issue and in particular the other factors which can be prayed in aid to explain the disparities, such as demographic mix, school exclusions, unemployment, and recording procedures, there remains, in our judgment, a clear core conclusion of racist stereotyping;

c)   countrywide in the significant under-reporting of "racial incidents" occasioned largely by a lack of confidence in the police and their perceived unwillingness to take such incidents seriously. Again we are conscious of other factors at play, but we find irresistible the conclusion that a core cause of under-reporting is the inadequate response of the Police Service which generates a lack of confidence in victims to report incidents; and

d)   in the identified failure of police training: as evidenced by the HMIC Report, "Winning the Race" and the Police Training Council Report, and the clear evidence in part 1 of this Inquiry which demonstrated that not a single officer questioned before us in 1998 had received any training of significance in racism awareness and race relations throughout the course of his or her career.

In reaching our conclusions, we do not accept the contention of the Commissioner of the Metropolitan Police Service that:-

"...if this Inquiry labels my Service as institutionally racist the average police officer, the average member of the public will assume the normal meaning of those words. They will assume a finding of conscious, wilful or deliberate action or inaction to the detriment of ethnic minority Londoners. They will assume the majority of good men and women who come into policing... go about their daily lives with racism in their minds and in their endeavour. I actually think that use of those two words in a way that would take on a new meaning to most people in society would actually undermine many of the endeavours to identify and respond to the issues of racism which challenge all institutions and particularly the police because of their privileged and powerful position."

We hope and believe that the average police officer and average member of the public will accept that we do not suggest that all police officers are racist and will both understand and accept the distinction we draw between overt individual racism and the pernicious and persistent institutional racism which we have described.

Nor do we say that in its policies the MPS is racist. Nor do we share the fear of those who say that in our finding of institutional racism, in the manner in which we have used that concept, there may be a risk that the moral authority of the MPS may be undermined. Already by the establishment under Deputy Assistant Commissioner John Grieve of the MPS Racial and Violent Crime Task Force the signs are that the problem is being recognised and tackled.

NOTE: it is important to be aware that there can also be **REVERSE RACISM**. This is when people from ethnic minority groups discriminate against those who are from majority groups. This is also unacceptable and illegal.

Racially Aggravated Offences

According to section 28 (1) Crime and Disorder Act 1998, an offence is racially aggravated if:-

a)   at the time of committing the offence, or immediately before or after doing so, the offender demonstrates towards the victim of the offence hostility based on the victim's membership (presumed membership) of a racial group; or

b)   the offence is motivated (wholly or partly) by hostility towards members of a racial group based on their membership of that group.

It is immaterial for the purposes of paragraph (a) or (b) of subsection (1) above whether or not the offender's hostility is also based, to any extent, on:-

a)   the fact or presumption that any person or group of persons belongs to any religious group; or

b)   any other factor not mentioned in that paragraph

Furthermore, it is an offence under section 32 (1) Crime and Disorder Act 1998, if a person commits:-

a)   an offence under section 2 of the Protection from Harassment Act 1997 (offence of harassment); or

b)   an offence under section 4 of that Act (putting people in fear of violence), which is racially aggravated for the purposes of this section.

By virtue of section 32 (3), a person guilty of an offence falling within subsection (1) (a) above shall be liable:-

a)   on summary conviction, to imprisonment for a term not exceeding six months or to a fine or to both;

b)   on conviction on indictment, to imprisonment for a term not exceeding two years or to a fine, or to both.

A person guilty of an offence falling within subsection (1) (b) above shall be liable:

a)   on summary conviction, to imprisonment for a term not exceeding six months or to a fine, or to both;

b)   on conviction on indictment, to imprisonment for a term not exceeding seven years or to a fine, or both.

Race Relations (Amendment) Act 2000

By virtue of this legislation, the provisions of the Race Relations Act 1976 have been extended to the Police and, with a few exceptions, to other public authorities.

According to section 19B Race Relations Act 1976 [this section was created by section 1 Race Relations (Amendment) Act 2000],

> *"it is unlawful for a public authority in carrying out any functions of the authority to do any act which constitutes discrimination.*

> *In this section, 'public authority' includes any person whose functions are of a public nature."*

The enactment of the Race Relations (Amendment) Act 2000 was precipitated by the public outcry that resulted from the Stephen Lawrence inquiry.

5. Sex Discrimination

This deals with discrimination on grounds of sex or marriage and applies to both men and women. The requirement for equal pay is contained in the Equal Pay Act 1970. In addition, if you are a citizen of the European Union and hold the nationality of a member state, you are entitled when you work to receive the same pay as another worker of the opposite sex performing the same work as yours, provided you both have the same employer.

Equal Opportunities Commission

The Equal Opportunities Commission (EOC) is a body created by Parliament in 1976 with 3 main tasks:

i) Working to end discrimination

ii) Promoting equal opportunities for women and men

iii) Reviewing and suggesting improvements to the Sex Discrimination Act and the Equal Pay Act

It also exists to advise individuals of their rights regarding employment, equal pay, education, provision of housing, goods, facilities and services, advertising and victimisation.

The Equal Opportunities Commission provides the following statistics relating to gender differences:

- 67% of women and 77% of men of working age were employed (1996)

- 45% of women employees and 8% of men employees work part-time

- Women employees working full-time earn on average only 80% of the average hourly earnings of men full-time employees. There is a gender pay gap of 20%.

- The average personal income of women aged 65 and over is only 58% of the average personal income of men aged 65 and over. There is a gender gap in post-retirement income of 42%

- *Women are less likely than men to get a degree or to get a vocational qualification*

- *Part-timers are much less likely to get training. As nearly half of women work part-time and many more will do so at some point in their careers, this leaves them at a considerable disadvantage to men.*

1. Discrimination against Women

Under Section 1(1) Sex Discrimination Act 1975, a person discriminates against a woman in any circumstances relevant for the purposes of any provision of this Act if:-

a)   on the ground of her sex he treats her less favourably than he treats or would treat a man, or

b)   he applies to her a requirement or condition which he applies or would apply equally to a man but:-

   i)   which is such that the proportion of women who can apply with it is considerably smaller than the proportion of men who can comply with it, and

   ii)   which he cannot show to be justifiable irrespective of the sex of the person to whom it is applied, and

   iii)   which is to her detriment because she cannot comply with it

Under section 1 (2), if a person treats or would treat a man differently according to the man's marital status, his treatment of a woman is for the purposes of subsection (1) (a), to be compared to his treatment of a man having the like marital status.

It is unlawful under section 6 (1) for a person, in relation to employment by him at an establishment in Great Britain, to discriminate against a woman:-

a)   in the arrangements he makes for the purpose of determining who shall be offered that employment, or

b)   in the terms on which he offers her that employment, or

c)   by refusing or deliberately omitting to offer her that employment

Furthermore, it is also unlawful under section 6 (2) for a person, in the case of a woman employed by him at an establishment in Great Britain, to discriminate against her:-

a)   in the way he affords her access to opportunities for promotion, transfer or training, or to any other benefits, facilities or services, or by refusing or deliberately omitting to afford her access to them,

b)   by dismissing her, or subjecting her to any other detriment.

Section 12 applies to an organisation of workers, an organisation of employers, or any other organisation whose members carry on a particular profession or trade for the purposes of which the organisation exists.

It is an offence under section 12 (2), for an organisation to which this section applies, in the case of a woman who is not a member of the organisation to discriminate against her:-

a)   in the terms on which it is prepared to admit her to membership, or

b)   by refusing, or deliberately omitting to accept, her application for membership

Furthermore, it is unlawful under section 12 (3), in the case of a woman who is a member of the organisation, to discriminate against her:-

a)   in the way it affords her access to any benefits, facilities or services, or by refusing or deliberately omitting to afford her access to them, or

b)   by depriving her of membership, or varying the terms on which she is a member, or

c)   by subjecting her to any other detriment.

Other areas covered by the rules are discrimination against women by:-

a)   Qualifying bodies,
b)   Vocational training bodies
c)   Educational establishments
d)   Local educational authorities, and
e)   Employment agencies

2. Discrimination Against Men

Section 2 (1) states that the provisions relating to sex discrimination against women are to be read as applying equally to the treatment of men, and for that purpose shall have effect with such modifications as are requisite.

However, according to section 2 (2), no account shall be taken of special treatment afforded to women in connection with pregnancy or childbirth as discrimination against men.

3. Discrimination against married persons in employment field and discrimination by way of victimisation.

Section 3 and 4 Sex Discrimination Act covers discrimination against married persons in employment field and discrimination by way of victimisation respectively. Such discrimination is also unacceptable.

4. Equal Pay

The sex discrimination rules also cover equal pay between men and women.

Thus, Equal Pay Act 1970 as amended by Sex Discrimination Act 1975 states that if the terms of a contract under which a woman is employed at an establishment in Great Britain do not include (directly or by reference to a collective agreement or otherwise) an equality clause they shall be deemed to include one [section 1 (1)].

An equality clause is a provision which relates to terms (whether concerned with pay or not) of a contract under which a woman is employed, and has the effect that:-

a)   where the woman is employed on like work with a man in the same employment:-

     i)   if (apart from the equality clause) any term of the woman's contract is or becomes less favourable to the woman than a term of similar kind in the contract under which that man is employed, that term of the woman's contract shall be treated as so modified as not to be less favourable, and

     ii)   if (apart from the equality clause) at any time the woman's contract does not include a term corresponding to a term benefiting that man included in the contract under which he is employed, the woman's contract shall be treated as including such a term:

b)   where the woman is employed on work rated as equivalent with that of a man in the same employment:-

i)   if (apart from the equality clause) any term of the woman's contract determined by the rating of the work is or becomes less favourable to the woman than a term of a similar kind in the contract under which that man is employed, that term of the woman's contract shall be treated as so modified as not to be less favourable, and

ii)   if (apart from the equality clause) at any time the woman's contract does not include a term corresponding to a term benefiting that man included in the contract under which he is employed and determined by the rating of the work, the woman's contract shall be treated as including such a term [section 1 (2) Equal Pay Act 1970 as amended].

5. Discriminatory Practice

Under section 37 (1) Sex Discrimination Act 1975, discriminatory practice means the application of a requirement or condition which results in an act of discrimination or is likely to result in such an act of discrimination if the persons to whom it is applied were not all of one sex.

According to section 37 (2), a person acts in contravention of this section if and so long as:-

a)   he applies a discriminatory practice, or

b)   he operates practices or other arrangements which in any circumstances would call for the application by him of a discriminatory practice.

Exceptions

There are some areas where the Sex Discrimination Acts do not apply.

a)   **Work Outside the UK**

The Sex Discrimination Acts do not apply to employees who work totally outside the UK, for example employees working on a British Ship where the work is entirely outside the territorial waters of Great Britain.

b)   **Genuine Occupational Qualifications**

In certain limited circumstances, sex may be a Genuine Occupational Qualification (GOQ) for a job. Examples are:

i)   Where a man or woman is needed because of physical appearance – e.g. for a job as a model – or to be authentic, e.g. as an actor playing a certain role

ii)   A man or woman is required to preserve decency or privacy e.g. lavatory attendant

iii)   The job is likely to involve the holder of the job doing his work, or living in a private home and needs to be held by a man because objection might reasonably be taken to allowing a woman to do this role (for example if the degree of physical or social contact with a person living in the home or knowledge of a person's intimate details will be made available to the holder of the job)

iv)   The holder of the job would have to 'live in' because of the nature of the job and there are no separate sleeping or toilet arrangements for men and women.

v)   The job is in a single sex establishment (or part of a single sex establishment), which provides special care, supervision or attention e.g. jobs in a women's refuge or single sex psychiatric unit in a mixed hospital

vi)   The employee provides people with personal services promoting their welfare or education – which can be provided most effectively by a person of the same sex, e.g. counselling

vii)   Part of the job is, or is likely to be, in a country where the laws and customs prevent a woman doing the job effectively

viii) The job is one of two to be held by a married couple.

Note: each time a job falls vacant, it is necessary to determine whether or not the GOQ still applies.

c)   Pregnancy, Childbirth, Retirement or Death

It is not unlawful to give different treatment to men and women in the following circumstances:

ii)   By giving special treatment to women in respect of pregnancy and childbirth, e.g. maternity leave

iii)   In the provision made regarding retirement or death, except that it is unlawful to discriminate against a woman as regards age of retirement. Occupational Pension Schemes must be open to both men and women on terms which are the same

d)   Other Special Cases

There are special provisions for the police, prison officers, ministers of religion and for competitive sports.

6. Disability Discrimination

According to recent figures, there are approximately six million disabled adults in Britain and about 14 per cent of the adult population have at least one impairment which causes disability.

The way 'disability' is defined will obviously affect the exact figures, as it covers a wide range of functional limitations, which could be physical, intellectual or sensory in nature. They could also be linked to a medical condition or mental illness, or to explain the complete or partial loss of a person's ability to participate in the life of the community on equal terms with the rest of the population.

Examples of disabilities include:

- Hearing impairments (total or partial deafness)

- Visual impairments (blind or partially sighted, short sightedness, colour blindness)

- Mobility problems (includes wheelchair users)

- Learning difficulties

- Mental Disorders (Emotional distress, anxiety and depression)

- Severe Disfigurement

- HIV/AIDS infection

However, it is important to realise that not everyone who has a disability is prevented from participating on equal terms with other members of society – indeed, many people with such disabilities do not consider themselves to be disabled and would not necessarily be regarded by others as disabled either.

Consider the following statistics:

- Disabled people are 4 times more likely to be officially unemployed (20.5%) as opposed to non-disabled people (5.4%) Source: Office of Population Censuses Survey

- 23% are disabled due to accident – half of which are work related (11.5%) Source: Social and Community Planning Research

- 20% are disabled due to illness. Source: Social and Community Planning Research

- 27% have been disabled since 19 years of age. Source: Social and Community Planning Research

- 70% of economically active disabled people become disabled during their working lives. Source: Social and Community Planning Research

- There are 6.8 million people caring for someone with a disability. Source: Social and Community Planning Research

- 51% of young people with disabilities don't find work or get on to a Youth Training Scheme as opposed to 17% non-disabled. Source: Scope Research

Disability Discrimination Act 1995

This Act deals with discrimination against people with disabilities. Discrimination would be when someone treats a person with disabilities less favourably than someone else, without justification, for a reason related to their disability. Discrimination also occurs if, without justification, a 'reasonable adjustment' is not made. The Act applies to all those who provide goods, facilities and services (including buying or renting of land or property) to the public. The employment provisions of the Act apply to employers with 15 or more employees.

The Act also requires schools, colleges and universities to provide information for disabled people and allows the government to set minimum standards so that disabled people have easier access to public transport.

Under the Act, the following provisions apply to various groups:

a.   **People with Disabilities**

The Act gives rights to disabled people who have difficulty in carrying out daily activities. Their disability must be substantial and have a long-term effect (i.e. last or be expected to last for at least 12 months).

b.   **Employers and Service Providers**

Employers and people who provide public services must take reasonable measures to make sure they are not discriminating against such people. Employers must not treat a person with a disability less favourably than someone else unless there is a good reason. They must also make any changes to the workplace which are reasonable.

c.   **Landlords and others who are responsible for letting or selling property**

People who sell or let property will have to ensure that they do not reasonably discriminate against disabled people.

1. Meaning of Disability

Section 1 (1) Disability Discrimination Act 1995 states that a person has a disability if he has a physical or mental impairment which has a substantial and long-term adverse effect on his ability to carry out normal day-to-day activities.

2. Meaning of Disability Discrimination

For this purpose of part II of the legislation, section 5 (1) states that an employer discriminates against a disabled person if:-

a)   for a reason which relates to the disabled person's disability, he treats him less favourably than he treats or would treat others to whom that reason does not or would not apply; and

b)   he cannot show that the treatment in question is justified.

Furthermore, an employer also discriminates against a disabled person, according to section 5 (2), if:-

a)   he fails to comply with a section 6 duty imposed (see below) on him in relation to the disabled person; and

b)   he cannot show that his failure to comply with the duty is justified

3. Duty of Employer to make adjustments

Under section 6 (1), where:-

a)   any arrangements made by or on behalf of an employer, or

b)   any physical feature of the premises occupied by the employer,

place the disabled person concerned at a substantial disadvantage in comparison with persons who are not disabled, it is the duty of the employer to take such steps as it is reasonable, in all the circumstances of the case, for him to have to take in order to prevent the arrangements or feature having that effect.

The following, according to section 6 (3), are examples of steps which an employer may have to take in relation to a disabled person in order to comply with subsection (1) above-

a)   making adjustments to premises;

b)   allocating some of the disabled person's duties to another person;

c)   transferring him to fill an existing vacancy;

d)   altering his working hours

e)   assigning him to a different place of work;

f)   allowing him to be absent during working hours for rehabilitation, assessment and treatment;

g)   giving him, or arranging for him to be given training;

h)   acquiring or modifying equipment;

i)   modifying instructions or reference manuals;

j)   modifying procedures for testing or assessment;

k)   providing a reader or interpreter;

l)   providing supervision

According to section 6 (4), in determining whether it is reasonable for an employer to have to take a particular step in order to comply with subsection (1) above, regard shall be had, in particular to:-

a)   the extent to which taking the step would prevent the effect in question;

b)   the extent to which it is practicable for the employer to take the step;

c)   the financial and other costs which would be incurred by the employer taking the step and the extent to which taking it would disrupt any of his activities;

d)   the extent of the employer's financial and other resources;

e)   the availability to the employer of financial or other assistance with respect to taking the step.

Under section 7 (1), an employer who has fewer than 20 employees is exempt from the employee requirements in section 6 (1) above.

4. Unlawful

Under section 4 (1), it is unlawful for an employer to discriminate against a disabled person:-

a)   in the arrangements which he makes for the purpose of determining to whom he should offer employment;

b)   in the terms on which he offers that person employment; or

c)   by refusing to offer, or deliberately not offering, him employment

It is also unlawful under section 4 (2) for an employer to discriminate against a disabled person whom he employs:-

a)   in the terms of employment which he affords him;

b)   in the opportunities which he affords him for promotion, a transfer, training or receiving any other benefit;

c)   by refusing to afford him, or deliberately not affording him, any such opportunity; or

d)   by dismissing him, or subjecting him to any other detriment

By virtue of section 8 (1), a complaint by a disabled person that he has been discriminate against may be presented to an industrial tribunal.

5. Other areas of disability discrimination

Though only discrimination by employers has so far been discussed, the Disability Discrimination legislation covers several other areas such as:-

a)   discrimination against contract workers [section 12]

b)   discrimination by trade organisations [section 13]

c)   discrimination in relation to goods, facilities and services [section 19]

d)   discrimination in relation to disposal of premises [section 22]

e)   taxi accessibility regulations [section 32]

f)   carrying of passengers in wheelchairs [section 36]

g)   carrying of guide dogs and hearing dogs [section 37].

7. Age Discrimination – Coming 2006

Age discrimination law will become effective in the UK by 2006. It is a European Union (EU) Council Employment Directive 2000/78/EC which establishes a general framework for equal treatment in employment and vocational training and guidance.

The directive is designed to outlaw discrimination at work and training on grounds of age, sexual orientation, disability and religion or belief. It sets the framework, which will ensure that there are minimum standards for combating discrimination throughout the European Union.

Future Legislation

In October 2000 the Government signed the EC Directive on Equal Treatment in Employment and Occupation with a commitment to implementing age discrimination legislation covering employment, vocational training and guidance by December 2006.

The Directive applies to both the public and the private sector and covers the following areas:

- access to employment, to self employment or to occupation

- access to all types and levels of vocational guidance, training, re-training and work experience

- employment and working conditions, including dismissals and pay

- access to membership of and involvement in a workers' or employment organisation and the accompanying benefits

7. Conclusion: (Discrimination)

Being discriminated against can be a painful experience. Discriminating against a person on the grounds of race, sex or disability is not only a breach of UK law but also International Law.

Article 14 of the European Convention on Human Rights (which is enforceable in countries on the European continent) states:

"The enjoyment of the rights and freedoms set forth in this convention shall be secured without discrimination on any ground such as sex, race, colour, language, religion, political or other opinion, national or social origin, association with a national minority, property or other status"

Furthermore, it is also a violation of article 7 of the Universal Declaration of Human Rights by the United Nations which states:

"All are equal before the law and are entitled without any discrimination to equal protection of the law. All are entitled to equal protection against any discrimination in violation of this declaration and against any incitement to such discrimination".

Basically, with a few exceptions as seen above, any form of discrimination against a particular person or set of people is unacceptable. As such, the victim can seek legal redress and possible compensation from the perpetrators.

B) EQUAL OPPORTUNITIES

1. Introduction

As discussed above, there is legislation in place to ensure that everyone has 'equality of opportunity', but what does Equal Opportunities really mean?

It is much more than treating everybody in the same way and is more about fairness. For example, if a building can only be entered via a flight of stairs, then everyone who goes into the building has to use the flight of stairs, so they are treated the **same**. However, this is not **fair** to wheelchair users, who could not reasonably be expected to get their wheelchair up stairs. In order to give them fair (or equal) access, then there should be some sort of alternative arrangement – perhaps a ramp or lift – so that they have just as good access into the building as a non-wheelchair user.

The following outline some of the main principles of equal opportunity:

2. Recognise that people are different

Society is made up of a mixture of different people. We are all from different backgrounds, races, cultures, religions and social groups. There is also a mixture of men and women, heterosexual and homosexual people, young, old able-bodied and disabled people.

It would be impossible to exist in a society where everyone is the same, because we all have different experiences and, through the circumstances of our birth, we all begin life in a different way.

Even in a small isolated island community where there is little contact with the outside world (perhaps with only a tiny indigenous population) the individuals in that community are still different from one another. People have different personalities and different life experiences from one another. If you were to ask two people from such a community to tell their life story, you could guarantee that they would have very different tales to tell. It therefore follows that in a country like the UK - with a large population - contains people with a wide range of differences between individuals.

3. Recognise that discrimination has taken place in the past and still takes place

Most people will either have experienced some sort of discrimination themselves or will know someone who has experienced it.

There is a vast amount of factual information which proves that people have experienced discrimination. In countries like South Africa and the United States of America, people from different races used to be separated from one another by government policy (Apartheid in South Africa and segregation in the southern states of the United States of America). These two systems actively discriminated against black people and gave white people many more advantages in terms of education, employment and access to services. Although both these systems no longer exist, they have still had an effect on how black people are perceived and treated in these countries and it will take some time, particularly in South Africa for them to 'catch up' with the advantages white people previously took for granted.

Another example of discrimination occurred in the UK where it was only as recently as the early twentieth century that women were allowed to vote. Previously, only men had that right by law. Women also had many restrictions placed upon them in terms of what jobs they could do and many were made to give up work as soon as they got married. Today, women still suffer discrimination in other ways, for example through men's attitudes and the belief that 'a woman's place is in the home'. There is also the phenomenon of the 'glass ceiling' at work where some women are unable to get to the top jobs because the predominately male senior members of staff will block their promotion.

Disabled people have only recently been protected by law but still suffer in particular through people's negative perceptions, and through lack of physical access to buildings and/or services.

It would be impossible to believe in the ideal of equal opportunities without a belief in this particular principle, particularly as the overwhelming evidence shows that discrimination has been taking place in so many areas of society.

4. Recognise the value of diversity

Different people have different skills, knowledge and experiences. When this diversity comes together, for example to solve a problem, meet an objective or to gather information, then the more diverse a group, the more likely they are to consider a broad range of options and eventually reach a more balanced result, possibly to a higher standard or faster than a group with less diversity. This is an area where businesses should be particularly keen to make the most of a varied workforce, because this diversity will enable a business to achieve greater productivity.

For example, if a company wanted to develop a product for women, it would make sense not to try and get ideas from a group of people that did not include a woman.

Similarly, if there is a problem to be solved, the more people were involved in the problem solving process, the more ideas are likely to be generated, because people have different life experiences they can call upon.

5. Commitment to the fair provision of goods, services and employment to all

This means that no person should be discriminated against when they try to buy items in a shop, obtain services (for example, welfare benefits, housing or utilities) or when they are applying for jobs.

We would not expect to try and use the bus, train or public transport and be told that we were the wrong race or the wrong sex and so we could not use the transport. In the same way, it would be wrong for an assistant in a shop to refuse to sell goods to a male customer because they preferred women, or to a wheelchair user because they took up too much space. In a civilised society we should all have fair access to the things we need to enjoy a good quality of life.

General Conclusion

An awareness of the different types of discrimination and an understanding of the principles of equal opportunities will be essential to a society seeking to be fair to all its individuals. Ultimately, it is to everyone's benefit that we are all treated fairly.

Self-Assessment Questions

1. *What are the 3 main types of discrimination?*

2. *How would you define 'victimisation'?*

Chapter 22

Universal Declaration of Commitment on HIV/AIDS

Contents of this Chapter

1. *Introduction*
2. *The Preamble*
3. *The Declaration*
4. *Conclusion*
5. *Self-Assessment Questions*

1. Introduction

In response to the ever-increasing rate of HIV/AIDS infection in the world, the General Assembly of the United Nations proclaimed the Universal Declaration of Commitment on HIV/AIDS on 27 June 2001.

2. The Preamble

1. We, Heads of State and Government and Representatives of States and Governments, assembled at the United Nations, from 25 to 27 June 2001, for the twenty-sixth special session of the General Assembly convened in accordance with resolution 55/13, as a matter of urgency, to review and address the problem of HIV/AIDS in all its aspects as well as to secure a global commitment to enhancing coordination and intensification of and international efforts to combat it in a comprehensive manner;

2. Deeply concerned that the global HIV/AIDS epidemic, through its devastating scale and impact, constitutes a global emergency and one of the most formidable challenges to human life and dignity as well as to the effective enjoyment of human rights, which undermines social and economic development throughout the world and affect levels of society - national, community, family and individual;

3.   Noting with profound concern, that by the end of the year 2000, 36.1 million people worldwide were living with HIV/AIDS, 90 per cent in developing countries and 75 per cent in sub-Saharan Africa;

4.   Noting with grave concern that all people, rich and poor, without distinction of age, gender or race are affected by the HIV/AIDS epidemic, further noting that people in developing countries are the most affected and that women, young adults and children, in particular girls are the most vulnerable;

5.   Concerned also that the continuing spread of HIV/AIDS will constitute a serious obstacle to the realisation of the global development goals we adopted at the Millennium Summit;

6.   Recalling and confirming our previous commitments on HIV/AIDS made through:

- The United Nations Millennium Declaration of 8 September 2000

- The Political Declaration and Further Actions and Initiatives to Implement the Commitments made at the World Summit for Social Development of 1 July 2000

- The Political Declaration and Further Action and Initiatives to implement the Beijing Declaration and Platform for Action of 10 June 2000;

- Key Actions for the Further Implementation of the Programme of Action of the International Conference on Population and Development of 2 July 1999;

- The regional call for action to fight HIV/AIDS in Asia and the Pacific of 25 April 2001;

- The Abuja Declaration and Framework for Action for the Fight Against HIV/AIDS, Tuberculosis and other Related Infectious Diseases in Africa, 27 April 2001;

- The Declaration of the Ibero-America Summit of Heads of State of November 2000 in Panama;

- The Caribbean Partnership Against HIV/AIDS, 14 February, 2001;

- The European Union Programme for Action: Accelerated Action on HIV/AIDS, malaria and Tuberculosis in the Context of Poverty Reduction of 14 May 2000;

- The Baltic Sea Declaration on HIV/AIDS Prevention of 4 May 2000;

- The Central Asian Declaration on HIV/AIDS of 18 May 2001;

7.   Convinced of the need to have an urgent, coordinated and sustained response to the HIV/AIDS epidemic, which will build on the experience, lessons learned over the past 20 years;

8.   Noting with grave concern that Africa, in particular sub-Saharan Africa, is currently the worst affected region where HIV/AIDS is considered as a state of emergency, which threatens development, social cohesion, political stability, food security and life expectancy and imposes a devastating economic burden and that the dramatic situation on the continent needs urgent and exceptional national, regional and international action;

9.   Welcoming the commitments of African Heads of State or Government, at the Abuja Special Summit in April 2001, particularly their pledge to set a target of allocating at least 15 per cent of their annual national budgets for the improvement of the health sector to help address the

HIV/AIDS epidemic; and recognizing that action to reach this target, by those countries whose resources are limited, will need to be complemented by increased international assistance;

10. Recognizing also that other regions are seriously affected and confront similar threats, particularly the Caribbean region, with the second highest rate of HIV infection after sub-Saharan Africa, the Asia Pacific region where 7.5 million people are already living with HIV/AIDS, the Latin America region with 1.5 million people living with HIV/AIDS, and the Central and Eastern European region with very rapidly rising infection rates; and that the potential exists for a rapid escalation of the epidemic and its impact throughout the world if no specific measures are taken;

11. Recognizing that poverty, underdevelopment and illiteracy are among the principal contributing factors to the spread of HIV/AIDS and noting with grave concern that HIV/AIDS is compounding poverty and is now reversing or impeding development in many countries and should therefore be addressed in an integrated manner;

12. Noting that armed conflicts and natural disasters also exacerbate the spread of the epidemic;

13. Noting further that stigma, silence, discrimination, and denial, as well as lack of confidentiality, undermine prevention, care and treatment efforts and increase the impact of the epidemic on individuals, families, communities and nations and must also be addressed;

14. Stressing that gender equality and the empowerment of women are fundamental elements in the reduction of the vulnerability of women and girls to HIV/AIDS;

15. Recognizing that access to medication in the context of pandemics such as HIV/AIDS is one of the fundamental elements to achieve progressively the full realization of the right of everyone to the enjoyment of the highest attainable standard of physical and mental health;

16. Recognizing that the full realization of human rights and fundamental freedoms for all is an essential element in a global response to the HIV/AIDS and prevents stigma and related discrimination against people living with or at risk of HIV/AIDS;

17. Acknowledging that prevention of HIV infection must be the mainstay of the national, regional and international response to the epidemic; and that prevention, care, support and treatment for those infected and affected by HIV/AIDS are mutually reinforcing elements of an effective response and must be integrated in a comprehensive approach to combat the epidemic;

18. Recognizing the need to achieve the prevention goals set out in this Declaration in order to stop the spread of the epidemic and acknowledging that all countries must continue to emphasize widespread and effective prevention, including awareness- raising campaigns through education, nutrition, information and health-care services;

19. Recognizing that care, support and treatment can contribute to effective prevention through increased acceptance of voluntary and confidential counselling and testing, and by keeping people living with HIV/AIDS and vulnerable groups in close contact with health-care systems and facilitating their access to information, counselling and preventive supplies;

20. Emphasizing the important role of cultural, family, ethical and religious factors in the prevention of the epidemic, and in treatment, care and support, taking into account the particularities of each country as well as the importance of respecting all human rights and fundamental freedoms;

21. Noting with concern that some negative economic, social, cultural, political, financial and legal factors are hampering awareness, education, prevention, care, treatment and support efforts;

22. Noting the importance of establishing and strengthening human resources and national health and social infrastructures as imperatives for the effective delivery of prevention, treatment, care and support services;

23. Recognizing that effective prevention, care and treatment strategies will require behavioural changes and increased availability of and non-discriminatory access to, inter alia, vaccines, condoms, microbicides, lubricants, sterile injecting equipment, drugs including anti-retroviral therapy, diagnostics and related technologies as well as increased research and development;

24. Recognizing also that the cost availability and affordability of drugs and related technology are significant factors to be reviewed and addressed in all aspects and that there is a need to reduce the cost of these drugs and technologies in close collaboration with the private sector and pharmaceutical companies;

25. Acknowledging that the lack of affordable pharmaceuticals and of feasible supply structures and health systems continue to hinder an effective response to HIV/AIDS in many countries, especially for the poorest people and recalling efforts to make drugs available at low prices for those in need;

26. Welcoming the efforts of countries to promote innovation and the development of domestic industries consistent with international law in order to increase access to medicines to protect the health of their populations; and noting that the impact of international trade agreements on access to or local manufacturing of, essential drugs and on the development of new drugs needs to be further evaluated.

27. Welcoming the progress made to contain the epidemic, particularly through: strong political commitment and leadership at the highest levels, including community leadership; effective use of available resources and traditional medicines; successful prevention, care support and treatment strategies; education and information initiatives; working in partnership with communities, civil society, people living with HIV/AIDS and vulnerable groups; and the active promotion and protection of human rights; and recognizing the importance of sharing and building on our collective and diverse experiences, through regional and international co-operation including North/South, South/South cooperation and triangular cooperation;

28. Acknowledging that resources devoted to combating the epidemic both at the national and international levels are not commensurate with the magnitude of the problem;

29. Recognizing the fundamental importance of strengthening national, regional and subregional capacities to address and effectively combat HIV/AIDS and that this will require increased and sustained human, financial and technical resources through strengthened national action and cooperation and increased regional, subregional and international cooperation.

30. Recognizing that external debt and debt-servicing problems have substantially constrained the capacity of many developing countries, as well as countries with economies in transition, to finance the fight against HIV/AIDS;

31. Affirming the key role played by the family in prevention, care, support and treatment of persons affected and infected by HIV/AIDS, bearing in mind that in different cultural, social and political systems various forms of the family exist;

32. Affirming that beyond the key role played by communities, strong partnerships among Governments, the United Nations system, intergovernmental organizations, people living with HIV/AIDS and vulnerable groups, medical, scientific and educational institutions, non-governmental organizations, the business sector including generic and research-based pharmaceutical companies, trade unions, medic, parliamentarians, foundations, community organizations, faith- based organizations and traditional leaders are important;

33. Acknowledging the particular role and significant contribution of people living with HIV/AIDS, young people and civil society actors in addressing the problem of HIV/AIDS in all its aspects and recognizing that their full involvement and participation in design, planning, implementation and evaluation of programmes is crucial to the development of effective responses to the HIV/AIDS epidemic;

34. Further acknowledging the efforts if international humanitarian organizations combating the epidemic, including among others the volunteers of the International Federation of Red Cross and Red Crescent Societies in the most affected areas all over the world;

35. Commending the leadership role on HIV/AIDS policy and coordination in the United Nations system of the UNAIDS Programme Coordinating Board; noting its endorsement in December 2000 of the Global Strategy Framework for HIV/AIDS, which could assist, as appropriate, Member States and relevant civil society actors in the development of HIV/AIDS strategies, taking into account the particular context of the epidemic in different parts of the world;

3. The Declaration

36. Solemnly declare our commitment to address the HIV/AIDS crisis by taking action as follows, taking into account the diverse situations and circumstances in different regions and countries throughout the world;

Leadership

Strong leadership at all levels of society is essential for an effective response to the epidemic

Leadership by Governments in combating HIV/AIDS is essential and their efforts should be complemented by the full and active participation of civil society, the business community and the private sector

Leadership involves personal commitment and concrete actions

At the national level

37. By 2003, ensure the development and implementation of multisectoral national strategies and financing plans for combating HIV/AIDS that: address the epidemic in forthright terms; confront sigma, silence and denial; address gender and age-based dimensions of the epidemic; eliminate discrimination and marginalization; involve partnerships with civil society and the business sector and the full participation of people living with HIV/AIDS, those in vulnerable groups and people mostly at risk, particularly women and young people; are resourced to the extent possible from national budgets without excluding other sources, inter alia international cooperation; fully promote and protect all human rights and fundamental freedoms, including the right to the highest attainable standard of physical and mental health; integrate a gender

perspective; and address risk, vulnerability, prevention, care, treatment and support and reduction of the impact of the epidemic; and strengthen health, education and legal system capacity;

38. By 2003, integrate HIV/AIDS prevention, care, treatment and support and impact mitigation priorities into the mainstream of development planning, including in poverty eradication strategies, national budget allocations and sectoral development plans;

At the regional and subregional level

39. Urge and support regional organizations and partners to: be actively involved in addressing the crisis; intensify regional, subregional and interregional cooperation and coordination; and develop regional strategies and responses in support of expanded country level efforts;

40. Support all regional and subregional initiatives on HIV/AIDS including: the International Partnership against AIDS in Africa (IPAA) and the ECA-African Development Forum Consensus and Plan of Action: Leadership to Overcome HIV/AIDS; the Abuja Declaration and Framework for Action for the Fight Against HIV/AIDS, Tuberculosis and Other Diseases; the CARICOM Pan-Caribbean Partner Against HIV/AIDS; the ESCAP Regional Call for Action HIV/AIDS·in Asia and the Pacific; the Baltic Sea Initiative and Action Plan. The Horizontal Technical Cooperation Group on HIV/AIDS in Latin America and the Caribbean; the European Union Programme for Action: Accelerated Action on HIV/AIDS, Malaria and Tuberculosis in the context of poverty reduction;

41. Encourage the development of regional approaches and plans to address HIV/AIDS;

42. Encourage and support local and national organizations to expand and strengthen regional partnerships, coalitions and networks;

43. Encourage the United Nations Economic and Social Council to request the regional commissions within their respective mandates and resources to support national efforts in their respective regions in combating HIV/AIDS.

At the global level

44. Support greater action and coordination by all relevant United Nations system organizations, including their full participation in the development and implementation of a regularly updated United Nations strategic plan for HIV/AIDS, guided by the principles contained in this Declaration;

45. Support greater cooperation between relevant United Nations system organizations and international organizations combating HIV/AIDS;

46. Foster stronger collaboration and the development of innovative partnerships between the public and private sectors and by 2003, establish and strengthen mechanisms that involve the private sector and civil society partners and people living with HIV/AIDS and vulnerable groups in the fight against HIV/AIDS;

Prevention

Prevention must be the mainstay of our response

47. By 2003, establish time-bound national targets to achieve the internationally agreed global prevention goal to reduce by 2005 HIV prevalence among young men and women aged 15 to 24 in the most affected countries by 25 per cent and by 25 per cent globally by 2010, and

to intensify efforts to achieve these targets as well as to challenge gender stereotypes and attitudes, and gender inequalities in relation to HIV/AIDS, encouraging the active involvement of men and boys;

48. By 2003, establish national prevention targets, recognizing and addressing factors leading to the spread of the epidemic and increasing people's vulnerability, to reduce HIV incidence for those identifiable groups, within particular local contexts, which currently have high or increasing rates of HIV infection, or which available public health information indicates are at the highest risk for new infection;

49. By 2005, strengthen the response to HIV/AIDS in the world of work by establishing and implementing prevention and care programmes in public, private and informal work sectors and take measures to provide a supportive workplace environment for people living with HIV/AIDS;

50. By 2005, develop and begin to implement national, regional and international strategies that facilitate access to HIV/AIDS prevention programmes for migrants and mobile workers, including the provision of information on health and social services;

51. By 2003, implement universal precautions in health-care settings to prevent transmission of HIV infection;

52. By 2005, ensure: that a wide range of prevention programmes which take account of local circumstances, ethics and cultural values, is available in all countries, particularly the most affected countries, including information, education and communication, in languages most understood by communities and respectful of cultures, aimed at reducing risk-taking behaviour and encouraging responsible sexual behaviour, including abstinence and fidelity; expanded access to essential commodities, including male and female condoms and sterile injecting equipment; harm reduction efforts related to drug use; expanded access to voluntary and confidential counselling and testing; safe blood supplies; and early and effective treatment of sexually transmittable infections;

53. By 2005, ensure that at least 90 per cent, and by 2010 at least 95 per cent of young men and women aged 15 to 24 have access to the information, education, including peer education and youth- specific HIV education, and services necessary to develop the life skills required to reduce their vulnerability to HIV infection; in full partnership with youth, parents, families, educators and health-care providers;

54. By 2005, reduce the proportion of infants infected with HIV by 20 per cent, and by 50 per cent by 2010, by: ensuring that 80 per cent of pregnant women accessing antenatal care have information, counselling and other HIV prevention services available to them, in the availability of and by providing access for HIV-infected women and babies to effective treatment to reduce mother-to-child transmission of HIV, as well as through effective interventions for HIV-infected women, including voluntary and confidential counselling and testing, access to treatment, especially anti-retroviral therapy and, where appropriate, breast milk substitutes and the provision of a continuum of care;

Care, support and treatment

Care, support and treatment are fundamental elements of an effective response

55. By 2003, ensure that national strategies, supported by regional and international strategies, are developed in close collaboration with the international community, including Governments and relevant intergovernmental organizations as well as with civil society and the business sector, to strengthen health care systems and address factors affecting the provision of HIV-

related drugs, including anti-retroviral drugs, inter alia affordability and pricing, including differential pricing, and technical and health care systems capacity. Also, in an urgent manner make every effort to: provide progressively and in a sustainable manner, the highest attainable standard of treatment for HIV/AIDS, including the prevention and treatment of opportunistic infections, and effective use of quality-controlled anti-retroviral therapy in a careful and monitored manner to improve adherence and effectiveness and reduce the risk of developing resistance; to cooperate constructively in strengthening pharmaceutical policies and practices, including those applicable to generic drugs and intellectual property regimes, in order further to promote innovation and the development of domestic industries consistent with international law;

56.   By 2005, develop and make significant progress in implementing comprehensive care strategies to: strengthen family and community-based care including that provided by the informal sector, and health care systems to provide and monitor treatment to people living with HIV/AIDS including infected children, and to support individuals, households, families and communities affected by HIV/AIDS; improve the capacity and working conditions of health care personnel, and the effectiveness of supply systems, financing plans and referral mechanisms required to provide access to affordable medicines, including anti-retroviral drugs, diagnostics and related technologies, as well as quality medical, palliative and psycho social care;

57.   By 2003, ensure that national strategies are developed in order to provide psycho-social care for individuals, families, and communities affected by HIV/AIDS;

HIV/AIDS and human rights

Realization of human rights and fundamental freedoms for all is essential to reduce vulnerability to HIV/AIDS

Respect for the rights of people living with HIV/AIDS drives an effective response

58.   By 2003, enact, strengthen or enforce as appropriate legislation, regulations and other measures to eliminate all forms of discrimination against, and to ensure the full enjoyment of all human rights and fundamental freedoms by people living with HIV/AIDS and members of vulnerable groups; in particular to ensure their access to, inter alia education, inheritance, employment, health care, social and health services, prevention, support, treatment, information and legal protection, while respecting their privacy and confidentiality; and develop strategies to combat sigma and social exclusion connected with the epidemic;

59.   By 2005, bearing in mind the context and character of the epidemic and that globally women and girls are disproportionately affected by HIV/AIDS, develop and accelerate the implementation of national strategies that: promote the advancement of women and women's full enjoyment of all human rights; promote shared responsibility of men and women to ensure safe sex; empower women to have control over and decide freely and responsibly on matters related to their sexuality to increase their ability to protect themselves from HIV infection;

60.   By 2005, implement measures to increase capacities of women and adolescent girls to protect themselves from the risk of HIV infection, principally through the provision of health care and health services, including sexual and reproductive health, and through prevention education that promotes gender equality within a culturally and gender sensitive framework;

61.   By 2005, ensure development and accelerated implementation of national strategies for women's empowerment, promotion and protection of women's full enjoyment of all human rights and reduction of their vulnerability to HIV/AIDS through the elimination of all forms of

discrimination, as well as all forms of violence against women and girls, including harmful traditional and customary practices, abuse, rape and other forms of sexual violence, battering and trafficking in women and girls;

Reducing vulnerability

The vulnerable must be given priority in the response

Empowering women is essential for reducing vulnerability

62. By 2003, in order to complement prevention programmes that address activities which place individuals at risk of HIV infection, such as risky and unsafe sexual behaviour and injecting drug use, have in place in all countries strategies, policies and programmes that identify and begin to address those factors that make individuals particularly vulnerable to HIV infection, including underdevelopment, economic insecurity, poverty, lack of empowerment of women, lack of education, social exclusion, illiteracy, discrimination, lack of information and/or commodities for self-protection, all types of sexual exploitation of women, girls and boys, including for commercial reasons; such strategies, policies and programmes should address the gender dimension of the epidemic, specify the action that will be taken to address vulnerability and set targets for achievement;

63. By 2003, develop and/or strengthen strategies, policies and programmes, which recognize the importance of the family in reducing vulnerability, inter alia, in educating and guiding children and take account of cultural, religious and ethical factors, to reduce the vulnerability of children and young people by: ensuring access of both girls and boys to primary and secondary education, including on HIV/AIDS in curricula for adolescents; ensuring safe and secure environments, especially for young girls; expanding good quality youth-friendly information and sexual health education and counselling service; strengthening reproductive and sexual health programmes; and involving families and young people in planning, implementing and evaluating HIV/AIDS prevention and care programmes, to the extent possible;

64. By 2003, develop and/or strengthen national strategies, policies and programmes, supported by regional and international initiatives, as appropriate, through a participatory approach, to promote and protect the health of those identifiable groups which currently have high or increasing rates of HIV infection or which public health information indicates are at greatest risk of and most vulnerable to new infection as indicated by such factors as the local history of the epidemic, poverty, sexual practices, drug using behaviour, livelihood, institutional location, disrupted social structures and population movements forced or otherwise;

Children orphaned and made vulnerable by HIV/AIDS

Children orphaned and affected by HIV/AIDS need special assistance

65. By 2003, develop and by 2005 implement national policies and strategies to: build and strengthen governmental, family and community capacities to provide a supportive environment for orphans and girls and boys infected and affected by HIV/AIDS including by providing appropriate counselling and psych-social support; ensuring their enrolment in school and access to shelter, good nutrition, health and social services on an equal basis with other children; to protect orphans and vulnerable children from all forms of abuse, violence, exploitation, discrimination, trafficking and loss of inheritance;

66. Ensure non-discrimination and full and equal enjoyment of all human rights through the promotion of an active and visible policy of de-stigmatisation of children orphaned and made vulnerable by HIV/AIDS.

67. Urge the international community, particularly donor countries, civil society, as well as the private sector to complement effectively national programmes to support programmes for children orphaned or made vulnerable by HIV/AIDS in affected regions, in countries at high risk and to direct special assistance to sub-Saharan Africa;

Alleviating social and economic impact

To address HIV/AIDS is to invest in sustainable development

68. By 2003, evaluate the economic and social impact of the HIV/AIDS epidemic and develop multisectoral strategies to: address the impact at the individual, family, community and national levels; develop and accelerate the implementation of national poverty eradication strategies to address the impact of HIV/AIDS on household income, livelihoods, and access to basic social services, with special focus on individuals, families and communities severely affected by the epidemic; review the social and economic impact of HIV/AIDS at all levels of society especially on women and the elderly, particularly in their role as caregivers and in families affected by HIV/AIDS and address their special needs adjust and adapt economic and social development policies, including social protection policies, to address the impact of HIV/AIDS on economic growth, provision of essential economic services, labour productivity, government revenues, and deficit-creating pressures on public resources;

69. By 2003, develop a national legal and policy framework that protects in the workplace the rights and dignity of persons living with and affected by HIV/AIDS and those at the greatest risk of HIV/AIDS in consultation with representatives of employers and workers, taking account of established international guidelines on HIV/AIDS in the workplace;

Research and development

With no cure for HIV/AIDS yet found, further research and development is crucial

70. Increase investment and accelerate research on the development of HIV vaccines, while building national research capacity especially in developing countries, and especially for viral strains prevalent in highly affected regions; in addition, support and encourage increased national and international investment in HIV/AIDS-related research and development including biomedical, operations, social, cultural and behavioural research and in traditional medicine to: improve prevention and therapeutic approaches; accelerate access to prevention, care and treatment and care technologies for HIV/AIDS (and its associated opportunistic infections and malignancies and sexually transmitted diseases), including female controlled methods and microbicides, and in particular, appropriate, safe and affordable HIV vaccines and their delivery, and to diagnostics, tests, methods to prevent mother-to child transmission; and improve our understanding of factors which influence the epidemic and actions which address it, inter alia, through increased funding and public/private partnerships; create a conducive environment for research and ensure that it is based on highest ethical standards;

71. Support and encourage the development of national research infrastructure, laboratory capacity, improved surveillance systems, data collection, processing and dissemination, and training of basic and clinical researchers, social scientists, health-care providers and technicians, with a focus on the countries most affected by HIV/AIDS, particularly developing countries and those countries experiencing or at risk of rapid expansion of the epidemic;

72. Develop and evaluate suitable approaches for monitoring treatment efficacy, toxicity, side effect, drug interactions, and drug resistance, develop methodologies to monitor the impact of treatment on HIV transmission and risk behaviours;

73. Strengthen international and regional cooperation in particular North/South, South/South and triangular cooperation related to transfer of relevant technologies, suitable to the environment in prevention and care of HIV/AIDS, the exchange of experiences and best practices, researchers and research findings and strengthen the role of UNAIDS in this process. In this context, encourage that the end results of these cooperative research findings and technologies be owned by all parties to the research, reflecting their relevant contribution and dependent upon their providing legal protection to such findings; and affirm that all such research should be free from bias;

74. By 2003, ensure that all research protocols for the investigation of HIV-related treatment including anti-retroviral therapies and vaccines based on international guidelines and best practices are evaluated by independent committees of ethics, in which persons living with HIV/AIDS and caregivers for anti-retroviral therapy participate;

HIV/AIDS in conflict and disaster affected regions

Conflicts and disasters contribute to the spread of HIV/AIDS

75. By 2003, develop and begin to implement national strategies that incorporate HIV/AIDS awareness, prevention, care and treatment elements into programmes or actions that respond to emergency situations, recognizing that populations destabilized by armed conflict, humanitarian emergencies and natural disasters, including refugees, internally displaced persons and in particular, women and children, are at increased risk of exposure to HIV infection; and, where appropriate, factor HIV/AIDS components into international assistance programmes;

76. Call on all United Nations agencies, regional and international organizations, as well as non-governmental organizations involved with the provision and delivery of international assistance to countries and regions affected by conflicts, humanitarian crises or natural disasters, to incorporate as a matter of urgency HIV/AIDS prevention, care and awareness elements into their plans and programmes and provide HIV/AIDS awareness and training to their personnel;

77. By 2003, have in place national strategies to address the spread of HIV among national uniformed services, where this is required, including armed forces and civil defence force and consider ways of using personnel from these services who are educated and trained in HIV/AIDS awareness and prevention to assist with HIV/AIDS awareness and prevention activities including participation in emergency, humanitarian, disaster relief and rehabilitation assistance;

78. By 2003, ensure the inclusion of HIV/AIDS awareness and training, including a gender component, into guidelines designed for use by defence personnel and other personnel involved in international peacekeeping operations while also continuing with ongoing education and prevention efforts, including pre deployment orientation, for these personnel;

Resources

The HIV/AIDS challenge cannot be met without new, additional and sustained resources

79. Ensure that the resources provided for the global response to address HIV/AIDS are substantial, sustained and geared towards achieving results;

80. By 2005, through a series of incremental steps, reach an overall target of annual expenditure on the epidemic of between US$ 7 billion in low and middle-income countries and those countries experiencing or at risk of experiencing rapid expansion for prevention, care,

treatment, support and mitigation of the impact of HIV/AIDS, and take measures to ensure that needed resources are made available, particularly from donor countries and also from national budgets, bearing in mind that resources of the most affected countries are seriously limited;

81. Call on the international community, where possible, to provide assistance for HIV/AIDS prevention, care and treatment in developing countries on a grant basis;

82. Increase and prioritise national budgetary allocations for HIV/AIDS programmes as required and ensure that adequate allocations are made by all ministries and other relevant stakeholders;

83. Urge the developed countries that have not done so to strive to meet the targets of 0.7 per cent of their gross national product for overall official development assistance and the targets of earmarking of 0.15 per cent to 0.20 per cent of gross national product as official development assistance for least developed countries as agreed, as soon as possible, taking into account the urgency and gravity of the HIV/AIDS epidemic;

84. Urge the international community to complement and supplement efforts of developing countries that commit increased national funds to fight the HIV/AIDS epidemic through increased international development assistance, particularly those countries most affected by HIV/AIDS, particularly in Africa, especially in sub-Saharan Africa, the Caribbean, countries at high risk of expansion of the HIV/AIDS epidemic and other affected regions whose resources to deal with the epidemic are seriously limited;

85. Integrate HIV/AIDS actions in development assistance programmes and poverty eradication strategies as appropriate and encourage the most effective and transparent use of all resources allocated;

86. Call on the international community and invite civil society and the private sector to take appropriate measures to help alleviate the social and economic impact of HIV/AIDS in the most affected developing countries;

87. Without further delay implement the enhanced Heavily Indebted Poor Country (HIPC) Initiative and agree to cancel all bilateral official debts of HIPC countries as soon as possible, especially those most affected by HIV/AIDS, in return for their making demonstrable commitments to poverty eradication and urge the use of debt service savings to finance poverty eradication programmes, particularly for HIV/AIDS prevention, treatment, care and support and other infections;

88. Call for speedy and concerted action to address effectively the debt problems of least developed countries, low-income developing countries, and middle-income developing countries, particularly those affected by HIV/AIDS, in a comprehensive, equitable, development-oriented and durable way through various national and international measures designed to make their debt sustainable in the long term and thereby to improve their capacity to deal with the HIV/AIDS epidemic, including, as appropriate, existing orderly mechanisms for debt reduction, such as debt swaps for projects aimed at the prevention, care and treatment of HIV/AIDS;

89. Encourage increased investment in HIV/AIDS-related research, nationally, regionally and internationally, in particular for the development of sustainable and affordable prevention technologies, such as vaccines and microbicides, and encourage the proactive preparation of financial and logistic plans to facilitate rapid access to vaccines when they become available;

90. Support the establishment, on an urgent basis, of a global HIV/AIDS and health fund to finance an urgent and expanded response to the epidemic based on an integrated approach to prevention, care, support and treatment and to assist Governments inter alia in their efforts to combat HIV/AIDS with due priority to the most affected countries, notably in sub Saharan Africa and the Caribbean and to those countries at high risk, mobilize contributions to the fund from public and private sources with a special appeal to donor countries, foundations, the business community including pharmaceutical companies, the private sector, philanthropists and wealthy individuals;

91. By 2002, launch a worldwide fund-raising campaign aimed at the general public as well as the private sector, conducted by UNAIDS with the support and collaboration of interested partners at all levels, to contribute to the global HIV/AIDS and health fund;

92. Direct increased funding to national, regional and subregional commissions and organizations to enable them to assist Governments at the national, subregional and regional level in their efforts to respond to the crisis;

93. Provide the UNAIDS co-sponsoring agencies and the UNAIDS secretariat with the resources needed to work with countries in support of the goals of this Declaration;

Follow-up

Maintaining the momentum and monitoring progress are essential at the national level

94. Conduct national periodic reviews involving the participation of civil society, particularly people living with HIV/AIDS, vulnerable groups and caregivers, of progress achieved in realizing these commitments and identify problems and obstacles to achieving progress and ensure wide dissemination of the results of these reviews;

95. Develop appropriate monitoring and evaluation mechanisms to assist with follow-up in measuring and assessing progress, develop appropriate monitoring and evaluation instruments, with adequate epidemiological data;

96. By 2003, establish or strengthen effective monitoring systems, where appropriate, for the promotion and protection of human rights of people living with HIV/AIDS;

At the regional level

97. Include HIV/AIDS and related public health concerns as appropriate on the agenda of regional meetings at the ministerial and Head of State and Government level;

98. Support data collection and processing to facilitate periodic reviews by regional commissions and/or regional organizations of progress in implementing regional strategies and addressing regional priorities and ensure wide dissemination of the results of these reviews;

99. Encourage the exchange between countries of information and experiences in implementing the measures and commitments contained in this Declaration, and in particular facilitate intensified South-South and triangular cooperation;

At the global level

100. Devote sufficient time and at least one full day of the annual General Assembly session to review and debate a report of the Secretary-General on progress achieved in realizing the commitments set out in this Declaration, with a view to identifying problems and constraints and making recommendations on action needed to make further progress;

101. Ensure that HIV/AIDS issues are included on the agenda of all appropriate United Nations conferences and meetings;

102. Support initiatives to convene conferences, seminars, workshops, training programmes and courses to follow up issues raised in this Declaration and in this regard encourage participation in and wide dissemination of the outcomes of: the forthcoming Dakar Conference on Access to Care for HIV Infection; the Sixth International Congress on AIDS in Asia and the Pacific; the XI International Conference on AIDS and Sexually Transmitted Infections in Africa; the XIV International Conference on AIDS, Barcelona; the Xth International Conference on People Living with HIV/AIDS, Port of Spain; the II Forum and III Conference of the Latin American and the Caribbean Horizontal Technical Cooperation on HIV/AIDS and Sexually Transmitted Infections, Loa Habana; the Vth International Conference on Home and Community Care for Persons Living with HIV/AIDS, Changmai, Thailand;

103. Explore, with a view to improving equity in access to essential drugs, the feasibility of developing and implementing, in collaboration with non-governmental organizations and other concerned partners, systems for voluntary monitoring and reporting of global drug prices;

We recognize and express our appreciation to those who have led the effort to raise awareness of the HIV/AIDS epidemic and to deal with its complex challenges;

We look forward to strong leadership by Governments, and concerted efforts with full and active participation of the United Nations, the entire multilateral system, civil society, the business community and private sector

And finally, we call on all countries to take the necessary steps to implement this Declaration, in strengthened partnership and cooperation with other multilateral and bilateral partners and with civil society.

Conclusion

It is hoped by the United Nations that a whole-hearted implementation of the Declaration by all nations will lead to better prevention and reduction of HIV/AIDS infections and related deaths.

Self-Assessment Questions

1.   *Why do you think a Universal Declaration of Commitment on HIV/AIDS was needed?*

2.   *"Global Emergency" is one of the phrases used when describing the impact of HIV/AIDS. How accurate do you think this phrase is? Do you think the emergency will get worse? Give reasons for your answer.*

3.   *In your opinion, how likely is it that the broad aims of the Declaration will be achieved. Explain your reasoning.*

Chapter 23

Abuja Declaration on HIV/AIDS, Tuberculosis & Other Related Infectious Diseases

Contents of this Chapter

1. Introduction
2. The Declaration – Recognition of the Problem
3. Declaration: Expression of Commitment
4. Conclusion
5. Self-Assessment Questions

1. Introduction

There are now several regional declarations on HIV/AIDS prevention. However, the Abuja Declaration by African leaders deserves particular attention because of the disproportionate impact HIV/AIDS has had on Africa.

The catastrophe that HIV/AIDS is unleashing to the world particularly to Africa pulled African leaders to Abuja, the Nigerian capital in April 2001 to formally recognise the problem and to make firm commitment to fight HIV/AIDS and other related infectious diseases.

Thus, in the presence of the UN Secretary General Kofi Annan, former US presidents Jimmy Carter and Bill Clinton and several other international figures, the African leaders made the Abuja declaration as shown below.

2. The Declaration – Recognition of the Problem

We, the Heads of State and Government of the Organisation of African Unity (OAU) met in Abuja, Nigeria from 26-27 April 2001, at a Special Summit devoted specifically to address the exceptional challenges of HIV/AIDS, Tuberculosis and Other Related Infectious Diseases, at the invitation of H.E. Present Olusegun Obasanjo of the Federal Republic of Nigeria and in accordance with the agreement reached at the Thirty-Sixth Ordinary Session of our Assembly in Lome, Togo from 10 to 12 July 2000.

2. We gathered in Abuja to undertake a critical review and assessment of the situation and the consequences of these diseases in Africa, and to reflect further on new ways and means whereby we, the leaders of our Continent, can take the lead in strengthening current successful interventions and developing new and more appropriate policies, practical strategies, effective implementation mechanisms and concrete monitoring structures at national, regional and continental levels with a view to ensuring adequate and effective control of HIV/AIDS, Tuberculosis and Other Related Infectious Diseases in our Continent.

3. We are deeply concerned about the rapid spread of HIV infection in our countries and the millions of deaths caused by AIDS, Tuberculosis and other related infectious diseases throughout the Continent, in spite of the serious efforts being made by our countries to control these diseases. Africa is exceptionally afflicted by the HIV/AIDS epidemic. This generalised epidemic is affecting a wide cross-section of our people, thus decimating the adult population, the most productive group, and leaving in its wake millions of orphans, and disrupted family structures.

4. We recognize the role played by poverty, poor nutritional conditions and underdevelopment in increasing vulnerability. We are concerned about the millions of African children who have died from AIDS and other preventable infectious diseases. We are equally concerned about the particular and severe impact that these diseases have on children and youth who represent the future of our continent, the plight of millions of children orphaned by AIDS and the impact on the social system in our countries.

5. We are particularly concerned about the high incidence of mother to child transmission, especially given the challenges of infant breastfeeding in the context of HIV infection on the continent.

6. We recognize that special efforts are required to ensure that Africa's children are protected from these pandemics and their consequences and that the full and effective participation of young people in prevention and control programmes is essential to their success.

7. We recognise that biologically, women and girls are particularly vulnerable to HIV infection. In addition, economic and social inequalities and traditionally accepted gender roles leave them in a subordinate position to men.

8. We appreciate the special needs and challenges of the HIV/AIDS pandemic for the youth that make them vulnerable to infection and adverse impacts of the epidemic.

9. We recognise that the practice of injectable drug abuse with sharing of contaminated needles in some African countries is a major concern. The abuse of alcohol, marijuana and other mind-altering drugs, which is on the increase among the youth further enhances their vulnerability to HIV infection.

10. We recognise the essential place that education, in its widest sense has played and will continue to play in the fight against HIV/AIDS in Africa. Education constitutes the most powerful, cost effective tool for reaching the largest number of people with information and personal development strategies that promote long-term behaviour change.

11. We acknowledge that forced migrations due to war, conflicts, natural disasters and economic factors including unilateral sanctions imposed on some African countries, lead to an increased vulnerability and the spread of the disease; we note that special attention should be given to the problem trafficking in human beings and its impact on HIV/AIDS.

12. We are aware that stigma, silence, denial and discrimination against people living with HIV/AIDS (PLWA) increase the impact of the epidemic and constitute a major barrier to an effective response to it. We recognise the importance of greater involvement of people living with HIV/AIDS.

13. We recognise that the epidemic of HIV/AIDS, Tuberculosis and other related infectious diseases, constitute not only a major health crisis, but also an exceptional threat to Africa's development, social cohesion, political stability, food security as well as the greatest global threat to the survival and life expectancy of African peoples. These diseases, which are themselves exacerbated by poverty and conflict situations in our continent, also entail a devastating economic burden, through the loss of human capital, reduced productivity and the diversion of human and financial resources to care and treatment.

14. We recognise the need to intensify our efforts in all areas of research such as traditional medicines and vaccine development.

15. We are fully convinced that containing and reversing the HIV/AIDS epidemic, tuberculosis and other infectious diseases should constitute our top priority for the first quarter of the 21st century. We are equally convinced that tackling these epidemics should constitute an integral part of our continental agenda for promoting poverty reduction, sustainable development and ensuring durable peace and political security and stability consistent with the Millennium African Recovery Programme.

16. We recognise and commend the efforts by our respective national Governments, our Continental Organisation and its Regional Economic Communities (REC), the national and international NGOs, the civil society, including youth, women, people with disability, religious organisations, sport organizations, Trade Unions, Employers organizations, Traditional Health Practitioners, Traditional Rulers, people living with HIV/AIDS and individuals, who care for, support and sensitise our people to the threat of HIV/AIDS and the associated opportunistic infections including Sexually Transmitted Infections (STIs).

17. We acknowledge the support that the International Community, including the United Nations System, its Specialised Agencies and programmes, bilateral agencies, private sector and other communities and stakeholders have provided in raising awareness about and combating the scourge of HIV/AIDS, Tuberculosis and Other Related Infectious Diseases in Africa.

18. We further acknowledge that, to successfully implement a comprehensive and multisectoral approach and campaign to overcome HIV/AIDS, Tuberculosis and other related infectious thee is a need to secure adequate financial and human resources at national and international levels.

19. We recognise the need to establish a sustainable source of income to fund HIV/AIDS programmes.

20. We recognise the importance of leadership at all levels in the fight against HIV/AIDS, Tuberculosis and Other Related Infectious Diseases in our continent. We, therefore, acknowledge the special importance of the "African Consensus and Plan of Action: Leadership to overcome HIV/AIDS" adopted at the African Development Forum 2000 as the outcome of a wide-ranging process of consultation with all stakeholders.

21. In this regard, we recall and reaffirm our commitment to all relevant decisions, declarations and resolutions in the area of health and development and on HIV/AIDS, particularly the "Lome Declaration on HIV/AIDS in Africa" (July 2000) and the "Decision on the adoption of the International Partnership against HIV/AIDS" (Algiers 1999).

22. We consider AIDS as a State of Emergency in the continent. To this end, all tariff and economic barriers to access to funding of AIDS related activities should be lifted.

3. Declaration: Expression of Commitment

23. To place the fight against HIV/AIDS at the forefront and as the highest priority issue in our respective national development plans. To that end, **WE ARE RESOLVED** to consolidate the foundations for the prevention and control of the scourge of HIV/AIDS, Tuberculosis and Other Related Infectious Diseases through a comprehensive multisectoral strategy which involves all appropriate development sectors of our governments as well as a broad mobilisation of our societies at all levels, including community level organisations, civil society, NGOs, the private sector, trade unions, the media, religious organisations, schools, youth organisations, women organisations, people living with HIV/AIDS organisations and individuals who care for, support and sensitise our population to the threat of HIV/AIDS and associated opportunistic infections and also to protect those not yet infected, particularly the women, children and youth through appropriate and effective prevention programmes.

24. To that effect, **WE COMMIT OURSELVES TO TAKE PERSONAL RESPONSIBILITY AND PROVIDE LEADERSHIP** for the activities of the National **AIDS** commissions/Councils. **WE THEREFORE RESOLVE** to lead from the front the battle against HIV/AIDS, Tuberculosis and Other Related Infectious Diseases by personally ensuring that such bodies were properly convened in   mobilizing our societies as a whole and providing focus for unified national policy-making and programme implementation, ensuring coordination of all sectors at all levels with a gender perspective and respect for human rights, particularly to ensure equal rights for people living with HIV/AIDS (PLWA).

25. **WE ALSO COMMIT OURSELVES TO ENSURE** that leadership role is exercised by everyone in his/her area of responsibility in the fight against HIV/AIDS and Other Related Diseases. **WE THEREFORE ENDORSE** "African Consensus and Plan of Action: Leadership to overcome HIV/AIDS" adopted during the Second African Development Forum on "AIDS: The Greatest Leadership Challenge" organised by the United Nations Economic Commission for Africa (UNECA) in collaboration with the OAU, UNAIDS and ILO (Addis Ababa, 3-7 December 2000).

26. **WE COMMIT OURSELVES** to take all necessary measures to ensure that the needed resources are made available from all sources and that they are efficiently and effectively utilised. In addition, **WE PLEDGE** to set a target of allocating at least 15% of our annual budget to the improvement of the health sector. **WE ALSO PLEDGE** to make available the necessary resources for the improvement of the comprehensive multi-sectoral response, and that an appropriate and adequate portion of this amount is put at the disposal of the National Commissions/Councils for the fight against HIV/AIDS, Tuberculosis and Other Related Infectious Diseases.

27. **WE REQUEST** the OAU Secretariat, in collaboration with ADB, ECA, and all other partner institutions, especially WHO AND UNAIDS, to assist member States in formulating a continental-wide policy for an international assistance strategy for the mobilisation of additional financial resources.

28. **WE CALL UPON** Donor countries to complement our resources mobilisation efforts to fight the scourge of HIV/AIDS, Tuberculosis and Other Related Infectious Diseases. Bearing in mind that Africa cannot, from its weak resource base, provide the huge financial resources needed. In this regard, **WE URGE** those countries to, among others, fulfil the yet to be met target of 0.7% of their GNP as Official Development Assistance (ODA) to developing countries.

29. We support the creation of a Global AIDS Fund capitalised by the donor community to the tune of US $5 – 10 billion accessible to all affected countries to enhance operationalisation of Action Plans, including accessing Anti-retroviral programmes in favour of the populations of Africa.

30. **WE UNDERTAKE** to mobilise all the human, material and financial resources required to provide **CARE** and **SUPPORT** and quality treatment to our populations infected with HIV/AIDS, Tuberculosis

and Other Related Infections, and to organise meetings to evaluate the status of implementation of the objective of access to care.

31. **WE RESOLVE** to enact and utilise appropriate legislation and international trade regulations to ensure the availability of drugs at affordable prices and technologies for treatment, care and prevention of HIV/AIDS, Tuberculosis and Other Infectious Diseases. **WE ALSO RESOLVE** to take immediate action to use tax exemption and other incentives to reduce the prices of drugs and all other inputs in health care services for accelerated improvement of the health of our populations.

32. **WE COMMIT OURSELVES** to explore and further develop the potential of traditional medicine and traditional health practitioners in the prevention, care and management of HIV/AIDS, Tuberculosis and Other Related Infectious Diseases.

33. **WE COMMIT OURSELVES** to support the development of effective affordable, accessible HIV vaccine relevant to Africa. We, therefore, support "The Africa; AIDS Vaccine Programme" (AAVO), its collaborative partners, International partners and Institutions committed to the facilitation of HIV vaccine research and testing in Africa.

34. **WE COMMIT OURSELVES** to documenting and sharing these successful and positive experiences with a view to sustaining and scaling them up for wider coverage; mindful that there are still challenges that confront us, particularly in the area of infant feeding.

35. **WE COMMIT OURSELVES** to scaling up the role of education and information in the fight against HIV/AIDS in recognition of the essential role education, in its widest sense plays as a cost-effective tool for reaching the largest number of people.

36. **WE COMMIT OURSELVES** to the strengthening and development of special youth programmes to ensure an AIDS-free generation.

37. **WE,** within the framework and spirit of our Sirte Declaration of 9 September 1999, **RENEW THE MANDATE** of our brothers, President Bouteflika of Algeria, President Mbeki of South Africa and President Obasanjo of Nigeria to continue discussion with our debt creditors, on our behalf, with the view to securing the total cancellation of Africa's external debt in favour of increased investment in the social sector.

38. **WE ENDORSE** the Abuja Declaration on HIV/AIDS, Tuberculosis and Other Related Infectious Diseases; and **WE PLEDGE** to promote advocacy at the national, regional and international levels; and **WE ALSO PLEDGE** to ensure massive participation of Heads of State and Government at the United Nations General Assembly Special Session (UNGASS) on HIV/AIDS slated for 25-27 June 2001 so as to ensure that the session comes up with concrete and urgent decisions for the fight against HIV/AIDS in Africa including the fight against poverty and deduction of Africa's debt.

39. **WE REQUEST** the OAU Secretary General, in collaboration with ECA, ADB, UNAIDS, WHO, UNICEF, UNDP, ILO, UNFPA, FAO, UNESCO, UNIFEM, IOM, UNDCP and other partners, to follow up on the implementation of the outcome of this Summit and submit a report to the Ordinary Sessions of our Assembly.

40. **WE MANDATE** the Government of the Federal Republic of Nigeria to submit a report on the outcome of this African Summit on HIV/AIDS, Tuberculosis and Other Related Infectious Diseases to the next Ordinary OAU Summit, which will be held in Lusaka, Zambia in July 2001.

Conclusion

While this is a very laudable effort, the question everyone seems to be asking is: Will all the leaders be totally committed to making the provisions of the declaration a reality? Only time will tell.

Self-Assessment Questions

1. *Do you think leaders have the will power and commitment to implement the provisions of The Declaration? Give full reasoning for your answer.*

Chapter 24

Elimination Of Discrimination Against Women

Contents of this Chapter

1. **Overview**
2. **Introduction**
3. **The Preamble**
4. **The Convention**
5. **Conclusion**
6. **Self-Assessment Questions**

1. Introduction

Women are victims of discrimination in every part of the world, but this is particularly worse in developing countries where women, in some countries can only be seen in the shadow of men, with no proper rights in their own right.

In the developing world, women are disproportionally affected by the HIV/AIDS epidemic as they are more prone to infection.

Part of the problem is caused by the fact that in many countries, women are discriminated against and have very low social, educational and economic status, therefore are heavily dependent on men.

Thus, the men have the final say in almost all areas of human endeavour including matters relating to sex. This economic dependency drives some women to engage in sexual activities that they would otherwise not engage in, thereby, compounding the problem of HIV transmission.

This Convention on the Elimination of all forms of Discrimination Against Women was adopted by the United Nations to bring to an end discrimination against women and to give them equal status alongside men.

On 18 December 1979, the Convention on the Elimination of All Forms of Discrimination against Women was adopted by the United Nations General Assembly. It entered into force as an international treaty on 3 September 1981 after the twentieth country had ratified it. By the tenth anniversary of the Convention in 1989, almost one hundred nations have agreed to be bound by its provisions.

2. *The Preamble*

The States Parties to the present Convention,

Noting that the Charter of the United Nations reaffirms faith in fundamental human rights, in the dignity and worth of the human person and in the equal rights of man and women,

Noting that the Universal Declaration of Human Rights affirms the principle of the inadmissibility of discrimination and proclaims that all human beings are born free and equal in dignity and rights and that everyone is entitled to all the rights and freedoms set forth therein, without distinction of any kind, including distinction based on sex,

Noting that the States Parties to the International Covenants on Human Rights have the obligation to ensure the equal right of men and women to enjoy all economic, social, cultural, civil and political rights,

Considering the international conventions concluded under the auspices of the United Nations and the specialized agencies promoting equality of rights of men and women,

Noting also the resolutions, declarations and recommendations adopted by the United Nations and the specialized agencies promoting equality of rights of men and women,

Concerned, however, that despite these various instruments extensive discrimination against women continues to exist,

Recalling that discrimination against women violates the principles of equality of rights and respect for human dignity, is an obstacle to the participation of women, on equal terms with men, in the political, social, economic and cultural life of their countries, hampers the growth of the prosperity of society and the family and makes more difficult the full development of the potentialities of women in the service of their countries and of humanity,

Concerned that in situations of poverty women have the least access to food, health, education, training and opportunities for employment and other needs,

Convinced that the establishment of the new international economic order based on equity and justice will contribute significantly towards the promotion of equality between men and women,

Emphasizing that the eradication of apartheid, of all forms of racism, racial discrimination, colonialism, neo-colonialism, aggression, foreign occupation and domination and interference in the internal affairs of States is essential to the full enjoyment of the rights of men and women,

Affirming that the strengthening of international peace and security, relaxation of international tension, mutual co-operation among all States irrespective of their social and economic systems, general and complete disarmament, and in particular nuclear disarmament under strict and effective international control, the affirmation of the principles of justice, equality and mutual benefit in relations among countries and the realization of the right of peoples under alien and colonial domination and foreign occupation to self-determination and independence, as well as respect for national sovereignty and territorial integrity, will promote social progress and development and as a consequence will contribute to the attainment of full equality between men and women,

Convinced that the full and complete development of a country, the welfare of the world and the cause of peace require the maximum participation of women on equal terms with men in all fields,

Bearing in mind the great contribution of women to the welfare of the family and to the development of society, so far not fully recognized, the social significance of maternity and the role of both parents in the family and in the upbringing of children, and aware that the role of women in procreation should not be a basis for discrimination but that the upbringing of children requires a sharing of responsibility between men and women and society as a whole,

Aware that a change in the traditional role of men as well as the role of women in society and in the family is needed to achieve full equality between men and women,

Determined to implement the principles set forth in the Declaration on the Elimination of Discrimination against Women and, for that purpose, to adopt the measures required for the elimination of such discrimination in all its forms and manifestations,

3. The Articles

Have agreed on the following:

PART I

Article 1

For the purposes of the present Convention, the term "discrimination against women" shall mean any distinction, exclusion or restriction made on the basis of sex which has the effect or purpose of impairing or nullifying the recognition, enjoyment or exercise by women irrespective of their marital status, on a basis of equality of men and women, of human rights and fundamental freedoms in the political, economic, social, cultural, civil or any other field.

Article 2

States Parties condemn discrimination against women in all its forms, agree to pursue by all appropriate means and without delay a policy of eliminating discrimination against women and, to this end, undertake:

(a) To embody the principle of the equality of men and women in their national constitutions or other appropriate legislation if not yet incorporated therein and to ensure, through law and other appropriate means, the practical realization of this principle;

(b) To adopt appropriate legislative and other measures, including sanctions where appropriate, prohibiting all discrimination against women;

(c) To establish legal protection of the rights of women on an equal basis with men and to ensure through competent national tribunals and other public institutions the effective protection of women against any act of discrimination;

(d)　To refrain from engaging in any act or practice of discrimination against women and to ensure that public authorities and institutions shall act in conformity with this obligation;

(e)　To take all appropriate measures to eliminate discrimination against women by any person, organization or enterprise;

(f)　To take all appropriate measures, including legislation, to modify or abolish existing laws, regulations, customs and practices which constitute discrimination against women;

(g)　To repeal all national penal provisions which constitute discrimination against women.

Article 3

States Parties shall take in all fields, in particular in the political, social, economic and cultural fields, all appropriate measures, including legislation, to ensure the full development and advancement of women, for the purpose of guaranteeing them the exercise and enjoyment of human rights and fundamental freedoms on a basis of equality with men.

Article 4

1. Adoption by States Parties of temporary special measures aimed at accelerating de facto equality between men and women shall not be considered discrimination as defined in the present Convention, but shall in no way entail as a consequence the maintenance of unequal or separate standards; these measures shall be discontinued when the objectives of equality of opportunity and treatment have been achieved.

2. Adoption by States Parties of special measures, including those measures contained in the present Convention, aimed at protecting maternity shall not be considered discriminatory.

Article 5

States Parties shall take all appropriate measures:

(a)　To modify the social and cultural patterns of conduct of men and women, with a view to achieving the elimination of prejudices and customary and all other practices which are based on the idea of the inferiority or the superiority of either of the sexes or on stereotyped roles for men and women;

(b)　To ensure that family education includes a proper understanding of maternity as a social function and the recognition of the common responsibility of men and women in the upbringing and development of their children, it being understood that the interest of the children is the primordial consideration in all cases.

Article 6

States Parties shall take all appropriate measures, including legislation, to suppress all forms of traffic in women and exploitation of prostitution of women.

PART II

Article 7

States Parties shall take all appropriate measures to eliminate discrimination against women in the political and public life of the country and, in particular, shall ensure to women, on equal terms with men, the right:

(a)   To vote in all elections and public referenda and to be eligible for election to all publicly elected bodies;

(b)   To participate in the formulation of government policy and the implementation thereof and to hold public office and perform all public functions at all levels of government;

(c)   To participate in non-governmental organizations and associations concerned with the public and political life of the country.

Article 8

States Parties shall take all appropriate measures to ensure to women, on equal terms with men and without any discrimination, the opportunity to represent their Governments at the international level and to participate in the work of international organizations.

Article 9

1. States Parties shall grant women equal rights with men to acquire, change or retain their nationality. They shall ensure in particular that neither marriage to an alien nor change of nationality by the husband during marriage shall automatically change the nationality of the wife, render her stateless or force upon her the nationality of the husband.

2. States Parties shall grant women equal rights with men with respect to the nationality of their children.

PART III

Article 10

States Parties shall take all appropriate measures to eliminate discrimination against women in order to ensure to them equal rights with men in the field of education and in particular to ensure, on a basis of equality of men and women:

(a)   The same conditions for career and vocational guidance, for access to studies and for the achievement of diplomas in educational establishments of all categories in rural as well as in urban areas; this equality shall be ensured in preschool, general, technical, professional and higher technical education, as well as in all types of vocational training;

(b)   Access to the same curricula, the same examinations, teaching staff with qualifications of the same standard and school premises and equipment of the same quality;

(c)   The elimination of any stereotyped concept of the roles of men and women at all levels and in all forms of education by encouraging coeducation and other types of education which will help to achieve this aim and, in particular, by the revision of textbooks and school programmes and the adaptation of teaching methods;

(d)   The same opportunities to benefit from scholarships and other study grants;

(e) The same opportunities for access to programmes of continuing education including adult and functional literacy programmes, particularly those aimed at reducing, at the earliest possible time, any gap in education existing between men and women;

(f) The reduction of female student drop-out rates and the organization of programmes for girls and women who have left school prematurely;

(g) The same opportunities to participate actively in sports and physical education;

(h) Access to specific educational information to help to ensure the health and well-being of families, including information and advice on family planning.

Article 11

1. States Parties shall take all appropriate measures to eliminate discrimination against women in the field of employment in order to ensure, on a basis of equality of men and women, the same rights, in particular:

(a) The right to work as an inalienable right of all human beings;

(b) The right to the same employment opportunities, including the application of the same criteria for selection in matters of employment;

(c) The right to free choice of profession and employment, the right to promotion, job security and all benefits and conditions of service and the right to receive vocational training and retraining, including apprenticeships, advanced vocational training and recurrent training;

(d) The right to equal remuneration, including benefits, and to equal treatment in respect of work of equal value, as well as equality of treatment in the evaluation of the quality of work;

(e) The right to social security, particularly in cases of retirement, unemployment, sickness, invalidity and old age and other incapacity to work, as well as the right to paid leave;

(f) The right to protection of health and to safety in working conditions, including the safeguarding of the function of reproduction.

2. In order to prevent discrimination against women on the grounds of marriage or maternity and to ensure their effective right to work, States Parties shall take appropriate measures:

(a) To prohibit, subject to the imposition of sanctions, dismissal on the grounds of pregnancy or of maternity leave and discrimination in dismissals on the basis of marital status;

(b) To introduce maternity leave with pay or with comparable social benefits without loss of former employment, seniority or social allowances;

(c) To encourage the provision of the necessary supporting social services to enable parents to combine family obligations with work responsibilities and participation in public life, in particular through promoting the establishment and development of a network of child-care facilities;

(d) To provide special protection to women during pregnancy in types of work proved to be harmful to them.

3. Protective legislation relating to matters covered in this article shall be reviewed periodically in the light of scientific and technological knowledge and shall be revised, repealed or extended as necessary.

Article 12

1. States Parties shall take all appropriate measures to eliminate discrimination against women in the field of health care in order to ensure, on a basis of equality of men and women, access to health care services, including those related to family planning.

2. Notwithstanding the provisions of paragraph 1 of this article, States Parties shall ensure to women appropriate services in connexion with pregnancy, confinement and the post-natal period, granting free services where necessary, as well as adequate nutrition during pregnancy and lactation.

Article 13

States Parties shall take all appropriate measures to eliminate discrimination against women in other areas of economic and social life in order to ensure, on a basis of equality of men and women, the same rights, in particular:

(a)   The right to family benefits;

(b)   The right to bank loans, mortgages and other forms of financial credit;

(c)   The right to participate in recreational activities, sports and all aspects of cultural life.

Article 14

1. States Parties shall take into account the particular problems faced by rural women and the significant roles which rural women play in the economic survival of their families, including their work in the non—monetized sectors of the economy, and shall take all appropriate measures to ensure the application of the provisions of this Convention to women in rural areas.

2. States Parties shall take all appropriate measures to eliminate discrimination against women in rural areas in order to ensure, on a basis of equality of men and women, that they participate in and benefit from rural development and, in particular, shall ensure to such women the right:

(a)   To participate in the elaboration and implementation of development planning at all levels;

(b)   To have access to adequate health care facilities, including information, counselling and services in family planning;

(c)   To benefit directly from social security programmes;

(d)   To obtain all types of training and education, formal and non-formal, including that relating to functional literacy, as well as, inter alia, the benefit of all community and extension services, in order to increase their technical proficiency;

(e)   To organize self-help groups and co-operatives in order to obtain equal access to economic opportunities through employment or self-employment;

(f)   To participate in all community activities;

(g)   To have access to agricultural credit and loans, marketing facilities, appropriate technology and equal treatment in land and agrarian reform as well as in land resettlement schemes;

(h)   To enjoy adequate living conditions, particularly in relation to housing, sanitation, electricity and water supply, transport and communications.

PART IV

Article 15

1. States Parties shall accord to women equality with men before the law.

2. States Parties shall accord to women, in civil matters, a legal capacity identical to that of men and the same opportunities to exercise that capacity. In particular, they shall give women equal rights to conclude contracts and to administer property and shall treat them equally in all stages of procedure in courts and tribunals.

3. States Parties agree that all contracts and all other private instruments of any kind with a legal effect which is directed at restricting the legal capacity of women shall be deemed null and void.

4. States Parties shall accord to men and women the same rights with regard to the law relating to the movement of persons and the freedom to choose their residence and domicile.

Article 16

1. States Parties shall take all appropriate measures to eliminate discrimination against women in all matters relating to marriage and family relations and in particular shall ensure, on a basis of equality of men and women:

(a)   The same right to enter into marriage;

(b)   The same right freely to choose a spouse and to enter into marriage only with their free and full consent;

(c)   The same rights and responsibilities during marriage and at its dissolution;

(d)   The same rights and responsibilities as parents, irrespective of their marital status, in matters relating to their children; in all cases the interests of the children shall be paramount;

(e)   The same rights to decide freely and responsibly on the number and spacing of their children and to have access to the information, education and means to enable them to exercise these rights;

(f)   The same rights and responsibilities with regard to guardianship, wardship, trusteeship and adoption of children, or similar institutions where these concepts exist in national legislation; in all cases the interests of the children shall be paramount;

(g)   The same personal rights as husband and wife, including the right to choose a family name, a profession and an occupation;

(h)   The same rights for both spouses in respect of the ownership, acquisition, management, administration, enjoyment and disposition of property, whether free of charge or for a valuable consideration.

2. The betrothal and the marriage of a child shall have no legal effect, and all necessary action, including legislation, shall be taken to specify a minimum age for marriage and to make the registration of marriages in an official registry compulsory.

PART V

Article 17

1. For the purpose of considering the progress made in the implementation of the present Convention, there shall be established a Committee on the Elimination of Discrimination against Women (hereinafter referred to as the Con consisting, at the time of entry into force of the Convention, of eighteen and, after ratification of or accession to the Convention by the thirty—fifth State Party, of twenty-three experts of high moral standing and competence in the field covered by the Convention. The experts shall be elected by States Parties from among their nationals and shall serve in their personal capacity, consideration being given to equitable geographical distribution and to the representation of the different forms of civilization as well as the principal legal systems.

2. The members of the Committee shall be elected by secret ballot from a list of persons nominated by States Parties. Each State Party may nominate one person from among its own nationals.

3. The initial election shall be held six months after the date of the entry into force of the present Convention. At least three months before the date of each election the Secretary-General of the United Nations shall address a letter to the States Parties inviting them to submit their nominations within two months. The Secretary-General shall prepare a list in alphabetical order of all persons thus nominated, indicating the States Parties which have nominated them, and shall submit it to the States Parties.

4. Elections of the members of the Committee shall be held at a meeting of States Parties convened by the Secretary-General at United Nations Headquarters. At that meeting, for which two thirds of the States Parties shall constitute a quorum, the persons elected to the Committee shall be those nominees who obtain the largest number of votes and an absolute majority of the votes of the representatives of States Parties present and voting.

5. The members of the Committee shall be elected for a term of four years. However, the terms of nine of the members elected at the first election shall expire at the end of two years; immediately after the first election the names of these nine members shall be chosen by lot by the Chairman of the Committee.

6. The election of the five additional members of the Committee shall be held in accordance with the provisions of paragraphs 2, 3 and 4 of this article, following the thirty-fifth ratification or accession. The terms of two of the additional members elected on this occasion shall expire at the end of two years, the names of these two members having been chosen by lot by the Chairman of the Committee.

7. For the filling of casual vacancies, the State Party whose expert has ceased to function as a member of the Committee shall appoint another expert from among its nationals, subject to the approval of the Committee.

8. The members of the Committee shall, with the approval of the General Assembly, receive emoluments from United Nations resources on such terms and conditions as the Assembly may decide, having regard to the importance of the Committee's responsibilities.

9. The Secretary- of the United Nations shall provide the necessary staff and facilities for the effective performance of the functions of the Committee under the present Convention.

Article 18

1. States Parties undertake to submit to the Secretary—General of the United Nations, for consideration by the Committee, a report on the legislative, judicial, administrative or other measures which they have adopted to give effect to he provisions of the present Convention and on the progress made in this respect:

(a)   Within one year after the entry into force for the State concerned; and

(b)   Thereafter at least every four years and further whenever the Committee so requests.

2. Reports may indicate factors and difficulties affecting the degree of fulfilment of obligations under the present Convention.

Article 19

1. The Committee shall adopt its own rules of procedure.

2. The Committee shall elect its officers for a term of two years.

Article 20

1. The Committee shall normally meet for a period of not more than two weeks annually in order to consider the reports submitted in accordance with article 18 of the present Convention.

2. The meetings of the Committee shall normally be held at United Nations Headquarters or at any other convenient place as determined by the Committee.

Article 21

1. The Committee shall, through the Economic and Social Council, report annually to the General Assembly of the United Nations on its activities and may make suggestions and general recommendations based on the examination of reports and information received from the States Parties. Such suggestions and general recommendations shall be included in the report of the Committee together with comments, if any, from States Parties.

2. The Secretary-General shall transmit the reports of the Committee to the Commission on the Status of Women for its information.

Article 22

The specialized agencies shall be entitled to be represented at the consideration of the implementation of such provisions of the present Convention as fall within the scope of their activities. The Committee may invite the specialized agencies to submit reports on the implementation of the Convention in areas falling within the scope of their activities.

PART VI

Article 23

Nothing in this Convention shall affect any provisions that are more conducive to the achievement of equality between men and women which may be contained:

(a)   In the legislation of a State Party; or

(b)   In any other international convention, treaty or agreement in force for that State.

Article 24

States Parties undertake to adopt all necessary measures at the national level aimed at achieving the full realization of the rights recognized in the present Convention.

Article 25

1. The present Convention shall be open for signature by all States.

2. The Secretary-General of the United Nations is designated as the depositary of the present Convention.

3. The present Convention is subject to ratification. Instruments of ratification shall be deposited with the Secretary-General of the United Nations.

4. The present Convention shall be open to accession by all States. Accession shall be effected by the deposit of an instrument of accession with the Secretary-General of the United Nations.

Article 26

1. A request for the revision of the present Convention may be made at any time by any State Party by means of a notification in writing addressed to the Secretary-General of the United Nations.

2. The General Assembly of the United Nations shall decide upon the steps, if any, to be taken in respect of such a request.

Article 27

1. The present Convention shall enter into force on the thirtieth day after the date of deposit with the Secretary-General of the United Nations of the twentieth instrument of ratification or accession.

2. For each State ratifying the present Convention or acceding to it after the deposit of the twentieth instrument of ratification or accession, the Convention shall enter into force on the thirtieth day after the date of the deposit of its own instrument of ratification or accession.

Article 28

1. The Secretary-General of the United Nations shall receive and circulate to all States the text of reservations made by States at the time of ratification or accession.

2. A reservation incompatible with the object and purpose of the present Convention shall not be permitted.

3. Reservations may be withdrawn at any time by notification to this effect addressed to the Secretary-General of the United Nations, who shall then inform all States thereof. Such notification shall take effect on the date on which it is received.

Article 29

1. Any dispute between two or more States Parties concerning the interpretation or application of the present Convention which is not settled by negotiation shall, at the request of one of them, be submitted to arbitration. If within six months from the date of the request for arbitration the parties are unable to agree on the organization of the arbitration, any one of those parties may refer the dispute to the International Court of Justice by request in conformity with the Statute of the Court.

2. Each State Party may at the time of signature or ratification of this Convention or accession thereto declare that it does not consider itself bound by paragraph 1 of this article. The other States Parties shall not be bound by that paragraph with respect to any State Party which has made such a reservation.

3. Any State Party which has made a reservation in accordance with paragraph 2 of this article may at any time withdraw that reservation by notification to the Secretary-General of the United Nations.

Article 30

The present Convention, the Arabic, Chinese, English, French, Russian and Spanish texts of which are equally authentic, shall be deposited with the Secretary-General of the United Nations.

IN WITNESS WHEREOF the undersigned, duly authorized, have signed the present Convention.

Conclusion

Women for so long have been victims of all sorts of discrimination, oppression and brutality all over the world. This convention is intended to bring to an end any such treatment against women.

Nevertheless, despite the good intentions expressed in the Convention, many women continues to be victims of such unacceptable behaviour.

Self-Assessment Questions

1.   *Why do you think there was a need for this Convention?*

2.   *What are some of the specific problems faced by women?*

3.   *How would you define discrimination against women?*

4.   *How far does this Convention go towards protecting women from discrimination? Justify your answer.*

Chapter 25

HIV/AIDS and Human Rights

Contents of this Chapter

1. Introduction

The rapid spread of HIV/AIDS in the world has raised all sorts of human rights issues. There is now clear evidence that there exists a big relationship between human rights and the spread of HIV/AIDS infection.

In relation to HIV/AIDS and human rights, the UN Declaration of commitment on HIV/AIDS (June 2001) states:

"The full realization of human rights and fundamental freedoms for all is an essential element in a global response to the HIV/AIDS pandemic, including in the areas of prevention, care, support and treatment, and that it reduces vulnerability to HIV/AIDS and prevents stigma and related discrimination against people living with or at risk of HIV/AIDS".

Despite these declarations and those contained in both the Universal Declaration of Human Rights and the European Convention on Human Rights, abuse of human rights continues to be perpetrated in many countries of the world. The abuse may be from governments, organisations or individuals.

2. *Human Rights Abuse and HIV/AIDS*

There has always been abuse of human rights in many countries. However, HIV/AIDS has raised some special human rights issues that are worth identifying.

According to Human Rights Watch, an International Human Rights Charity, abuses in relation to HIV/AIDS would include the following:

a) Human Rights Abuses that facilitate the spread of HIV/AIDS

Human rights violations that help spread the HIV/AIDS infection include:

* Sexual assault on women and girls.

* Forced unprotected sex on women and girls.

* Refusal of the right to have information on HIV transmission.

* Lack of access to protective measures (e.g. condoms).

* Stigmatisation of the infected person, who then refuses to seek help, thereby spreading the disease further.

* Violence against sex workers and intravenous drug users.

* Lack of available harm reduction measure increases the spread.

* Fear of possible discrimination and stigmatisation prevents people at risk from HIV infection seeking HIV tests.

* Discrimination and stigmatisation of men who have sex with men, who may be driven underground, and so may not have access to prevention information and assistance.

b) Human Rights Abuses that follow HIV infection

There is also abuse of human rights after a person has been infected with HIV/AIDS, namely:

* Economic deprivation of the infected persons, their family and friends.

* Denial of healthcare and other services to infected persons.

* Discrimination at work or denial of employment.

* Physical abuse of infected person, which in some cases may lead to death.

* Breach of their confidentiality.

* Stigmatisation, ostracisation and social exclusion of the infected person, family and friends.

* Confining infected persons to institutions and prisons without help, which will further spread the disease.

3. The Relationship Between HIV/AIDS & Human Rights

The Office of the United Nations High Commission for Human Rights (OHCHR) states that the relationship between HIV/AIDS and human rights appear in three areas, namely:

a)   Increased vulnerability

Certain groups are more vulnerable to contracting the HIV virus because they are unable to realise their civil and political, economic, social and cultural rights. Individuals who are denied the rights to freedom of association and access to information may be precluded from discussing issues related to HIV/AIDS, participating in AIDS service organisations and self-help group, and taking other preventative measures to protect themselves from HIV infection.

Women - and particularly young women - are more vulnerable to infection if they lack access to information, education and the services necessary to ensure sexual and reproductive health and prevention of infection. People living in poverty often are unable to access HIV care and treatment, including anti-retrovirals and other medications for opportunistic infections.

c)   Discrimination and Stigma

The rights of people living with HIV/AIDS are often violated because of their presumed or known HIV status, causing them to suffer both the burden of the disease and the consequential loss of other rights.

Stigmatisation and discrimination may obstruct their access to treatment and may affect their employment, housing and other rights. This, in turn, contributes to vulnerability of others to infection, since HIV-related stigma and discrimination discourages individuals infected with and affected by HIV from contacting health and social services. The result is that those most needing information, education and counselling will not benefit even where such services are available.

d)   It Impedes an Effective Response

Effective HIV prevention, treatment, support and care strategies are hampered in an environment where human rights are not respected.

4. Human Rights, Women and HIV/AIDS

There is clear evidence that women are disproportionally disadvantaged in the HIV/AIDS infection rate, particularly in developing countries; most of which is as a result of human rights abuses. Women and HIV/AIDS has therefore, become a huge human rights issue in recent times.

Regarding human rights, women and HIV/AIDS, the World Health Organisation (Fact sheet no 247 – June 2000) comments:

"Women's right to safe sexuality and to autonomy in all decisions relating to sexuality is respected almost nowhere.

As it is intimately related to economic independence, this right is most violated in those places where women exchange sex for survival as a way of life.

And we are not talking about prostitution but rather a basic social and economic arrangement between the sexes which results on the one hand from poverty affecting men and women and on the other hand, from male control over women's lives in a context of poverty.

By and large, most men, however poor can choose when, with whom and with what protection if any, to have sex. Most women cannot.

As such, our basic premise has to be that unless and until the scope of human rights is fully extended to economic security (i.e. the right not to live in abject poverty in a world of immense riches), women's right to safe sexuality is not going to be achieved...

...The Major Issues

- *Lack of control over own sexuality and sexual relationships.*

- *Poor reproductive and sexual health, leading to serious morbidity and mortality. Rates of infection in young (15-19) women are between 5 and 6 times higher than in young men (recent studies in various African populations).*

- *Neglect of health needs, nutrition, medical care, etc. women's access to care and support for HIV/AIDS is much delayed (if it arrives at all) and limited. Family resources nearly always devoted to caring for the man. Women, even when infected themselves, are providing all the care.*

- *Clinical management based on research on men. This year we plan to update guidance and start with module on clinical management of HIV/AIDS in women.*

- *All forms of coerced sex – from violent rape to cultural/economic obligations to have sex when it is not really wanted, increases risk of microlesions and therefore of STI/HIV infection.*

- *Harmful cultural practices: from genital mutilation to practices such as 'dry' sex.*

- *Stigma and discrimination in relation to AIDS (and all STDs): much stronger against women who risk violence, abandonment, neglect (of health and material needs), destitution, ostracism from family and community. Furthermore, women, are often blamed for spread of disease, always seen as the 'vector' even though the majority have been infected by only partner/husband.*

- *Adolescents: access to education for prevention, (in and out of school and through media campaigns), condoms, and reproductive health services before and after they are sexually active. Promotion and protection of adolescent reproductive rights (particularly girls). Obstacles in terms of laws and policies, health service provision, cultural attitudes and expectations of girls and boys' sexual behaviour, cultural practices, and educational and employment opportunities.*

- *Sexual abuse: there is now evidence that this is an underestimated mode of transmission of HIV infection in children (even very small children). Adult men seek ever younger female partners (younger than 15 years of age) in order to avoid HIV infection, or if already infected, in order to be 'cured'.*

- *Disclosure of status, partner notification, confidentiality: These are all more difficult issues for women than for men for the reasons disclosed above – negative consequences; and the fact that women have usually been infected by their only partner/husband.*

- *Because disclosure is more difficult, women's access to care and support is further decreased. VCT as an entry point for care and prevention is vital. Protection for women when they disclose status must be assured. We have this year worked intensively with UNAIDS on issues of disclosure and confidentiality...*

...Human Rights Issues relating to mother to child transmission

Informed Consent

To testing during pregnancy
To the intervention itself
To termination/continuing with the pregnancy

- *Provision of adequate pre-test counselling, pre-intervention counselling/information; infant feeding counselling; contraceptive advice especially if not breastfeeding.*

- *Protection of confidentiality, including shared confidentiality in the interests of care and support; and the problem of not breastfeeding when this amounts to 'public disclosure' of positive serostatus. Legal provisions, health service practices and community NGO support.*

- *Provision of family planning services, alternative infant feeding/breastmilk substitutes, material support for fuel, water etc. in addition to the intervention itself.*

- *Involvement of partner/husband at all stages, positive and negative consequences.*

- *Potential adverse effects of taking antiretrovirals (ARVs) especially in repeat pregnancies of an HIV infected woman.*

- *Women's access to care and treatment apart from the MTCT intervention, woman as vessel for the baby.*

- *Generation of orphans. Parents likely to die. On mother's death, baby's survival chances much reduced. Should woman herself be treated, at least for common HIV related illness.*

- *Selection of women to benefit from MTCT."*

5. Human Rights Approach to HIV/AIDS

Following on the relationship between HIV/AIDS and human rights mentioned above, the OHCHR's suggested human rights approach to HIV/AIDS is stated below.

The OHCHR states:

"There is clear evidence that where individuals and communities are able to realize their rights – to education, free association, information and, most importantly, non-discrimination – the personal and societal impact of HIV and AIDS are reduced. The protection and promotion of human rights are therefore essential to preventing the spread of HIV and to mitigating the social and economic impact of the pandemic. The reasons for this are threefold. The promotion and protection of human rights reduces vulnerability to HIV infection by addressing its root causes; lessens the adverse impact on those infected and affected by HIV; and empowers individuals and communities to respond to the pandemic. An effective international response to the pandemic therefore must be grounded in respect for all civil, cultural, economic, political, and social rights as well as the right to development, in accordance with international human rights principles, norms and standards.

States' obligations to promote and protect HIV/AIDS-related human rights are defined in existing international treaties. HIV/AIDS-related human rights include the right to life; the right to liberty and security of the person; the right to the highest attainable standard of mental and physical health; the right to non-discrimination, equal protection and equality before the law; the right to freedom of movement; the right to seek and enjoy asylum; the right to privacy; the right to freedom of expression and opinion and the right to freely receive and impart information; the right to freedom of association; the right to marry and found a family; the right to work; the right to equal access to education; the right to an adequate standard of living; the right to social security, assistance and welfare; the right to share in scientific advancement and its benefits; the right to participate in public and cultural life; the right to be free from torture and other cruel, inhuman or degrading treatment or punishment.

The United Nations human rights instruments and mechanisms provide the normative legal framework as well as the necessary tools for ensuring the implementation of HIV-related rights. Through their consideration of States reports, concluding observations and recommendations, and general comments, the UN treaty bodies provide States with direction and assistance in the implementation of HIV-related rights".

6. International Guidelines on HIV/AIDS and Human Rights

Considering the huge and complicated human rights issues that are involved in dealing with HIV/AIDS, the United Nations Commission on Human Rights (UNCHR) in its document res. 1997/33, U.N. Doc. E/CN.4/1997/150 (1997), provided the following guidelines for the protection of human rights in the context of HIV and AIDS.

"The commission on Human Rights.

Recalling its resolution 1996/43 of 19 April 1996 and other relevant resolutions and decisions adopted by organizations of the United Nations system, as well as by other competent forums.

Emphasizing in view of the continuing challenges presented by HIV/AIDS, the need for intensified efforts to ensure universal respect for and observance of human rights and fundamental freedoms for all, reduces vulnerability to HIV/AIDS and to prevent HIV/AIDS-related discrimination and stigma.

Welcoming the report of the secretary-General on the Second International Consultation on HIV/AIDS and Human Rights (E/CN.4/1997/37), which presents the outcome of the Consultation, including the Guidelines recommended by the expert participants for States on the promotion and protection of fundamental rights and freedoms in the context of HIV/AIDS, and strategies for their dissemination and implementation.

1)   *Invites all States to consider the Guidelines recommended by the experts who participated in the Second International Consultation on HIV/AIDS and Human Rights, as contained in documents E/CN.4/1997/37 and summarized in the annex to the present resolution*

2)   *Calls upon the United Nations High Commissioner for Human Rights, the Joint United Nations Programme on HIV/AIDS (UNAIDS), its co-sponsors and the other partners to provide technical cooperation to States, upon the request of Governments when required, from within existing resources, for the promotion and protection of human rights in the context of HIV/AIDS*

3)   *Requests the Secretary-General to solicit the opinion of Governments, specialized agencies and international and non-governmental organizations and to prepare for consideration by the Commission at its fifty-fifth session a progress report on the follow-up to the present resolution*

Annex

Guideline 1: States should establish an effective national framework for their response to HIV/AIDS, which ensures a coordinated, participatory, transparent and accountable approach, integrating HIV/AIDS policy and programme responsibilities across all branches.

Guideline 2: States should ensure, through political and financial support, that community consultation occurs in all phases of HIV/AIDS policy design, programme implementation and evaluation and that community organizations are enabled to carry out their activities, including in the field of ethics, law and human rights effectively.

Guideline 3: States should review and reform public health laws to ensure that they adequately address public health issues raised by HIV/AIDS, that their provisions applicable to casually transmitted diseases are not inappropriately applied to HIV/AIDS and that they are consistent with international human rights obligation.

Guideline 4: States should review and reform criminal laws and correctional systems to ensure that they are consistent with international human rights obligations and are not misused in the context of HIV/AIDS or targeted against vulnerable groups.

Guideline 5: States should enact or strengthen anti-discrimination and other protective laws that protect vulnerable groups, people living with HIV/AIDS *and people living with disabilities from discrimination in both the public and private sectors, ensure privacy and confidentiality and ethics in research involving human subjects, emphasize education and conciliation, and provide for speedy and effective administrative and civil remedies.*

Guideline 6: States should enact legislation to provide for the regulation of HIV-related goods, services and information, so as to ensure widespread availability of qualitative prevention measures and services, adequate HIV prevention and care information and safe and effective medication at an affordable price.

Guideline 7: States should implement and support legal support services that will educate people affected by HIV/AIDS about their rights, provide free legal services to enforce those rights, develop expertise on HIV-related legal issues and utilize means of protection in addition to the courts, such as offices of ministries of justice, ombudsmen, health complaint units and human rights commissions.

Guideline 8: States, in collaboration with and through the community, should promote a supportive and enabling environment for women, children and other vulnerable groups by addressing underlying prejudices and inequalities through community dialogue, specially designed social and health services and support to community groups.

Guideline 9: States should promote the wide and ongoing distribution of creative education, training and media programmes explicitly designed to change attitudes of discrimination and stigmatization associated with HIV/AIDS to understanding and acceptance.

Guideline 10: States should ensure that government and private sectors develop codes of conduct regarding HIV/AIDS issues that translate human rights principles into codes of professional responsibility and practice, with accompanying mechanisms to implement and enforce those codes.

Guideline 11: States should ensure monitoring and enforcement mechanisms to guarantee the protection of HIV-related human rights, including those of people living with HIV/AIDS, their families and communities

Guideline 12: States should cooperate through all relevant programmes and agencies of the United Nations system, including the Joint United Nations Programme on HIV/AIDS, to share knowledge and experience concerning HIV-related human rights issues and should ensure effective mechanisms to protect human rights in the context of HIV/AIDS at the international level.

Nevertheless, these important and noble guidelines have been completely ignored by several governments and organisations.

Conclusion

Respect for human rights is essential, +++ if the spread of HIV/AIDS is to be curtailed in the world, particularly in developing countries.

Critical questions that have always disturbed some human rights commentators are:

a)   How useful are human rights if people do not know that they have such rights?; and

b)   How useful are human rights if there are no effective remedies when the rights are breached?

Nevertheless, the existence of human rights laws can have great persuasive effects on many governments, organizations and individuals.

Self-Assessment Questions

1. Is there any relationship between HIV/AIDS and human rights? Justify your answer.

2. In which area can human rights abuse occur in relation to HIV/AIDS?

3. What is the relationship between human rights, women and HIV/AIDS?

4. What is the recommended human rights approach to HIV/AIDS?

5. What international guidelines exist in relation to HIV/AIDS and human rights?

Chapter 26

Strategic Planning in HIV & AIDS Prevention

Contents of this Chapter

1. Introduction

The successful prevention, management and control of HIV/AIDS will require enormous and skilful planning. However, a "ducking and diving" short-term approach will not work; rather, a strategic approach is necessary for the effective curtailment of the menace of HIV and AIDS.

Strategic Planning means long-term planning. Thus, it can involve planning over a range of 5-15 years or more.

This chapter will examine the fundamental principles of Strategic Management and Planning in relation to HIV and AIDS prevention. It is important that decision/policy makers in HIV/AIDS prevention, management and control should have knowledge of this area.

2. Situation

In decision-making language, the huge pandemic of HIV/AIDS in the world is referred to as the 'Situation'. It is not referred to as a 'problem' as some might think. Basically, a situation has arisen.

3. The Problem

From the Situation mentioned above, we can now diagnose the 'Problem', if there is any. On closer examination of the situation, it shows that part of the problem includes:

a)   HIV/AIDS killing millions of people,

b)   The huge death rate is leading to huge manpower loss,

c)   This manpower loss could have negative effects on economic and social development,

d)   HIV/AIDS is also creating an unprecedented number of orphans,

e)   All of the problems mentioned above can lead to political, economic and social instability in the country.

Thus, we surely do have a problem. The problems diagnosed so far, are only examples. You can easily identify many more problems in addition to those listed.

4. Mission Statement

A mission statement is necessary as part of the process of strategic planning and problem-solving. Mission statements should not be narrow and restrictive, but should be fairly broad.

Thus, in this case, a country's mission statement might be:

> "To improve the sexual and reproductive health of the people in order to improve economic development and social cohesion."

5. Situation/Environmental Analysis

To facilitate proper strategic planning, we need to carry out what is known as an environmental analysis of an imaginary country.

A proper environmental analysis should reveal the country's state of affairs in relation to its ability and preparedness in the prevention, management and control of HIV/AIDS. It should, in particular, enable us to answer the following questions:

- Where are we now in relation to HIV/AIDS prevention?
- Where do we want to go from here? and
- How do we get there?

Two of the most commonly used tools of environmental analysis are PEST and SWOT analysis, which are discussed below.

a) PEST Analysis

PEST, as we have heard, is one of the environmental analysis tools. PEST is an analysis of the country's:

Political

Economic

Socio-Legal, and

Technological

environment, (in this example) in relation to HIV/AIDS and STD prevention. Thus, a PEST analysis is an examination of the following:

The Political Environment

This may look at the:

- Management strength of the government.

- Level of political stability.

- The political system itself and its workings.

- The structure of decision-making and the decision-making process.

- Level of government commitment in HIV/AIDS prevention.

- Existence of government agencies and pressure groups in HIV/AIDS prevention.

- Appropriate laws that exist in this area. Also, which laws need to be exacted, to better facilitate HIV/AIDS prevention.

The Economic Environment

Analysis in this area should include an examination of:

- The state of the economy.

- The country's financial position.

- How much of the finances could be used for the prevention of HIV/AIDS.

- How much in actual fact, is the government willing to commit in the fight against HIV/AIDS.

- The possibility of external financial assistance to combat the disease.

- The possibility of raising the funds internally.

- Is there likely to be economic instability in the future, caused by mismanagement, inflation, interest rate rises, exchange rate fluctuations, etc?

- Are there natural resources available?

The Socio-Legal Environment

Socio-Legal environmental analysis should include:

- Level of HIV/AIDS awareness of the population.

- Expected level of willingness of the population to accept the prevention message.

- The level of literacy and ignorance of the people.

- Those more likely to be infected with HIV/AIDS.

- How many HIV/AIDS prevention experts are in existence?

- The amount of community-based resources that are available for the prevention, management and control of HIV/AIDS.

- A thorough appreciation of cultural and religious effects on HIV/AIDS prevention.

- Is there likely to be resistance against some forms of prevention tools, (e.g. condoms), which are objected to by some groups, on the grounds of religious or cultural beliefs?

- Are there existing laws to aid prevention education? If not, what type of law(s) are necessary and when?

- How many NGOs are involved in HIV/AIDS prevention and which are the most efficient and effective ones?

- Are there existing laws to aid effective HIV/AIDS prevention?

- If there are none, which laws should we enact?

The Technological Environment

Analysis of the technological environment should include:

- The existing appropriate infrastructure.

- Level and type of healthcare services in existence in the country.

- Effectiveness of existing communication medium (e.g. TV, radio, print media, mail, etc).

- How many people have access to a particular media?

- The effectiveness of the transportation system.

- The most effective local communication tools in existence; which can be used to get to the widest possible audience

- Who are likely to be the most effective communicators to spread the HIV/AIDS prevention message?

- How many people have access to the Internet?

Such frank environmental analysis will assist decision-makers to appreciate the enormity of the problem and take much more sensible action.

Some writers may now describe PEST analysis as PELST or PESTL analysis, as they seek to separate the 'Legal' from the Socio-Legal Environment.

b) SWOT Analysis

A SWOT Analysis, as mentioned, is another tool in environmental analysis. Once a PEST analysis is done, then a detailed SWOT analysis is carried out to examine the following:

Strengths,
Weaknesses,
Opportunities,
Threats,

in the prevention, management and control of HIV/AIDS.

For it to be useful, a SWOT analysis has to be realistic.

As you will appreciate, the following SWOT analysis is an imaginary one.

Strengths

In our proposed fight against HIV/AIDS and other STDs, what are the strengths of the country? Our analysis shows that we have the following strengths:

a)   Capable leadership.

b)   Political stability.

c)   Strong government commitment in HIV/AIDS prevention.

d)   Natural resources.

e)   Access to funds.

f)   Good communication/media infrastructure.

Weaknesses

The analysis also showed that the country has the following weaknesses:

- Acute shortage of trained personnel in HIV/AIDS prevention education.

- Very few HIV testing and counselling centres.

- Little or no hygiene and public health education.

- Lack of HIV/AIDS prevention books/pamphlets and information centres.

- Huge numbers of the population are ignorant about HIV/AIDS.

- Bad healthcare system and infrastructure.

- Very low percentage of the GDP spent on healthcare, particularly in HIV/AIDS prevention.

Opportunities

This heading seeks to identify the possible opportunities the country has in the prevention, management and control of the diseases. Thus, the country's opportunities might include:

- Majority of the population are not yet infected with HIV/AIDS.

- It is now possible to properly train many people on HIV/AIDS prevention within a relatively short period of time. This has been made possible by institutions such as the College of Venereal Disease Prevention, London, UK.

- There is the possibility of financial assistance by the World Bank, IMF and other international NGOs in the fight against HIV/AIDS.

- The population seems to be willing to learn how to prevent HIV/AIDS prevention.

- There are many organizations (NGOs) that are now involved in HIV/AIDS prevention activities.

- There are now cheaper anti-retroviral drugs available for the treatment of HIV/AIDS.

- The government's willingness and promise of an increase in healthcare spending, particularly in relation to HIV/AIDS.

Threats

Some of the possible threats that the country faces are:

- Millions already infected and many more are likely to be infected.

- Potential manpower loss.

- Organisations and companies will suffer financially as a result of huge loss of manpower.

- Threat to economic progress and development.

- The potentially huge financial costs to the government for the control and treatment of HIV/AIDS. Money that could have been used in other areas of the economy (such as education and employment) is diverted to fight HIV/AIDS.

- Potential orphans problem.

- Some people or groups (particularly some religious groups) may be against certain prevention methods.

- It could lead to a demoralized society.

- It could destabilize the country and become a threat to national security.

6. Objectives

Once the mission statement is written, and the situation analysis done, we then need to formulate our objectives. Some of the objectives might therefore be:

a)   to achieve 50% improvement in public health and hygiene by 2007,

b)   to achieve 80% reduction in the HIV/AIDS infection rate by 2008,

c)   to achieve 50% improvement in the treatment and management of HIV/AIDS and other sexually transmitted diseases by 2008.

While there can be more objectives, it is advisable to minimise them to a specific number.

Furthermore, objectives should always relate to the acronym SMART:

(i)   **S**pecific
(ii)   **M**easurable
(iii)   **A**chievable
(iv)   **R**ealistic
(v)   **T**imescale (there should always be one)

7. Strategies

The next step in strategic planning, after the objectives have been established and an environmental analysis completed, is to identify the strategies required. These are the means by which the objectives will be achieved. Basically, strategies should answer the question: 'How do we achieve these objectives?'

Thus, some of the likely strategies to be adopted are:

a) Formulation of national and regional HIV/AIDS policies, which will aid a coherent application of the strategies nationwide.

b) To improve HIV/AIDS prevention education and training.

c) To increase the number of those trained in HIV/AIDS prevention education.

d) To improve prevention education of STDs other than HIV/AIDS.

e) To facilitate and improve the treatment and management of HIV/AIDS.

f) To increase HIV test and counselling centres.

g) To increase HIV/AIDS information and counselling centres.

h) To increase the nation's healthcare expenditure.

i) To improve human rights and empower women.

j) To reduce the level of poverty, by adopting viable poverty reduction and job and investment creation programmes.

8. Tactics

A derivative of the strategies to be adopted are the tactics to be applied in implementing the strategies. Thus, the possible tactics in this section might include:

a) Create a body or committee that will be responsible for the strategic planning in the prevention of HIV/AIDS. These may be National AIDS Councils or strategic committees which will formulate and aid the implementation of prevention policies and strategies

b) Incorporating HIV/AIDS and STD prevention into the education curriculum of schools and colleges.

c) Production of prevention education books, booklets and pamphlets to be distributed to the people.

d) Translation of these education materials into local languages in order to reach the widest possible audience.

e) Localisation of

    i) HIV test/counselling centres
    ii) Prevention education centres
    iii) Treatment centres

f) Formation of community based HIV/AIDS prevention initiatives.

g) Promotional campaigns using:

- Employers
- Trade unions
- Community representatives
- Community leaders
- Women's' groups and associations
- Boy Scouts groups
- Girl Guide groups
- Employee groups and associations
- Youth workers
- Youth service schemes
- Tenants associations
- Trade associations
- Teachers, nurses, midwives, doctors and social workers
- Local or national celebrities
- Religious personnel
- Comedians and musicians
- Persons already infected with HIV

h)   Promotion of sexual abstinence; particularly for underaged children.

i)   Promote against promiscuity.

j)   Distribution of free condoms to those who choose to be sexually active. This is particularly necessary for those who are too poor to afford condoms. Hospital, clinic and HIV test, information, advice and counselling centres may all be used for the distribution of such free condoms.

k)   By providing local vocational training programmes and rural business initiatives to create viable employment, in order to reduce poverty.

l)   By using qualified and experienced consultants to assist in the planning and the implementation of programmes and strategies. The College of Venereal Disease Prevention provides comprehensive consultancy services in this area. The College has extensive knowledge and experience in HIV/AIDS and STD prevention education.

9. Promotion

A beautifully written strategic plan could fail woefully if it was not promoted properly. Thus, promotion is one of the most important tools in strategic management.

Remember that the HIV/AIDS prevention information has to be communicated to the people. Both information and strategies need to be promoted, if it is to work. Effective marketing will make people much more trusting to accept the prevention message.

The traditional promotional mix in marketing is:

a) Advertising
b) Sales promotion
c) Publicity; and
d) Personal selling

These promotional tools are briefly explained below:

Advertising

Advertising would include the use of:

- TV
- Radio
- Print media
- Billboards
- Internet
- Videos
- Cassettes
- Photos of those suffering from HIV or dying from AIDS

The advertising message should be translated into local languages, where required.

Sales Promotion

Sales promotion tools would include the following:

- Seminars, fairs and exhibitions
- Sponsorship
- Free giveaway condoms
- Shows, concerts and displays
- Lectures, conferences and debates

Publicity

Using publicity and public relations as a promotional tool in HIV/AIDS prevention would include:

- Media publicisation of high profile meetings or statements by officials involved in HIV/AIDS prevention.

- Publicising involvement or comments by celebrities or other respected persons.

- Lobbying decision-makers, politicians and healthcare professionals on the importance of HIV/AIDS prevention.

- Sponsorship

- Press releases

- In-house journals

- Exhibitions

- Organising special events

- Use of expert commentators

- Training programmes

Personal Selling

This would include:

- Face to face communication with a person or groups of people in the community on HIV/AIDS prevention.

- Doctors, nurses and midwives telling their patients of the need to prevent themselves becoming infected with HIV/AIDS.

- Health and public health professionals educating their clients on prevention.

- Community based persons and organisations that go from door to door to educate people on how to prevent HIV/AIDS.

- Teachers educating their pupils and students at schools and colleges on HIV/AIDS prevention.

- Employers training and educating their employees on the need to be prevented from HIV/AIDS infection.

- Trade unions and other institutions educating their members on HIV/AIDS prevention.

- Parents educating their children, relatives and friends on HIV/AIDS prevention.

Basically, every individual in the community is empowered and entrusted with the responsibility of preventing HIV/AIDS.

10. Budget

The implementation of the strategy, the promotion and the prevention campaign will, without doubt, cost a lot of money. Therefore, a budget needs to be allocated to meet the cost if the campaign is to be successful. There is no point in starting a campaign which has to be stopped halfway through lack of funds. A thorough and realistic budget had to be set aside to facilitate the campaign.

Some of the methods of setting such a budget are briefly described below:

a) Objective and Task Method

This is where a budget is allocated based on the objectives established and the calculation of the costs of the tasks to be performed, in order to achieve the objectives. Experts will be needed to arrive at the appropriate costs and budget.

This is a very pragmatic approach to setting the budget.

b) Percentage of GDP Method

Some countries may just decide to allocate a certain percentage of their GDP for healthcare and the prevention, management and control of HIV/AIDS and other sexually transmitted diseases. It is important that any percentage of the GDP that is allocated has to be both sensible and realistic.

c) Competitive Parity Method

Some countries may set their HIV/AIDS prevention budget to be on a par with the amount allocated by other competitor nations. Considering the fact that the HIV/AIDS problems and the strategies to be adopted differ from country to country, it may not be the wisest way to determine the budget.

d) Affordability Method

Some countries could only afford certain amount of money to improve healthcare and to fight HIV/AIDS. Basically, the amount allocated is the only amount it can afford because of the other many competing demands.

e) Arbitrary Method

This method has no basis at all, only that someone or a particular group of people decide to set aside a certain amount of money for HIV/AIDS prevention. This method is based on assumption and guesswork.

f) Funding from other Sources

A well-designed and implemented HIV/AIDS prevention strategic plan may also attract external funding from international institutions such as:

- The World Bank
- The United Nations
- UNAIDS
- The European Union
- USAIDS

- Foreign Governments; and
- Many international NGOs

11. Training

For the successful implementation of a project of this magnitude, proper training is required for those who will be involved in both the management and implementation of the strategies. In addition, proper and extensive training is needed for those who will be involved in the campaign.

Such training will enable participants to communicate efficiently and apply customer service skills in the implementation of the strategies and the delivery of the campaign. The importance of training cannot be overemphasised.

12. Pre-Launch Plan

This is where final arrangements and briefings are made for the successful launch of the strategy. This plan should also be promoted so that the population is aware of it and are eager to see the launch itself.

13. Launch and Implementation

This is where the programme is launched and the strategies implemented. Normally, the local, national and international media will be invited to attend the launch ceremony. The whole nation is also well aware of the launch.

14. Feedback and Control

It is important that the authorities keep a close eye on the possible successes or failures of the implementation. There should therefore be an effective monitoring and feedback system in place to inform government and other appropriate agencies as to the effectiveness of the campaign. This is important in order to effect remedial action, where necessary.

Such control and feedback mechanisms would include:

- Public surveys as to people's level of awareness of HIV/AIDS and its prevention.

- Opinion of doctors, nurses and other healthcare professionals.

- Teachers, pupils and students opinion.

- Community based opinion polls.

- Present level of infection compared to the level months, weeks or years ago.

- Extent of indifference of the population concerning HIV/AIDS prevention issues.

- Level of complaints from the public concerning the method(s) or nature of the campaign.

- Letters or statements of satisfaction made by members of the public.

The existence of control mechanisms should enable governments to ascertain the level of the effectiveness and success of the campaign.

15. Re-Enforcement of Prevention Message

It is a well-known fact that many people have short memories. Therefore, the prevention message should be re-enforced periodically (after the initially comprehensive campaign) as a reminder that HIV/AIDS continues to be a threat. This will ensure that people do not become complacent. However, the message should also include success stories, where there have been any, in order to make people feel that there is hope and it is worth persevering.

Marketing should try to vary the message by using different tools, styles, language and images, in order to avoid people becoming immune to it and bored from 'the same old story' syndrome.

15. Accountability

People or organisations entrusted with the HIV/AIDS prevention responsibility should be skilful and highly accountable and can account for their actions, deeds and expenditure.

Accountability is particularly important in developing countries, where many see public funds as an opportunity to enrich themselves without the need to provide the services that they are contracted to provide. This is in the belief that they can do this with impunity.

It will be absolutely unacceptable for funds allocated for HIV/AIDS prevention to be embezzled by an unaccountable person or organisation without the work being done properly. Such behaviour can be likened to "crimes against humanity".

Thus, authorities should devise mechanisms to ensure transparent accountability.

Conclusion

It is clear from the discussion so far, that effective strategic planning is required for the successful prevention of HIV/AIDS and other sexually transmitted diseases.

Self-Assessment Questions

1. Why is strategic planning so important in HIV/AIDS prevention?

2. In relation to strategic planning, what do you understand by the terms:

   - Situation
   - Problem
   - Mission statement

3. How important are objectives and strategies in strategic management?

4. Explain in detail the concept of environmental analysis in relation to strategic planning.

5. Is promotion really important in strategic planning? Justify your answer.

6. Why is it important to set aside a budget to implement the HIV/AIDS prevention strategic plan?

7. Why is training of personnel important in the implementation of the strategic plan?

8. With the knowledge that you have gained, write an HIV/AIDS prevention strategy for your own government.

9. Why is periodic re-enforcement of the prevention message necessary?

10. Why is accountability important in HIV/AIDS prevention?

Chapter 27

International AIDS Organisations

Contents of this Chapter

1. Introduction

There are very many organisations all over the world that are involved in HIV/AIDS prevention activities in one way or the other. This chapter seeks to identify and explain briefly the main activities of only a few of them.

2. AIDS Organisations

Briefly mentioned below are some of the main AIDS organisations in the world. This is by no means an exhaustive list at all, as there are just too many to mention all of them.

1. College of Venereal Disease Prevention

It is one of the very few educational institutions involved in HIV/AIDS prevention education that runs diploma and advanced diploma courses in the prevention of HIV/AIDS and Sexually Transmitted Diseases, by distance learning.

It was founded in 1999 in response to the ever-growing global epidemic of HIV/AIDS and other Sexually Transmitted Diseases.

The college provides extensive, simple, non-technical and non-political education as well as effective strategies in the prevention of HIV/AIDS and sexually transmitted infections (STI's).

There are diploma, advanced diploma and post-graduate courses which are delivered by distance learning, part-time and full-time basis.

The college provides comprehensive expert consultancy services to sovereign governments and other international organisations in the planning, strategy and control of HIV/AIDS and other sexually transmitted diseases. It also runs 1-5 day seminars, workshops, bespoke courses for organisations in both the public and private sectors. These courses are delivered by using many excellent videos that deal with HIV/AIDS, its prevention and related areas.

Thus, the college can provide training services both in the UK and on other locations in any country in the world. Anyone interested in such services should contact the college.

College of Venereal Disease Prevention
45 Vyner Street
London
E2 9DQ
United Kingdom.
Tel: + 44 (20) 8980 1000
Fax: + 44 (20) 8980 1110
E-mail: dcs@cvdp.co.uk
Website: www.cvdp.co.uk

2. Medical Foundation for AIDS & Sexual Health

The Medical Foundation for AIDS and Sexual Health works with policy makers and health professionals, to promote excellence in the prevention and management of HIV and other sexually transmitted infections.

It undertakes a range of projects and works in partnership with others, in order to influence policy and offer advice to doctors and other health professionals. Its activities include:

managing a major project to develop standards for National Health Service (NHS) HIV services and facilitate the further development of managed clinical networks for HIV, in support of key objectives in the government's national strategy for sexual health and HIV for England.

Developing materials to support health professionals, and particularly to help them respond to demands arising from new government policy and changing patient needs.

Providing authoritative responses and briefings to government and other policy-makers on current policy issues.

Medical Foundation for AIDS and Sexual Health
BMA House
Tavistock Square
London WC1H 9JP
United Kingdom.
Tel: + 44 (20) 7383 6345
Website: medfash.org.uk

3. Terrence Higgins Trust

The Terrence Higgins Trust was set up in 1982 by a group of Terrence's friends who wanted to prevent more people having to face the same illness as him.

Terrence Higgins was one of the first people in the UK to die of AIDS. He died aged 37, on 4th July 1982 at St. Thomas's Hospital, London. By naming the Trust after him, the founder members, who were his friends, hoped to personalise and humanise AIDS in a very public way.

The original objectives of the Trust were:

a)   to institute, promote, undertake, encourage and assist research into the causes, origins, transmission and treatment of AIDS, HIV, and apparently related conditions.

b)   To promote the welfare of those infected or affected by HIV or AIDS

c)   To alleviate the physical, mental or financial deprivation caused by AIDS or HIV

d)   To advance the education of the public, the medical and nursing professions, national and local public institutions in order to reduce or halt the spread of HIV or AIDS

However, the Trust's current aims are to:

a)   provide high quality services that are informed by and which meet the diverse needs of individuals and communities affected by HIV and AIDS;

b)   place at the core of the organisation's activities people with HIV, people using services and people in "at risk" communities, and to provide maximum opportunity for appropriate involvement,

c)   Reduce risk and rates of HIV transmission through health promotion programmes;

d)   Campaign, advocate and challenge the oppression and prejudice faced by people with HIV and AIDS;

e)   Develop and promote innovative models of good practice, sharing with and learning from other HIV and AIDS organisations nationally and internationally;

f)   Work in collaboration and partnership with other people and organisations;

g)   Ensure that the prevention, care and cure of HIV and the promotion of good sexual health continues to be a national priority;

h)   Maintain its independence by mobilising sufficient human and financial resources and using these appropriately to achieve the organisation's mission.

Terrence Higgins Trust
52-54 Gray's Inn Road
London
WC1X 8JU
United Kingdom
Tel: + 44 (20) 7831 0330
Fax: + 44 (20) 7242 0121
Website: www.tht.org.uk

4. UNAIDS

As the leading advocate for worldwide action against HIV/AIDS, the global mission of UNAIDS, the global mission of UNAIDS is to lead, strengthen and support an expanded response to the epidemic that will:

a)   prevent the spread of HIV;

b)   provide care and support for those infected and affected by the disease;

c)   reduce the vulnerability of individuals and communities to HIV/AIDS;

d)   alleviate the socio-economic and human impact of the epidemic

From 1986, the World Health Organisation (WHO) had the head responsibility on AIDS in the United Nations, helping countries to set up much-needed national AIDS programmes. But by the mid 1990's, it became clear that the relentless spread of HIV, and the epidemic's devastating impact on all aspects of human lives and on social and economic development, were creating an emergency that would require a greatly expanded United Nations effort. Nor could any single United Nations organisation provide the coordinated level of assistance needed to address the many factors driving the HIV epidemic, or help countries deal with the impact of HIV/AIDS on households, communities and local economies.

Addressing these challenges head-on, the United Nations took an innovative approach in 1996, drawing six organisations together in a joint and co-sponsored programme – the joint United Nations programme on HIV/AIDS (UNAIDS).

The goal of UNAIDS is to catalyse, strengthen and orchestrate the unique expertise, resources, and networks of influence that each of these organisations offers. Working together through UNAIDS, the co-sponsors expand their outreach through strategic alliances with other United Nations agencies, national governments, corporations, media, religious organisations, community-based groups, regional and country networks of people living with HIV/AIDS, and other non-governmental organisations.

UNAIDS
20, Avenue Appia
CH – 1211
Geneva 27
Switzerland
Tel: + (4122) 791 3666
Fax: + (4122) 791 4187
Website: www.unaids.org

5. International Association of Physicians in AIDS Care (IAPAC)

The IAPAC was established in 1995 by healthcare professionals and civic leaders who recognised an urgent need for a coordinated medical response to the HIV/AIDS pandemic.

IAPAC currently holds regional offices located in Johannesburg, and Paris, and represents a professional membership of physicians and other healthcare professionals in over 89 countries. Its activities are conducted by a professionally diverse staff, spanning three continents and are guided by an international Board of Trustees composed of highly esteemed medical, public health and advocacy professionals.

The mission of the IAPAC is to craft and implement global educational and advocacy strategies to improve the quality of care provided to all people living with HIV/AIDS and associated co-infectious diseases.

It vision is to make sure that people living with HIV/AIDS and associated co-infectious diseases may obtain the best healthcare available provided by physicians and allied health professionals armed with cutting-edge clinical expertise.

Headquarters
33 North Lasalle Street
Suite 1700
Chicago, Illinois
60602 – 2601
USA
Tel: + (312) 795 4930
Fax: + (312) 795 4938
Website: www.iapac.org

Southern Africa Regional Office
1st Floor, Broll Place
Sunnyside Office Park
Sunnyside Drive
Parktown
Johannesburg
Republic of South Africa

And

Suite 244
Postnet Killarney
P/Bag x2600
Houghton 2046
Republic of South Africa
Tel: + 27 11 484 2500
Fax: + 27 11 643 5990
E-mail: info@pac.org.za

6. European Union HIV/AIDS Programme in Developing Countries

The EU HIV/AIDS programme in developing countries aims to reduce the spread of HIV/AIDS. It co-operates with governments and non-governmental organisations (NGO's), international agencies and the United Nations, the private sector and people living with HIV/AIDS.

The programme was started in 1987 and has since implemented HIV/AIDS interventions at national, regional and international level in at least 90 developing countries. These include preventative and care measures, multi-sectoral support, studies and communication initiatives. HIV/AIDS policies are guided by the European Commission in Brussels, Belgium.

The EU HIV/AIDS programme in developing countries has developed policy principles and strategies to support activities that include the fields of:

a)   sexually transmitted diseases (STD's);

b)   multi-sectional HIV/AIDS interventions;

c)   HIV/AIDS and life-skills education for young people in and out of school;

d)   Media campaigns;

e)   Provision of safe blood and care

It has developed and run training courses concerning safe blood, planning and implementing STD management and laboratory testing. It has also supervised new data analysis and projection models to assess and/or predict the pandemic's impacts.

Administration and management of HIV/AIDS and population policies is carried out by the Common Service for External Relations (SCR).

EU HIV/AIDS Programme in Developing Countries

         DG Development
Unit A/2
Rue de La Loi 200
B – 1049
Brussels
Belgium
Tel: + 32 2 296 5592
Fax: + 32 2 296 7141
Website: www.europa.eu.int/comm/development/aids/htms

7. Family Health International

Established in 1971 and with 500 employees, Family Health International (FHI) serves its clients in over 40 countries. Through its global reach, it is committed to helping women and men obtain access to safe, effective, and affordable family planning services and methods; to preventing the spread of HIV/AIDS and sexually transmitted diseases (STD's); and to improving the health of women and children.

FHI operates in collaboration with a worldwide network of government agencies, research institutions, non-governmental organisations, and private sector entities, and offers a broad spectrum of technical services ranging from clinical research to advising governments on national health policy. FHI contributes to significant advances in public health through research, training and information to improve family planning and reproductive health service delivery and HIV/AIDS and STD prevention and care programmes.

FHI's primary objective is better public health. Its strengths lie in its technical expertise, effectiveness in managing complex programmes, achievements in contraceptive development and research, and more than a quarter century of collaboration with an international network of partners in health.

FHI
P.O. Box 13950
Research Triangle Park
North Caroline 27709
U.S.A
Tel: + (919) 544 7040
Fax: + (919) 544 7261
Website: www.fhi.org

FHI
HIV/AIDS Department
2101 Wilson Boulevard
Suite 700
Arlington, VA 22201
U.S.A.

Tel: + (703) 516 9779
Fax: + (703) 516 9781
Website: www.fhi.org

8. AVERT

AVERT, which was founded in 1986, is a leading UK based AIDS Education and Medical Research Charity. It is responsible for a wide range of education and medical research work with the overall aim of:

a)   preventing people from becoming infected with HIV.

b)   improving the quality of life of those already infected.

c)   through medical research working to develop a cure for AIDS.

Part of AVERT'S work is in the international AVERTING AIDS Grant Scheme. This scheme particularly supports projects in countries where there is a very high level of infection and several projects are currently supported in South Africa. One South African project is the Raphael Centre, one of the first South African Centres for people living with HIV and AIDS. The centre not only provides a range of care for people visiting the centre, but it also supports their children, other children orphaned by AIDS. As well as acting as a community education centre.

Currently AVERT is funding work at a number of leading establishments around the UK, including work at the University of Liverpool, University College London, and Oxford University. The work covers a number of different areas including the development of an AIDS vaccine, drug development including work on the side effects of the current drugs, as well as work on basic immunology and virology.

AVERT
4 Brighton Road
Horsham
West Sussex
RH13 5BA UK
Tel: +44 1403 210202
Website: www.avert.org

9. International Union Against Sexually Transmitted Infections

The International Union against Sexually Transmitted Infections (IUSTI), founded in 1923, is the oldest international organisation in the field whose object is the achievement of international cooperation in the control of sexually transmitted diseases, including HIV infection.

IUSTI is especially concerned not only with the medical aspects but the social and epidemiological aspects of the control of sexually transmitted diseases and increasingly HIV/AIDS.

Membership of IUSTI is open to both individuals and organisations involved in the study or prevention of sexually transmitted diseases. A medical qualification is not necessary to be a member.

The aims/objectives of the Union are to bring together (join/unify etc) all forces devoted to the fight against sexually transmitted diseases (STDs) including HIV/AIDS and the endemic traponematoses and to promote (and coordinate) throughout the world activities aimed at the research, prevention and control of the diseases and to encourage its members to contribute to public health programs for the control of STDs.

IUSTI
Department of GU
Royal South Hants Hospital
Brintons Terrace
Southampton
UK
Website: www.iusti.org

10. SIDALAC

SIDALAC is a regional AIDS initiative for Latin America and the Caribbean which was promoted by the World Bank in a similar fashion as previously experienced in Africa and in Asia. This initiative is now part of the United Nations Programme on AIDS (UNAIDS), co-sponsored by six of the system's agencies: the United Nations Children's Fund (UNICEF); the United Nations Development Programme (UNDP); the United Nations Fund for Population Activities (UNFPA); the United Nations Educational Scientific and Cultural Organisation (UNESCO); the World Health Organisation (WHO); and the World Bank.

This initiative's implementing agency is the Mexican Health Foundation.

This initiative is based on the conviction that the involvement of high ranking government officials, in and outside of health care systems, and the participation of diverse social groups is of the greatest importance to successfully modify the course of the AIDS and STDs epidemics and to provide adequate health care services to affected populations.

The overall objective of SIDALAC is to contribute to the mobilisation of national and international efforts against AIDS and other STDs in Latin America and the Caribbean through enhanced awareness of decision makers in the region, and the support and development of a new generation of control programmes with a specific scope for Latin America and the Caribbean.

SIDALAC is a regional initiative with the following general objectives:

a) To develop research projects that provide useful information for strategic planning in the prevention of HIV/AIDS and the provision of adequate health care for those affected.

b)   To widely disseminate the results of such projects, and promote the interchange of country experiences and lessons learned.

SIDALAC
Fundación Mexicana Para La Salud, A.C.
Periférico Sur 4809
Colonia El Arenal Tepapam
C.P. 14610 Mexico, D.F.
Tel: + (52) 56 55 90 11
Website: www.sidalac.org.mx

11. AIDS Foundation East – West

AIDS Foundation East-West (AFEW) is an international, humanitarian, public health non-governmental organisation whose mission is to contribute to the reduction of the impact of HIV/AIDS in the Newly Independent States (NIS) of the former Soviet Union. This new Dutch organisation intends to draw upon the knowledge, resources, experience, and expertise generated by the international and Russian national staff of the Moscow office of Medecins Sans Frontieres-Holland (MSF-H). AFEW intends to continue to develop and implement effective HIV/AIDS prevention, care and support interventions in the region.

AFEW works to accomplish its mission by developing, implementing and promoting tools for effective HIV/AIDS prevention, care and support designed for, and appropriate to, the scientific conditions of the NIS. By cooperating closely with national governmental and non-governmental structure, AFEW boosts local coping capacities, advocates for public health and legal reform in the fields of HIV and AIDS, and contributes to social justice in societies through its work practices. AFEW further endeavours to strengthen East-West engagement in the region by exchanging knowledge and people via its programme activities, promoting better understanding, stimulating an appropriate and committed response.

AIDS Foundation East-West
15-5, Chayonova Street
Moscow, 125267
Russia
Tel: +7 095 250 6377
Website: www. afew. org

12. Southern Africa AIDS Information Dissemination Service (SAFAIDS)

SAFAIDS is a regional HIV/AIDS resource (RHR) established in 1994 and based in Zimbabwe. The organisation's goal is to disseminate HIV/AIDS information in order to promote, inform and support appropriate responses to the epidemic in the fields of HIV prevention, care, long-term planning and coping with the impact.

Through its extensive networking and information collation, SAFAIDS endeavours to keep pace with the epidemic and its changing demands. SAFAIDS' work is responsive to client requests for policy development and evaluations.

However, SAFAIDS continues proactively to identify and meet information needs and will continue to seek greater strategic influence by prioritising partnerships with key players in the region.
This will be achieved by:

Building capacity for other NGOs to enhance a multiplier effort in good practices.

a)   information production, collection and dissemination to a wide audience using electronic and print media.

b)   provision of technical support and advice to NGO's, government bodies and other institutions.

c)   facilitation of easy access to appropriately targeted usable information on HIV/AIDS across a wide range of sectors.

d)   developing a consultant database: SAFAIDS is building up a resource list of easy identification and access to local and regional expertise.

SAFAIDS
17 Beveridge Road
P.O. Box A509
Avondale, Harere
Zimbabwe
Tel: + 263 4 336 193/4
Website: www.safaids.org.zw

13. AIDS Vaccine Advocacy Coalition

Founded in 1995, the AIDS Vaccine Advocacy Coalition's (AVAC) mission is to speed the ethical development and global delivery of preventive HIV vaccines. AVAC is a watchdog, education and advocate.

It addresses ethical issues, critiques the work of industry and government, provides education and mobilisation services, and speaks on behalf of affected communities with a credible, impartial, and objective voice. AVAC is a coalition of volunteer advocates and paid staff.

AVAC
101 West, 23rd Street No.2227
New York, NY 10011
USA
Tel: +1 212 367 1084
Website: www.avac.org

14. National AIDS Trust (NAT)

NAT is the UK's leading policy development and advocacy AIDS organisation working to ensure that people in power take action on HIV, both within the UK and internationally.

NAT works with others to develop informed responses to this growing epidemic. It advises and pressures for adoption of its policy proposals to achieve the best possible support for people with and affected by HIV.

In effect, NAT is an agent for change committed to advancing the human rights of people living with HIV and affected communities.

NAT
New City Cloisters
196 Old Street
London
EC1V 9FR
UK
Tel: + 44 (20) 7814 6767
Website: www.nat.org.uk

15. AIDS Information Switzerland

AIDS Information Switzerland was formed in 1989 by doctors from the whole of Switzerland as a politically and denominationally neutral association for the benefit of the public, in order to bring doctor's viewpoints increasingly into the AIDS discussion. On the basis of its strictly scientific-orientated activities more than 600 people, predominantly doctors, dentists and pharmacists, among whom are numerous professors and senior consultants, have joined the organisation. The association is additionally supported by a scientific advisory council which includes experts from various medical fields.

The main task of AIDS Information Switzerland, which the doctors fulfil voluntarily, consists in giving information to any questions connected with AIDS. In addition to the numerous publications for specialists, AIDS Information Switzerland has also issued various booklets and leaflets for the more general public written in language accessible to all. Furthermore, there are doctors available on an advisory telephone, three times a week in German part of Switzerland and daily in Ticino, to help with any questions on the subject of AIDS. Personal consultation is also offered on request. The association also supports children infected with HIV through a social fund.

AIDS Information Switzerland
P.O. Box 3176
CH- 8033
Zurich
Switzerland
Tel: + 41 1261 03 86
Website: www.aids-info.ch

16. Latino Commission on AIDS

The Latino Commission on AIDS is a non-profit membership organisation dedicated to improving and expanding AIDS prevention, research, treatment and other services in the Latino community the USA, through organising education, mode programme development and training.

Using its extensive network of members, the Commission works to mobilise and affect a Latino community response to the health crisis created by HIV/AIDS. Since 1990 the Commission had developed a series of education, advocacy and training programmes that respond to the needs of the Latino community.

Latino Commission on AIDS
24 West, 25th Street, 9th Floor
New York, NY 10010
USA
Tel: + 1 212 675 3288
Website: www.latinoaids.org

17. Positive Action

The Positive Action Society Lesotho was registered on the 24th of May 1999 under the Friendly Societies Act of Lesotho, with the aim of helping in the fight against HIV/AIDS in Southern Africa by actively involving infected and affected people.

It has over 200 signed up members in Lesotho and operates with a core group of approximately 20 volunteers on a daily basis from their rented premises in Maseru, the capital of Lesotho. The core group consists of people living with HIV/AIDS (60%), Peer Education and affected people (family member suffering from HIV/AIDS or already passed away).

Its vision is to provide opportunities and encourage as many people as possible to get actively involved to help in the fight against HIV/AIDS in Southern Africa until the population becomes AIDS free.

Its mission is to become a national and international model for a multi sector approach in the fight against HIV/AIDS by actively involving infected and affected people and providing a conducive environment to reduce the stigma attached to the epidemic. The organisation intends to utilise the marketing and communication skills of the private sector and create income generation opportunities for infected and affected people to lessen the impact of poverty on families and orphans in concerted actions with the government, religious, - traditional – community based and other non-governmental organisations.

Positive Action Society
Options Building
Pioneer Road
P.O. Box 1895
Maseru 100
Lesotho
Tel: +266 885 0069
Website: www.positive-action.org

18. Journalists Against AIDS - Nigeria

Journalists Against AIDS (JAAIDS) Nigeria is a media-based non-governmental organisation in Nigeria working in the field of HIV/AIDS and development.

Its mission is to contribute to the prevention and control of HIV/AIDS in Nigeria by improving the quality of HIV/AIDS communication messages and by strengthening the quality of policy response and interventions.

Its goals are:

a)   To improve the quality of media reporting of HIV/AIDS and reproductive health issues, through continuous training of journalists and provision of information resources for their use,

b)   To provide the HIV/AIDS information needs of the media and other members of the public through publications of news bulletins, reports and journals and utilisation of information communication technology,

c)   To encourage informed discourse on issues relating to HIV/AIDS in the media as well as the general public, through sensitisation programmes, seminars, workshops etc,

d)   To promote and ensure a culture of transparency, accountability and inclusiveness in the national response to HIV/AIDS and ensure the involvement of all stakeholders in the policy formation and implementation process,

e)   To defend and promote the rights of people infected or otherwise affected by HIV/AIDS through high-level advocacy and provision of access to information by PWLHA,

f)   To improve the quality of collaboration and networking among NGOs, Community Based Organisations (CBOs), governmental organisations and other agencies working in the area of HIV/AIDS in Nigeria and the West African sub-region.

Journalists Against AIDS – Nigeria
Media Resource Centre on HIV/AIDS and Reproductive Health
1st Floor, 42 Ijaye Road
Ogba Lagos
P.O. Box 56282, Falomo
Lagos, Nigeria
Tel: +234 1 773 1457
Website: www.nigeria-aids.org

19. International Council of AIDS Services Organisations (ICASO)

ICASO is a global network of non-governmental and community-based organisations. ICASO was formed in 1991 with secretariats in five geographic regions, and a central secretariat based in Canada 1995 ICASO was incorporated under Canadian law. However, it is a non-government organisation accredited to the United Nations Economic and Social Council (ECOSOC).

ICASO's vision is to ensure that:

a)   people living with, and affected by HIV/AIDS are free from stigma and discrimination, and have access to the highest quality education, treatment, care and support.

b)   All vulnerable people and communities living with or affected by HIV/AIDS have full access to the knowledge, means and support to prevent further HIV infections.

c)   All relevant policies and programmes are strategically designed with a focus on human rights.

d)   People living with, and affected by HIV/AIDS are fully involved in all aspects of prevention, treatment, care and support, and research.

e)   Communities and their organisations are mobilised and resourced to fully participate in the response to HIV/AIDS.

f)   The needs and concerns of communities and their organisations are clearly and strongly articulated.

ICASO
399 Church Street
4th Floor
Toronto, ON M5B 2J6
Canada
Tel: + 1 416 340 2437
Website: www.icaso.org

20. AIDS NGOs Network in East Africa (ANNEA)

ANNEA was established in 1994 by NGOs involved in HIV/AIDS related activities in Tanzania, Kenya and Uganda.

The founding members recognised that by networking, they were better placed to support each other in order to conduct AIDS work more efficiently and effectively. These concerns were especially heightened by the rapid rate of infection in the East African region.

By the end of 2000, ANNEA had more than 120 members; 46 from Kenya 38 from Tanzania and 36 from Uganda. Membership from organisations in other countries in the East African region i.e. Ethiopia, Sudan, Eritrea, Djibouti, Somalia, Rwanda, Burundi, and Seychelles is strongly encouraged by ANNAE.

The goal of ANNAE is to contribute to the reduction of the spread and impact of HIV/AIDS, while promoting and supporting the rights of people living with HIV/AIDS.

While its mission is to build solidarity among AIDS related NGOs in East Africa, strengthen and support them in their interventions to accelerate HIV/AIDS prevention, promote quality of care of people living with HIV/AIDS and mitigate impact.

ANNAE
Rebman House
Old Moshi Road
P.O. Box 6187
Arusha
Tanzania
Tel: + 255 27 254 8224
www.annea.or.tz

21. Asia Pacific Council of AIDS Service Organisations (APCASO)

APCASO is a network of non-governmental and community based organisations that provide HIV/AIDS services within the Asia Pacific region. Together with AfriCASO (Africa), EuroCASO (Europe), LACCASO (Latin/America and the Caribbean), and NACASO (North America), APCASO is part of the International Council of AIDS Service Organisations (ICASO).

The mission of APCASO is to promote the responses of non-governmental community-based AIDS organisations to the global challenge of HIV/AIDS, with particular emphasis on strengthening the response in communities with few resources and within affected communities.

Secretary APCASO
12 Jalan 13/48A
The Boulevard Shop Office
Off Jalan Sentul
51000 Kuala Lumpur
Malaysia
Email: valenmorg@pd.jaring.my
Website: www.apcaso.org

22. AIDS Foundation of South Africa

Based in Dublin, the AIDS Foundation of South Africa was founded in 1988 by a group of concerned individuals who saw their friends living with HIV/AIDS, with neither government nor community support. Its mission is to mobilise and manage resources for HIV/AIDS work in the country.

The Foundation is a non-governmental agency acting as an interface between donors and NGOs and CBOs working in the HIV/AIDS sector. It places donor funds strategically within selected NGOs and CBOs and provides ongoing technical support and skills building to those organisations.

In 1999, the Foundation formalised its granting making role with the establishment of the Grants and Technical Support Programme. The overall purpose of the Foundation's Grants and Technical Support Programme is to address two fundamental problems the AIDS Foundation has identified within smaller organisations working in the field of HIV/AIDS.

These are:

a)   the lack of available resources for NGOs and CBOs to carry out their work in a manner that allows them to get on with the job properly.

b)   The limited capacity of NGOs and CBOs to plan, implement, maintain and evaluate their interventions effectively.

The limitation of funding available for HIV/AIDS work in South Africa has forced the Foundation to concentrate its efforts in three of the country's worst affected provinces, Kwazulu Natal, Mpumalanga and the Free state.

AIDS Foundation of South Africa
P.O. Box 50582
Musgrave
4062
South Africa
Tel: + 27 31 202 9520
Website: www.aids.org.za

23. The Global Business Coalition on HIV and AIDS

The Global Business Coalition on HIV and AIDS (GBC) which was founded in 1997, is a rapidly-expanding coalition of international businesses dedicated to combating the AIDS epidemic through the business sector's unique skills and expertise. The GBC's first goal is to increase its membership significantly, before identifying and advocating for opportunities to improve business sector AIDS programmes, nationally and globally.

The GBC seeks to increase action by businesses significantly. In order to achieve this, it seeks to provide leadership on the positive impact business practices can have in fighting the disease, by combining advocacy, policy development and grassroots action with member companies and other stakeholders. The GBC works in four key priority areas:

a)   increased action by business
b)   Policy Development and Leadership
c)   Supporting National Business Action
d)   Change

HIV/AIDS has a pervasive impact on growth, income and poverty for nations heavily affected by the epidemic as well as for the global economy.

The national impact is devastating to all sectors of the economy; Health and development of human capital is compromised as the number of orphans rise and supply of teachers due to AIDS related illness decrease. Foreign exchange of domestic commodities and resources fall decline as productivity in the industrial sector falls. The epidemic discourages investment tourism and consumption in heavily affected countries as shareholders, tourists and consumers fear and suffer from the impact of HIV/AIDS.

GBC believe that HIV/AIDS has a clear impact on a company's profitability and productivity caused by

a) Increased costs
b) Declining markets
c) Threats to consumer base
d) Increased absenteeism
e) Staff turnover
f) Lower morale

In the face of this unprecedented challenge, businesses like the public sector and civil society must respond decisively. Yet despite the scale of the threat posed by HIV/AIDS, the business community has been slow to respond.

The mission of the Global Business Coalition on HIV/AIDS therefore, is to invigorate corporate attitudes and activities, making the business sector a recognised and valued partner in the war on AIDS.

Global Business Coalition on HIV/AIDS
1515 Broadway, 45th Floor
c/o Viacom
New York, NY 10036
Tel: + 1 212 846 5893
Website: www.businessfightsaids.org

24. The Global AIDS Interfaith Alliance

The Global AIDS Interfaith Alliance (GAIA) was founded in June 2000 to stop the transmission of the HIV virus from others to infants in sub-Saharan Africa. It is made up of top AIDS researchers and doctors, religious leaders, concerned benefactors and African medical officials, most of whom are associated with religiously-based clinics and hospitals.

GAIA relies on contributions to help fund the costs associated with all infrastructure planning and development pertaining to transportation and administering of medicine, conducting HIV testing and counselling, and undertaking appropriate prevention and self-care education.

GAIA is particularly concerned to help improve the status of women. New efforts are underway to organise and educate groups of women and female students. This includes training for access to clinical services and research related to the empowerment of women, educating women on how to remain healthy and respond effectively to unwanted sexual advances, and the consequent prevention of HIV mother-to-child transmission in sub-Saharan Africa.

The Global Interfaith Alliance
The Presidio of San Francisco
PO Box 29110
San Francisco, CA
USA
Tel: + 1415 461 9681
Website: www.thegaia.org

25. National AIDS Committee – Jamaica

The National AIDS Committee (NAC) is a private non-governmental organisation that was established in 1988 by the Minister of Health to co-ordinate the national multi-sectional response to the AIDS epidemic in Jamaica. The committee began with 18 members and now has over 100 member organisations.

The National AIDS Committee has four main functions:

a)   To advise the Minister of Health on policy issues relevant to HIV/AIDS/STIs.

b)   To involve all sectors of society in efforts to prevent and control HIV/AIDS/STIs.

c)   To act as a central body where ideas, experiences and questions about HIV/AIDS/STIs in Jamaica can be shared, discussed and addressed.

d)   To provide a sustainable means of supporting the initiatives of the NAC and member organisations by eliciting funds from fundraising activities, public and private sector participation.

The National AIDS Committee – Jamaica
2-4 King Street
4th Floor, Oceana Building
Kingston
Jamaica W.1
Tel: + 876 967 1100
Website: www.nacjamaica.com

26. Australasia Society for HIV Medicine

Australasian Society for HIV Medicine (ASHM) is Australia's peak organisation representing medical practitioners and health professionals working in HIV and related disease areas. The society was incorporated in 1990 and maintains a membership in the vicinity of 750. Over time the organisation has shifted from a focus on educating its members to focusing on the education of the broader health sector. In 2000 ASHM also became formally involved in the provision of hepatitis C education.

The society is governed by a voluntary national committee which is elected annually. Much of the policy direction of the society is carried out by standing committees which function in the following areas:

a)   International/development

b)   Treatments

c)   Education

d)   Hepatitis C

e)   Professional affairs

27. National AIDS Control Organisation – India

The National AIDS Control Organisation (NACO), is the model organisation for formulation of policy and implementation of programmes for prevention and control of HIV/AIDS in India.

In a scenario with no vaccine or drug for a cure in sight, NACO believe that information, awareness and education are the best ways to prevent the disease spreading.

National AIDS Control Organisation
Ministry of Health and Family Welfare
Government of India, 9th Floor
Chandralok Building,
36 Janpath,
New Delhi – 110 001
India.
E-mail: asec-mdg@hub.nic.in
Website: www.naco.nic.in

28. UNAIDS - China

The UNAIDS has had an office in China since early 1996.

The seven co-sponsoring agencies of UNAIDS (UNICEF, UNDP, UNDCP, UNFRA, UNESCO, WHO and World Bank) are all involved in some way or another in AIDS activities in China. In particular, WHO, UNDP and UNICEF have collaborated with the Chinese programme on a number of initiatives including surveillance, advocacy and training.

The Theme Group's terms of reference accord with the focus of UNAIDS, which is to strengthen national capacities to take action on HIV/AIDS and to ensure long-term sustainable response. To achieve these goals, key activities include increased collaboration and joint action by the six co-sponsors and joint monitoring and evaluation of the common UN response; facilitating and providing for technical support for national response to AIDS in order to disseminate international best practice; strengthening the capacity of Chinese leadership to co-ordinate and monitor the national response to HIV/AIDS; advocacy for political commitment and multi-sectional involvement and co-operation for resource mobilisation.

UNAIDS – China
No. 066, Golden Island Diplomatic Compound
No 1, Xibahe Nanlu
Beijing 100028, P.R. China
Tel: + 8610 8425 7172
Website: www.unchina.org/unaids

30. The Jerusalem AIDS Project (JAIP)

JAIP is an independent, international NGO in the area of professional training in HIV/AIDS both in the Middle East and in developing countries in Asia and Latin America. Teams of experts from the project were involved in 35 major community-based AIDS education interventions in 21 countries, in addition to the work done on a national scale in Israel.

JAIP's training programme in Israel has been implemented nationwide since September 1987. The organisation had specialised in school-based AIDS education, and its two curricula for elementary and high schools have been endorsed by the Ministry of Education in Israel. Over 2,700 teachers, physicians and nurses in the country had graduated JAIP's training since 1987. Also in the last 6 years, JAIP had initiated a peer AIDS education programme, using 2nd and 3rd year medical students, who were carefully chosen and trained – as AIDS educators in schools and the community at large. The programmes produced and distributed by JAIP are designed to be taught in the classroom and in other youth settings. They also make use and distribute the AIDS educational kit which is self contained and self explanatory. This educational kit uses the Immune System Approach or the ISYAP model in teaching about HIV/AIDS.

The Jerusalem AIDS Project
P.O.B. 7956
Jerusalem 91077
Israel
Tel: + 972 2 679 7677
Website: www.aidsnews.org.il

31. Albergues de Mexico

Albergues De Mexico is a private institution founded in 1991. It's activity was started in 1988 in Ermita Ajusco, South of Mexico city.

A group of volunteers led by Dr. Rene Garcia Felix started to help HIV/AIDS patients to ensure they receive proper medical care in hospitals and at home, to organise self-support groups for them and for their families, to initiate workshops and courses, to establish communities.

The institution was opened in Ajusco to host patients for short period of time. However, the institution has since grown constantly with means provided by its founders and by donators joining the institution.

Albergues de Mexico
Ermita Ajusco, en Santo Tomas Ajusco
Camino el Acueducto
Domicilio Conocido
C.P. 14700
Tel: + 52 5 2867336
Website: www.agora.stm.it/albergues

32. NAZ Project London

The NAZ Project London provides sexual health and HIV prevention and support services to the South Asian, Middle Eastern, North African, Horn of Africa and Latin American Communities in London.

It exists to challenge the myths and prejudices that exist about and within these socially excluded communities and to ensure that they have access to care, support and culturally and linguistically appropriate information.

The project is committed to service users playing an important role at all levels within the organisation.

NAZ Project London
Palingswick House
241 King Street
London
W6 9LP
UK
Tel: + 44 20 8741 1879
Website: www.nazorg.uk

33. Canadian Foundation for AIDS Research

CANFAR is a national charitable foundation created to raise awareness in order to generate funds for research into all aspects of HIV infection and AIDS. The role of CANFAR is to fund institution-based AIDS researchers at educational, hospital and health facilities, research institutes, and established community service organisations in Canada. CANFAR's Scientific Advisory Committee (SAC) is made up of experts from five areas of AIDS related research: fundamental and applied research, education and prevention, psycho-social, care, and community research. SAC members are aware of research already in progress and know what topics need exploring. Members are responsible for advising the Board on granting policy, establishing priorities for research funding, and evaluating proposals for funding.

The Canadian Foundation for AIDS Research is the only organisation operating in Canada for the sole purpose of privately funding research on AIDS and HIV infection. CANFAR's activities do not duplicate those of existing research programs, organisations or agencies. CANFAR augments and compliments existing research programs, providing additional funding to sustain or complete ongoing efforts. The Foundation also funds research in areas that have not received necessary funding, or require seed funding. Canadian AIDS researchers in the clinical, biological and social sciences desperately need more funding in order to answer some of the most important questions related to AIDS in Canada.

In addition to funding research, CANFAR undertakes local and national HIV/AIDS awareness programs. CANFAR co-founded the Red Ribbon Campaign, a community based (Toronto) program that offers for a donation a Red Ribbon – the internationally recognised symbol of HIV/AIDS support. This week long program commemorates the United Nations World AIDS Day (December1) with several hundred volunteers canvassing street corners, subway stations, office towers, theatres, bars and retail establishments.

CANFAR has developed a national bilingual HIV/AIDS youth awareness and fundraising program called "Have a Heart". With the average age of new HIV infections down from 32 to 23, we desperately need to make all Canadian teens HIV/AIDS smart. The program creates a fun outlet in which teens can become more aware of this often grim topic. With the support of the "Have a

Heart" sponsors, CANFAR supplies each school with all the campaign materials – chocolate Heart o'Grams, posters and HIV/AIDS awareness pamphlets.

CANFAR
165 University Avenue
Suite 901
Toronto, Ontario
Canada, M5H 3B8
Tel: + 1 (416) 361 6281
Website: www.canfar.com

34. PASCA

The Central American HIV/AIDS Prevention Project (Proyecto Accion SIDO de Centroamerica – PASCO) is an international program to strengthen Central America's capacity to respond to the AIDS epidemic. PASCA provides technical assistance to governments, Non-Governmental Organisations (NGOs), and to the private sector in HIV/AIDS/STD prevention in five Central American countries: Panama, Nicaragua, Honduras, El Salvador, Guatemala.

PASCA is financed by the United States Agency for International Development (USAID/G-CAP) and is operated by the Academy for Educational Development (AED) in collaboration with *The Futures Group International.* (TFGI).

PASCA's goal is to strengthen Central America's capacity to respond to the HIV/AIDS epidemic. PASCA was designed to meet this goal through interventions in the following three areas:

Policy Dialogue:

PASCA supports national and regional efforts to establish a positive policy environment for HIV/AIDS prevention. PASCA provides technical assistance to UNAIDS and National AIDS Prevention Programs, helping to improve the scientific basis for decision making (seroprevalence, behavioural, socio-economic studies, strategic planning) provided to those responsible for the development and implementation of laws and norms which impact HIV/AIDS prevention. PASCA also sponsors study tours and information dissemination activities at the national and regional level. The Policy Dialogue component works in a multi-sectoral fashion with National AIDS prevention programs, UNAIDS, national and regional legislatures, the media, as well as the NGO sector for advocacy issues. The Policy Dialogue component cosponsors research with the governments as well as with NGOs, strategic planning processes and biomedical conferences throughout the region.

NGO Strengthening

PASCO provides training, technical assistance and financial support to NGOs working in HIV/AIDS/STD prevention in Central America. The focus is on institutional strengthening, as opposed to directing interventions. PASCA helps NGOs improve their management capabilities and build technical skills. PASCA's working to improve NGOs ability to deliver quality programs, thus strengthening their role in HIV prevention.

PASCA's NGO Strengthening Component has three main strategies:

A.   Training and Technical Assistance.

PASCA has provided or will provide training and technical assistance in financial management, fund raising, cost recovery, counselling, individual counselling, advocacy, focus group training, project design, and in monitoring and evaluation of projects.

B.   Networking activities

Establishment of the Central American Information Center Network (Red de Información Proyecto de Accion en SIDA, REDAS). PASCA cosponsors networking activities throughout the region. PASCA, through small grants to several already established information centres, is helping to establish the Central American Information Centre Network which will allow the centres to electronically exchange information and holdings about HIV/AIDS/STD prevention.

PASCA
3a Avenida 20-96, Zona 10
01010 Guatemala, Guatemala C.A.
Telephone: (502) 363-3980
Website: www.pasca.org

35. International HIV/AIDS Alliance

The International HIV/AIDS Alliance (the Alliance) is an international development non-governmental organisation which was set up in 1993 by a consortium of international donors. The Alliance was established to respond to the need for a specialist, professional intermediary organisation which would work in effective partnerships with non-governmental and community-based organisations in developing countries, as well as with national governments, private and public donors and the UN system. The Alliance's mission is to support communities in developing countries to play a full and effective role in the global response to AIDS.

What has the Alliance Achieved?

Over the course of ten years, millions have benefited from the technical and financial support the Alliance has given to HIV prevention, AIDS care, and orphan projects. In 2002 alone, more than 825,000 people from the poorest and most vulnerable populations were reached directly and more than 91,000 were trained or supported through programmes for volunteers, peer educators and care givers. In addition, an estimated 4.9 million were reached indirectly.

In turn, the Alliance learns from these community partnerships and uses these experiences to more broadly promote effective AIDS strategies – encouraging both better programmes and better public policy. Research implemented by the Alliance and the Horizons Project has demonstrated both the importance of involving people with AIDS and how to do so effectively.

Alliance training materials have helped foster partnerships and referral systems between NGOs and governments in countries of Latin America, Africa and Asia. Needs assessments have helped articulate the priorities of children affected by AIDS, while programme design tools help increasing numbers of NGOs to link orphan support work to HIV prevention and AIDS care.

The Alliance has helped people with AIDS and other affected community members to influence laws and policies in several countries and to strengthen United Nations action declarations and programme frameworks.

Repeated external evaluations and the testimonies of people living with AIDS have demonstrated that the Alliance's work is effective and efficient.

- "a key player in the effort to slow the HIV/AIDS epidemic"

- "reducing the suffering of people living with HIV/AIDS and improving the quality of their lives and the lives of their families and caregivers"

- "donors have received outstanding return on investment"

- "after knowing that I am infected, I always ask all the clients to wear the condom."

Where does the Alliance work?

The Alliance works in countries heavily affected by AIDS to help people cope with the epidemic, and in less affected countries to stop HIV from becoming a serious problem. To date, the Alliance has provided technical assistance to NGOs and CBOs from more than 40 countries. As of June 2002, ongoing programmes are underway in 18 countries in addition to regional and international work.

The International HIV/AIDS Alliance
Queensbury House
104-106 Queens Road
Brighton
BN1 3XF, UK

Telephone: +44 1273 718 900
Fax: +44 1273 718 901

Email: mail@aidsalliance.org
Website: www.aidsalliance.org

36. Elton John AIDS Foundation

Vision

To provide national leadership and resources that will result in educational programmes on the prevention of HIV/AIDS and the improvement of care for individuals living with HIV/AIDS.

Mission

To provide funding for educational programs targeted at HIV/AIDS prevention and/or the elimination of prejudice and discrimination against HIV/AIDS-affected individuals, and for programmes that provide services to people living with or at risk for HIV/AIDS.

The Elton John AIDS Foundation, with offices in Los Angeles and London, is an international non-profit organisation funding prevention education programmes and direct patient-care services worldwide. The charity was established in 1992 by Sir Elton John, who serves as its Chairman.

Background

With offices in Los Angeles and London, the Elton John AIDS Foundation is an international non-profit organisation funding prevention education programmes and direct patient care services worldwide The charity was established in 1992 by Elton John, who serves as its Chairman.

In 1993, the North American-based Elton John AIDS Foundation established a collaborative effort with the National AIDS Fund, a Washington DC based organisation with Community Partnerships all across the United States. This collaboration was established in order to facilitate nationwide distribution of grants to communities and populations most impacted by HIV/AIDS. These grants are issued as a challenge to the National AIDS Fund's local Community Partnerships, which use the grants to leverage an additional 2 dollars of local money for every dollar provided by the Elton John AIDS Foundation – significantly increasing the impact of the Foundation's investment. Today, this represents 60% of the Foundation's grant-making. The new affiliation between the National AIDS Fund and the University of California San Francisco – AIDS Research Institute will raise the visibility and reach of the Elton John AIDS Foundation both domestically and internationally.

Funding from the Elton John AIDS Foundation encompasses a broad spectrum of services supporting men, women, young adults, children, infants, minorities and entire families living with or at risk for HIV/AIDS. Grants support programmes and services ranging from education outreach programmes, food banks, meal delivery programmes, hospice care and adoption services for children orphaned and/or living with HIV.

The Elton John AIDS Foundation in Los Angeles and London are pleased to announce that to date the total grant distribution has surpassed $30 million. From 1992 to 2001, the Elton John AIDS Foundation funded more than 2,028 grants in North America. The Foundation has distributed $17 million in grants in North America and $13 million internationally. In North America, over 80 per cent of all money raised goes directly to patient-care grants, making the Elton John AIDS Foundation one of the largest public non-profit organisations in the AIDS arena.

PO Box 17139
Beverly Hills
California,
90209-3139
Voice Mail: (310)535-1775
website: www.ejaf.org

37. Bill & Melinda Gates Foundation

The Bill & Melinda Gates Foundation is building upon the unprecedented opportunities of the 21st century to improve equity in global health and learning – because the life and potential of a child born in one place is as valuable as that in another.

The foundation was created in January 2000, through the merger of the Gates Learning Foundation, which worked to expand access to technology through public libraries, and the William H. Gates Foundation, which focused on improving global health. Led by Bill Gates' father, William H. Gates, Sr., and Patty Stonesifer, the Seattle-based foundation has an endowment of approximately $25 billion through the personal generosity of Bill and Melinda Gates.

The foundation's Global Health Program is focused on reducing global health inequities by accelerating the development, deployment and sustainability of health interventions that will save lives and dramatically reduce the disease burden in developing countries.

The Global Health Program directs its resources to:

- Promote research and development of health technologies that will accelerate prevention, elimination or eradication of diseases, as well as increase their affordability in low-resource setting

- Support programs that demonstrate effectiveness and feasibility of wide scale implementation of innovative health interventions, allowing other organisations and governments to confidently invest in similar models

- Encourage sustainable access by developing countries to existing and future health technologies interventions through catalytic financing mechanisms

- Increase visibility of effective public health approaches and strengthen support for public health leadership in developing countries.

Bill & Melinda Gates Foundation
PO Box 23350
Seattle, WA 98102, USA
Phone (206) 709-3140

E-mail: info@gatesfoundation.org
Website: www.gatesfoundation.org

38. International Federation of Red Cross and Red Crescent Societies

Mission and Role

The International Federation of Red Cross and Red Crescent Societies is the world's largest humanitarian organisation, providing assistance without discrimination as to nationality, race, religious beliefs, class or political opinions.

Founded in 1919, the International Federation comprises 178 member Red Cross and Red Crescent societies, a Secretariat in Geneva and more than 60 delegations strategically located to support activities around the world. There are more societies in formation. The Red Crescent is used in place of the Red Cross in many Islamic countries.

The Federation's mission is **to improve the lives of vulnerable people by mobilising the power of humanity**. Vulnerable people are those who are at greatest risk from situations that threaten their survival, or their capacity to live with an acceptable level of social and economic security and human dignity. Often, these are victims of natural disasters, poverty brought about by socio-economic crises, refugees and victims of health emergencies.

The role of the field delegations is to assist and advise National Societies with relief operations and development programmes, and encourage regional cooperation.

The Federation, together with National Societies and the International Committee of the Red Cross, make up the International Red Cross and Red Crescent Movement.

Federation HIV/AIDS Policy

Introduction:

The International Federation of Red Cross and Red Crescent Societies (International Federation) has a long tradition of working in the area of health and care. National Red Cross and Red Crescent Societies have been supporting individual HIV/AIDS projects since the mid-1980s. At its General Assembly in 2001, the International Federation took a truly global approach to the fight against HIV/AIDS and called for its 1987 HIV/AIDS policy, which had been reviewed in 1991 and 1993, to be updated. This policy provides a framework to support National Society implementation according to local needs and feasibility.

Scope:

The Policy addresses the strong recommitment of the International Federation to continuing and scaling-up prevention, destigmatization, advocacy and provision of health care and other services related to HIV/AIDS, in particular to vulnerable populations, noting:

- The close relationship between health and human rights and the importance of involving people living with HIV/AIDS (PLWHA) in the fight against AIDS expressed in the International Federation's HIV/AIDS policies since 1987;

- that prevention, care, treatment, support and fighting stigma and discrimination are closely interrelated interventions and are inseparable in successful community responses to HIV/AIDS, as underscored by the 13th session of the International Federation's General Assembly which took place in November 2001;

- the need for scaling up the above-mentioned approaches in order to curb the epidemic as expressed in the Ouagadougou Declaration adopted at the Red Cross and Red Crescent Pan-African Conference in 2000;

- the need to develop further the scale and effectiveness of programmes in order to really focus where the Red Cross Red Crescent can make a difference, including reaching out to those groups most vulnerable to HIV/AIDS, as expressed in the Berlin Declaration adopted at the 6th European Red Cross and Red Crescent Conference in 2002;

- the need for jointly and urgently addressing HIV/AIDS as a major global development and potential security problem as expressed in the Declaration adopted by the United Nations' General Assembly Special Session on AIDS in 2001 in which the International Federation is mentioned as one of the important players in the fight against HIV/AIDS (article 34);

- that health – which should be viewed as a state of complete physical, mental and social well-being and not merely the absence of disease and infirmity (World Health Organisation (WHO),1948) – is an inalienable right of all people without any regard to race, religion, colour, nationality, sex or origin. Health of the individual is fundamental and is an indispensable prerequisite to global, national and individual development, as expressed in the International Federation's health policy (1999);

- HIV/AIDS is a major development problem, which exacerbates other health problems such as tuberculosis (TB), malaria and other common health problems;

- That the HIV/AIDS epidemic affects all sectors of society and in extreme cases erodes the social fabric of society, leaving the elderly and young people to fend for themselves;

- Poverty, inequity, instability, the widening gap in social justice, gender inequity and lack of respect for human rights are important factors driving the HIV/AIDS epidemic.

International Federation of Red Cross and Red Crescent Societies
PO Box 372
CH-1211 Geneva 19
Switzerland

Telephone: +41 22 730 42 22
Fax: +41 22 733 03 95

E-mail: secretariat@ifrc.org
Website: www.ifrc.org

39. World Bank HIV/AIDS

The World Bank – in partnership with others – is working to roll back the spread of the HIV/AIDS global epidemic. As the largest long-term investor in prevention and mitigation of HIV/AIDS in developing countries, the World Bank Group is working with its partners to:

- Prevent the further spread of HIV/AIDS among vulnerable groups and in the general population;

- Promote countries' health policies and multi-sectoral approaches (e.g. by working in education, social safety nets, transport and other vital areas);

- Expand basic care and treatment activities for those affected by HIV/AIDS and their families, as well as for children whose parents have died of AIDS and other vulnerable children.

The World Bank is working with all regions in the developing world that are affected by HIV/AIDS. The Global HIV/AIDS Program and ACT Africa (AIDS Campaign Team for Africa) are both helping to coordinate this work.

The Global HIV/AIDS Program

The Global HIV/AIDS Program was created in 2002 to support the World Bank's efforts to address the HIV/AIDS pandemic from a cross-sectoral perspective. The program offers global learning and knowledge sharing on approaches and best practices to addressing HIV/AIDS. A key function of the Global HIV/AIDS Program is to lead the monitoring and evaluation efforts of UNAIDS (the Joint United Nations Programme on HIV/AIDS) partners at country level.

The Global HIV/AIDS Program supports the World Bank in its efforts to mainstream HIV/AIDS into all sectors. The Program is actively working to:

- Strengthen the Bank's capacity to respond to the needs of national governments, civil society and other stakeholders;

- Share and expand available knowledge about effective approaches to HIV/AIDS, and develop new approaches;

- Improve the quality of monitoring and evaluation, and build capacity in this area among partners working in AIDS-related projects and programs at country level.

As one of eight co-sponsors of UNAIDS, the Bank is playing a key role in shaping the global response to the HIV/AIDS epidemic. On January 1, 1996, UNAIDS began its expanded, multi-sectoral United Nations response to HIV/AIDS, which has since expanded to a partnership inclusive of governments, NGOs, and the private sector. The eight co-sponsoring organisations are the **United Nations Children's Fund** (UNICEF), the **United Nations Development Programme** (UNDP), the **United Nations Population Fund** (UNFPA), the **United Nations Education, Scientific and Cultural Organisation** (UNESCO), the **World Health Organisation** (WHO), the **United Nations International Drug Control Programme** (UNDCP), the **International Labor Organisation** (ILO) and the **World Bank**. This year the World Bank Chairs the Committee of Cosponsoring Organisations (CCO) of UNAIDS.

Global HIV/AIDS Program
1818 H Street, NW MSN # G6-082A
Washington DC 20433 USA

Telephone: (202) 202 473-9414
Fax: (202) 522-3235

E-mail: wbglobalhivaids@worldbank.org
www1.worldbank.org/hiv_aids/globalprogram.asp

HIV/AIDS in Africa

To support implementation of its HIV/AIDS strategy, the Bank has established a multisectoral AIDS Campaign Team for Africa (ACTafrica), based in the Office of the Regional Vice President for Africa. The high-level placement of ACTafrica underscores the Bank's commitment to HIV/AIDS prevention and care and enables the team to maximise collaboration among the various sector families. The team serves as the region's focal point and clearinghouse on HIV/AIDS and will provide a variety of services, including:

• Supporting implementation of the MAP;

• Supporting African countries through knowledge dissemination and exchange;

• Mainstreaming HIV/AIDS into the Bank's work in multiple sectors;

• Supporting Bank country teams in addressing HIV/AIDS in their country assistance strategies;

• Building HIV/AIDS impact assessment into existing environmental and/or social assessment processes;

• Strengthening and expanding the Bank's partnership with UNAIDS, as well as with key agencies, non-governmental organisations, and donors.

AIDS Campaign Team for Africa
Room J5-282
The World Bank
1818 H Street, N.W.
Washington D.C. 20433, USA

Tel: (202) 458-0606
Fax: (202) 522-7396

E-mail: actafrica@worldbank.org
www.worldbank.org/afr/aids

40. Care International

CARE is one of the world's largest independent, international relief and development organisations. Non-political and non-secretarian, it operates in more than 70 countries in Africa, Asia, Latin America, the Middle East and Eastern Europe.

Vision

The members of CARE International are united by a common vision:

It seeks a world of hope, tolerance and social justice, where poverty has been overcome and people live in dignity and security. CARE International hopes to be a global force and partner of choice within a worldwide movement dedicated to ending poverty.

Mission

CARE International's mission is to serve individuals and families in the poorest communities in the world. Drawing strength from its global diversity, resources and experience, it promotes innovative solutions and are advocates for global responsibility. It promotes lasting change by:

- Strengthening capacity for self-help
- Providing economic opportunity
- Delivering relief in emergencies
- Influencing policy decisions at all levels
- Addressing discrimination in all its forms

Core Activities

To fulfil its mission and progress towards its vision, CARE International pursues four inter-connected lines of activity:

- Development and rehabilitation programming that address the underlying causes of poverty and social injustice;

- Emergency response programming that provides rapid and effective support to victims of disasters;

- Influencing policy development and implementation at all levels to make significant positive changes in the lives of poor people and communities;

- Building diverse constituencies that support CI's vision and mission in all countries where we work

CARE's Work

CARE's projects either respond to immediate humanitarian need arising from disaster, or focus on more systematic causes of poverty and discrimination that threaten the lives of the poor in the longer term. In all cases, it seeks lasting solutions and improvements by working closely with the people it serves, and in partnership with local groups and organisations.

CARE's approach to poverty and discrimination means that its projects deal with a wide range of social and economic issues. These include: health; basic and girls' education; social protection; food security; economic activity development; agriculture and natural resource management; water and sanitation; HIV/AIDS; and local capacity building.

Agriculture: CARE helps farmers adopt measures to grow and sell crops more profitably, without the use of expensive and potentially dangerous equipment or pesticides. Women's programmes promote the cultivation of new vegetable varieties and help to increase the yield of traditional ones.

Education and training: CARE provides skills training to enable local individuals and families to make better decisions within their communities. Its train-the-trainers initiatives involve local farmers in sharing new methods of crop development, and the adult literacy programmes, bookkeeping and administration classes create new opportunities in business and financial management. Often the health programmes will also involve a training component, such as the prevention of HIV/AIDS or proper measures to avoid water-borne diseases.

Small business support: CARE provides small loans, business training and technical assistance to more than 50,000 people each year, more than half of whom are women, to help them finance their own enterprises and escape from poverty. When businesses become self-sufficient, CARE helps these entrepreneurs obtain credit and support from established financial institutions.

Gender and development: In all their projects, CARE strives to involve women as project participants, decision makers and beneficiaries. Of particular focus are women's issues such as reproductive health, family planning, income generation and girls' education. CARE provides schooling for young girls to encourage long-term health, self-sufficiency, strong family and community status, and parenting skills.

Primary health care: CARE health projects combat child mortality from preventable diseases by constructing wells, immunising children, teaching mothers how to prevent disease, and providing nourishing food to hungry families. CARE is known for innovative approaches to ensuring rural families have access to basic health care, such as the training of community health workers and the establishment of mobile clinics.

Rehabilitation: Following a humanitarian disaster, CARE International maintains a long-term commitment to the communities with which it works. It provides apprenticeships for young people in carpentry, stonemasonry, cooking, tailoring, mechanics and market gardening. It also offers counselling, medical and psychosocial assistance, help to establish or restructure social and health systems, build or rebuild health centres, and provides mobile clinics.

CARE International Secretariat
Boulevard du Regent, 58 box 10
B-1000, Brussels, Belgium

Telephone: 32 2 502 4333
Fax: 32 2 502 8202

Web: www.care-international.org

Conclusion

All the organisations mentioned above, play a vital role in the prevention and management of HIV and AIDS.

However, despite these commendable efforts, HIV/AIDS continue to plague humanity. Thus, education will continue to be vital in the fight against HIV/AIDS.

Self-Assessment Questions

1. What role or roles, in your opinion, should International AIDS Organisations play?

2. To what extent do you think they are likely to be successful?

3. What is the main legislation covering the following groups:

    a) Racial Discrimination
    b) Sex Discrimination
    c) Disability Discrimination

4. What racially motivated crime is also covered by the Criminal Law?

5. Why is the Stephen Lawrence Report so important in terms of racial discrimination in the UK?

6. What does G.O.Q. stand for and when does it apply?

7. What other categories are exempt from the Sex Discrimination Act?

8. Why is it difficult to establish the number of people who have a disability?

9. Explain the 4 main principles of Equal Opportunities

Books in the Simplified Series

Books available from October 2004

1. HIV and AIDS Prevention
2. Sexually Transmitted Disease Prevention (other than HIV/AIDS)
3. HIV/AIDS Prevention, Management and Strategy
4. Understanding and Preventing HIV/AIDS (a booklet for schools, colleges, teachers and advisers)
5. How to get your Dream Job in Social Housing
6. Management Principles
7. Monetary and Social Economics
8. Financial Principles
9. Management, Economics and Financial Principles (3 books in 1)

Books expected to be available from November 2004

10. Asylum and Refugee Law
11. Law of Mental Illness
12. Human Rights Law
13. Immigration Rules relating to Welfare & Employment (A practical guide for every employer & welfare adviser)
14. Tenancy Law and Security of Tenure
15. Housing Management and Practice
16. Introduction to Social Welfare and Benefits

Books expected to be available from December 2004

17. Housing law
18. Refugee Management
19. Law, Policy and Management of Homelessness
20. Business Law

Books expected to be available from February 2005

21. Housing Services Management
22. Social Care and Supported Housing
23. Law Relating to Social Care and Special Needs
24. Human Resource Management and Practice

Books expected to be available from March 2005

25. Mental Health Management – Volume 1
26. Mental Health Management – Volume 2
27. Citizen's Advice and Practice

Books expected to be available from May 2005

28. Medical and Healthcare Law
29. Prevention and Management of Drug & Alcohol Abuse
30. Immigration and Nationality Law

Books expected to be available from July 2005

31. Law of Care and Protection of Children
32. Law of Care and Protection of Animals

ISBN 141202672-5

9 781412 026727